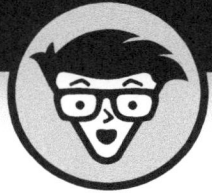

Men's Health

by Christine Adamec; Kimlin Tam Ashing, PhD;
Simon Atkins, MD; William E. Berger, MD, MBA;
LaReine Chabut; Megan Coffee, MD, PhD;
Patricia Corrigan; Sarah Densmore; Charles H. Elliott, PhD;
Humberto M. Fagundes, MD; Kevin Felner, MD;
Kristin Ferguson-Wagstaffe;
Marshalee George, PhD, MSPH, MSN, AOCNP®, CRNP;
Mary Kenan, PhD; Lane Kennedy;
Mark Edwin Kunik, MD, MPH; Clete A. Kushida, MD, PhD;
Paul H. Lange, MD; Pierre A. Lehu; Alan P. Lyss, MD;
Isabella Mainwaring, CDP, QLS, OCN; John R. Marler, MD;
Sarah McKay, PhD; Tamar Medford; Liz Neporent;
Sharon Perkins, RN; Dr. Simon Poole; Carol Ann Rinzler;
Amy Riolo; James M. Rippe, MD; Alan L. Rubin, MD;
Suzanne Schlosberg; Meg Schneider; Patricia Burkhart Smith;
Laura L. Smith, PhD; Richard W. Snyder, DO;
Michael Wasserman, MD; Dr. Ruth K. Westheimer;
and Tonya A. Winders, MBA.

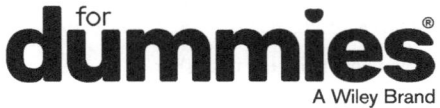

for dummies®
A Wiley Brand

Men's Health For Dummies®

Published by: **John Wiley & Sons, Inc.,** 111 River Street, Hoboken, NJ 07030-5774, www.wiley.com

For general information on our other products and services, please contact our Customer Care Department within the U.S. at 877-762-2974, outside the U.S. at 317-572-3993, or fax 317-572-4002. For technical support, please visit https://hub.wiley.com/community/support/dummies.

Wiley publishes in a variety of print and electronic formats and by print-on-demand. Some material included with standard print versions of this book may not be included in e-books or in print-on-demand. If this book refers to media that is not included in the version you purchased, you may download this material at http://booksupport.wiley.com. For more information about Wiley products, visit www.wiley.com.

Library of Congress Control Number is available from the publisher.

ISBN 978-1-394-36882-2 (pbk); ISBN 978-1-394-36884-6 (ebk); ISBN 978-1-394-36883-9 (ebk)

Printed and bound by CPI Group (UK) Ltd, Croydon, CR0 4YY

C9781394368822_041125

Contents at a Glance

Table of Contents

Introduction

M en don't live as long as women. That's not bad luck, it's a wake-up call. Men are dropping off earlier thanks to heart disease, cancer, accidents, and other heavy hitters. The bad news is that many of these diseases and conditions result from choices guys make. Genetics play a part, but behaviors and habits contribute substantially. The good news is, men can make different and better choices!

This book isn't about sugarcoating or scaring you. It's about giving you the information and tools to keep your body and mind sharp, protect the parts that matter, and outsmart the biggest threats to your health so you can share more cups of coffee with the people you love.

About This Book

We wrote this book because we don't think there should be a gap in the lifespans of men and women. The guys living in retirement homes may be having the best odds of their lives, but the ladies living there are likely wishing for a few more good men! We know plenty of daughters and sons (regardless of age) who would certainly like a few more years with their since-passed fathers or grandfathers, if given a chance. Consider the uncomplicated yet effective health practices in this book to be the fairy dust that can add that time.

We also wrote it because we think men have questions they don't even know to ask, because they think they're generally expected to "just figure it out," whatever that day's "it" is. No need to guess; we filled this book with the good stuff.

Because living a life of healthy habits can reduce men's chances of dying prematurely, we fill the first part of the book with the "what" — the good lifestyle habits that can promote joyful, easier, more comfortable living, and that can also slow disease progression or even prevent it from starting. Then we give you the "why" — information about the top diseases that disproportionately cause early deaths that men can avoid through better day-to-day choices.

This book is presented as a reference so you can grab it, get the information you need, and set it down as you get on with your life. Use the table of contents or the index to find a specific topic, or just open the book to any page and start reading. Dip in and out — there are no rules! But if you prefer to read books from the front cover to the back, start with Chapter 1.

And although the stats we include are current at the time of publication, in a couple of years they may not be. But the concepts in this book are evergreen, so you can come back anytime for a still-valuable refresher.

Foolish Assumptions

As we wrote this book, we made the assumption that you fit into one or more of the following groups:

>> You're a guy interested in figuring out what "healthy" means, and you're open to adopting some habits that can help get you there.

>> You want to avoid developing diseases that significantly impact how you live or how long you live.

>> You're age 18 or older — the concepts we present aren't generally particular to adults, but any specific instructions haven't been written for an adolescent's needs.

>> You're not reading the book for yourself, but because a man you care about isn't living a wholly healthful life and could stand to make a few changes.

>> You're curious to learn more about healthy habits that can help reduce the risk of sometimes-fatal diseases, and live longer as a result.

Icons Used in This Book

Throughout this book, icons in the margins highlight certain types of valuable information that call out for your attention. Here are the icons you'll encounter and a brief description of each.

TIP

This icon marks tips and shortcuts that can help you make smarter health decisions or save time or energy when working out.

REMEMBER

Remember icons mark the information that's especially important to know. To siphon off the most important information in each chapter, just skim through and find these icons.

TECHNICAL STUFF

This icon marks information that contains more detail than you *need* to know but might be interesting if you're an information junkie.

WARNING

Watch out! The Warning icon marks important information that could be a health risk if you ignore it.

Beyond the Book

In addition to the abundance of information and guidance related to men's health that we provide in this book, you get access to even more help and information online at Dummies.com. Check out this book's online Cheat Sheet. Just go to www.dummies.com and search for "Men's Health For Dummies Cheat Sheet."

Where to Go from Here

You can start reading this book wherever you have the biggest question. Want to learn why unintentional injuries (accidents) are disproportionately fatal to men? Start with Chapter 17. Have a question about sexually transmitted infections? See Chapter 13. Want to know how to set goals that can help you make and keep a plan? Off you go to Chapter 3. Begin where you want, and start planning that additional retirement vacation.

1

What's Going On Inside the Male Body

Find out the primary contributors to men's premature deaths and the changes you can make to live a healthier life.

Understand the lifespan gap between men and women and how modern lifestyles contribute to premature death.

Decide what lifestyle changes you want to make and create a game plan and goals so you succeed for life.

Chapter **1**

Keeping Your Body in the Game through Extra Innings

Here's a fun fact that's not actually fun at all: in 2023, American men lived on average 5.3 fewer years than women. That's an improvement from the COVID-19 pandemic peak of 5.8 years in 2021, but it's still a pretty sobering reality check. And this holds true globally — the gap's the same for 2023.

Women living longer than men isn't some unavoidable biological destiny. Sure, women have some built-in advantages. They have some protection from estrogen and their immune systems, they're less likely to drive 95 miles per hour in a 65 mph zone, and they probably don't think "chest pain" is something you can just walk off or rub some dirt on. And genetics is certainly a contributor to diseases men develop. But the real causes of this longevity gap aren't written in our DNA; they're largely written in our daily choices.

REMEMBER

Although the main causes of death are the same for men and women, men die more often from heart disease, cancer, and unintentional injuries (also called accidents). Men are more likely to skip doctor visits, ignore symptoms, and treat their bodies like they don't need regular maintenance.

The good news is, most of these deaths are preventable. And you're already ahead of the curve because you're reading this book. So let's dive into why men are checking out early and, more importantly, what you can do to change course.

Dodging the Big Killers

Although the leading causes of death for men have fluctuated a little since 2010, when the gap between men's and women's lifespans was smallest, the top three contributors have stayed steady — heart disease, cancer, and accidents. (Well, COVID-19 pushed in from 2019-2021, but the death rates plummeted after 2021, so we're focusing on diseases that have had a consistent and sustained impact on men's lifespans.)

The good news is, none of these three diseases (along with a few buddies that are also sending men to early graves) have to be death sentences if you get ahead of things early.

Avoiding heart disease

Heart disease kills more men than anything else — nearly 300,000 American men in 2021. Even guys in their 40s are having heart attacks at rates that would make your grandfather nervous. Although genetics are a component, men develop heart disease mostly because of their lifestyle choices. They're more likely to smoke cigarettes, eat a poor diet, get too little exercise, and ignore stress.

TIP

Here's a two-step action plan to help your heart right now:

>> Know your numbers. The American Heart Association (www.heart.org) sets blood pressure targets under 130/80, so check yours and see where you stand. If you don't own a home monitor, you can get one for less than $35, or head to your local drug store's pharmacy and use theirs for free. Check your blood pressure weekly, not obsessively. Find more about blood pressure in Chapter 15.

>> Move your body for 150 minutes per week, and walking counts. Find out what else counts in Chapter 5.

Take a look at Chapter 15 to get up to speed on heart disease and additional steps you can take to prevent it.

Reducing cancer risks

Cancer is the second leading killer, with close to 250,000 American men succumbing in 2021. Men often avoid health screenings, which prevent them from finding issues early enough for more successful treatment. Women get mammograms, pap smears, and regular checkups because they've normalized preventive care. Meanwhile, men treat colonoscopies like medieval torture. (Before you've had your first one, it certainly can appear that way.)

Some of the big cancers killing men are lung and prostate, and testicular cancer is the most common cancer in guys younger than 35. When screened and caught early, five-year survival rates for many cancers can be above 85 percent, but when caught late, the rates can be less than 35 percent.

TIP

You can also significantly reduce your cancer risk by not smoking, changing your diet, and getting enough moderate exercise. Take a look at Chapter 16 for more information about cancer and ways you can reduce your risks.

Steering clear of accidents

This category sounds easy to steer clear of, but in the United States it's actually the third leading contributor to men's deaths, claiming about 100,000 lives. *Unintentional injuries,* also known as accidents, is medical speak for drug overdoses, car accidents, falls, and workplace injuries — basically, all the ways men hurt themselves through risk-taking or poor judgment.

Drug overdoses are driving this trend; men are two to three times more likely to die from overdoses than women. Opioid addiction often starts legitimately — back surgery, injury, or dental work creates pain that needs a serious analgesic — but escalates quickly. If you're prescribed opioids, use them exactly as directed and dispose of leftovers immediately. If you're struggling with addiction, get help. This isn't a moral failing; it's a medical condition with effective treatments, and if left untreated, could literally kill you.

Vehicle accidents remain a major killer in part because men drive more aggressively and are involved in more fatal crashes than women. Some solutions are simple: slow down, buckle up, and put the phone away. Others are more difficult — if you're a truck driver, simply getting a lot more road time puts you at greater risk for fatal accidents.

Workplace safety matters too. The Bureau of Labor Statistics reports that men account for nearly 90 percent of workplace fatalities, many of them related to equipment operation or falls. If you work in construction, manufacturing, or any high-risk job, follow safety protocols religiously if you want to reduce your risk of dying early.

The bottom line on accident-driven causes of death? They're largely preventable. Chapter 17 has additional suggestions for how you can avoid becoming a statistic.

Rounding out the other fatal influencers

Overwhelmingly, heart disease, cancer, and accidents are the causes of men's deaths. To a much lesser degree, men die from stroke (Chapter 18), chronic respiratory diseases like COPD and asthma (Chapter 19), diabetes, and Alzheimer's disease (see Chapter 20 for both). Although genes have a stronger role in developing some conditions than others,in many cases you can meaningfully reduce your risks of developing each. Take a look at the chapters we've noted to get more information.

Addressing the Mental Health Elephant in the Room

Mental health issues are making men suffer and are contributing to shorter and less satisfying lives. A guy pretending everything's fine isn't a strategy that works. Every journey of a thousand miles starts with one step, though, and you reading this book is that step if mental health is a concern for you.

Stress

Chronic stress doesn't just make you irritable; it literally rewires your body for failure. Chronic stress increases heart attack and stroke risk.

WARNING

Men are particularly bad at managing stress because they're conditioned to "power through" instead of addressing the root causes.

Stress hormones such as cortisol wreck your cardiovascular system, suppress your immune function, and mess with your sleep. Men are more likely to cope with stress through drinking, smoking, or working longer hours — all strategies that make the problem worse and contribute to the development of other fatal diseases, too.

TIP

Even quick and easy stress reduction techniques can make a difference while you're sorting out and fixing the root causes. Next time you're feeling stressed or overwhelmed, try ten minutes of deep breathing, take a walk around the block, or call a friend. Even brief stress-reduction activities can lower cortisol levels significantly. Head to Chapter 7 for more on stress.

Anxiety and depression

Anxiety in men frequently shows up as physical symptoms, such as chest tightness, headaches, or stomach issues, making many guys think they have a medical problem rather than a mental health issue. Male depression shows up as anger, irritability, substance abuse, or emotional withdrawal — not what you expect to see for depression.

Compared to women, men are less likely to seek help for mental health symptoms, often because they don't recognize these signals for what they really are. The good news is that both depression and anxiety are highly treatable conditions, either on your own or with the help of a professional.

REMEMBER

Getting help isn't weakness; it's maintenance. Just like you'd see a mechanic for a broken transmission, you should see a mental health professional for a broken mood. We discuss several different types of therapy in Chapter 7, as well as self-help actions you can take.

Talking about Sexual Health

If you don't understand the basics of the male reproductive system, the rest of the conversation about sexual health is just guesswork.

Doing an equipment check

At its core, the male reproductive system includes the penis, testes (testicles), epididymis, vas deferens, seminal vesicles, prostate gland, and urethra. The testes produce sperm and testosterone, the prostate and seminal vesicles add fluids to create semen, and the penis delivers it to the outside world. Simple on paper — complex in reality. Chapter 11 goes into much more detail.

Making or avoiding babies

The male reproductive system is basically a production-and-delivery service for sperm. The system is designed to make babies and keep the human race going. But you may not want a little human (yet or at all), or you've been there, done that, and don't want more t-shirts. Enter contraceptives, which we talk about in detail in Chapter 12.

Avoiding sexually transmitted infections

Sexually transmitted infections, or STIs, spread through sexual activity. Some, like chlamydia and gonorrhea, can be cured with antibiotics. Others, like herpes or HIV, can be managed but not eliminated. Many can cause serious long-term health issues if untreated, including infertility.

TIP

You can generally avoid STIs with some basic precautions. Check out Chapter 13 for more.

Dealing with sexual and other system problems

A guy's reproductive health isn't just about avoiding infections or pregnancy. Issues like erectile dysfunction, premature ejaculation, prostate problems, or testicular cancer can all impact sexual function, fertility, and overall well-being. Take a look at Chapter 14 for explanations and pointers on how to approach any that you face.

Adjusting (or Overhauling) Your Lifestyle

In order to lead a healthy lifestyle, you don't need to transform into a CrossFit monk who drinks kale smoothies (although we'd like to see a face-off between that monk and Jackie Chan). You just need to make some smart adjustments that won't make you miserable.

Getting enough exercise

REMEMBER

After 40, your biceps matter less than your heart. Cardio exercise adds years to your life, while pure strength training mainly adds years to your mirror-gazing. As with many things in life, balance.

TIP

You want to hit (or exceed) 150 minutes of moderate exercise per week to get maximum health benefits. You could break this down to 30 minutes five days a week, or 37.5 minutes four days a week, or 25 minutes every day but Monday — the total minutes is what matters. And *moderate* means you can still hold a conversation while doing it. Walking counts. Gardening counts. Chapter 5 tells you what else counts.

Add strength training twice a week to maintain muscle mass and bone density as you age. You don't need to deadlift your body weight; even light resistance training helps retain muscle and support your metabolism as you age. Head to Chapter 6 for more.

Eating like an adult

Your college diet of pizza and energy drinks stops working when your metabolism hits the brakes around age 30. You don't need to eat like a rabbit, but you do need to eat like someone who wants to see 70.

TIP

The Mediterranean diet promotes longevity and tastes good, so it's easy to adopt. It offers lots of vegetables, lean proteins, healthy fats, and moderate wine consumption. Translation: more fish and olive oil, less processed garbage. If the Med's not your thing, you can take some other practical steps to improve your diet: Cook at home more often (you control the ingredients), eat vegetables with every meal (yes, every meal), and limit processed foods to weekends. See Chapter 4 for more nutrition tips.

Taking a reality check on smoking and drinking

There's no gentle way to say this — if you smoke, you need to quit. Smoking cuts years off your life expectancy and dramatically increases your risk of heart disease, stroke, lung cancer, and many other cancers. E-cigarettes and vaping aren't necessarily safer alternatives; they may just be different ways to damage your lungs and cardiovascular system.

REMEMBER

Quitting certainly isn't easy, but the benefits are immediate. Your body starts healing as soon as you quit. Within minutes, your heart rate drops. Within one to two days, carbon monoxide levels normalize. Within a year, your heart attack risk is cut dramatically. Chapter 9 gives you some resources if you're ready to toss your smokes.

Alcohol is more complicated. The Mediterranean diet includes moderate wine consumption, and some studies suggest light drinking might have cardiovascular benefits. But alcohol also increases risks for several cancers and accidents — two of the top killers of men.

The U.S. Centers for Disease Control and Prevention (www.cdc.gov) defines moderate drinking as two drinks per day for men. If you're consistently above that, you're moving into dangerous territory. Research from the prestigious medical journal *The Lancet* suggests that any potential benefits of light drinking are offset by increased cancer risk, particularly for men over 40.

In the face of evolving research, we say if you don't drink, don't start for health reasons. If you do drink, keep it moderate and honest about what "moderate actually means. That nightly "glass" of wine that's actually three glasses isn't helping your longevity.

Recovering via sleep

Sleep isn't laziness; it's when your body repairs itself. Men who sleep less than six hours nightly have lower testosterone levels and die earlier than men who get the recommended hours of snoozing.

REMEMBER

Most adults need 7-9 hours' sleep per night. If you're consistently getting less, you're not "getting by" — you're slowly degrading your health. Poor sleep increases heart disease risk, weakens your immune system, and makes you more likely to gain weight.

TIP

Keeping your bedroom cool (around 65–68°F or 18–20°C), avoiding screens for an hour before bed, and going to bed and waking up at the same times (even on weekends) are ways you can improve the quality of your sleep. Chapter 8 sheds light on sleep.

Making Changes That Stick

Big lifestyle changes such as modifying your diet or tripling your weekly workout sessions (or starting to get any at all) don't happen because you "feel motivated" one day. They happen because you commit, even when the changes feel inconvenient or difficult. The first step is mindset: stop waiting for the perfect moment and start acting like the healthy person you want to become. Small, consistent actions compound into big results over time.

TIP

Setting clear, specific goals can also help you adopt new habits. "Get healthier" is too vague. "Walk 30 minutes after work, five days a week" is actionable. Goals work best when you can measure them, track them, and celebrate small wins along the way. Progress fuels momentum, and who doesn't like a little celebration?

And if you build yourself an accountability network, you're more apt to sustain your new habits. This could be a workout partner, a coach, or a group chat that checks in daily. When someone else knows what you're aiming for, it's harder to quietly give up. Accountability also gives you a boost when you hit the inevitable slumps. Head to Chapter 3 for pointers on adopting changes in your life.

Keeping Tabs on Your Health

Here's an uncomfortable truth: men are not great patients. They often avoid doctors until something's actively bleeding or broken, and they're surprised when preventable problems become serious ones. If this sounds like you, hopefully we can help, both here and in Chapter 10.

TIP

Make sure you actually trust your primary-care doctor (PCP). Good doctors explain things in plain English, listen to your concerns without rushing, and involve you in decision-making. If your current doctor makes you feel uncomfortable if you ask questions or dismisses your concerns, find a new one. You're paying for this service; you deserve quality care.

Men are less likely than women to visit a doctor in any given year. Annual physicals aren't about finding problems — they're about preventing them. Your doctor can catch high blood pressure, diabetes, and early signs of heart disease years before you'd notice symptoms. And the appointments don't take a lot of time — usually just 30–45 minutes, not including paperwork, digital or otherwise (so much paperwork).

REMEMBER

Come prepared with questions, and write them down beforehand because you'll forget half of them once you're in the exam room. Ask about anything that's been bothering you, even if it seems minor. Most importantly, be honest. If you drink more than you should, say so. If you're stressed, anxious, or depressed, mention it. If you're having sexual health issues, bring them up. Your doctor has heard it all before and can't provide good care without accurate information.

Chapter **2**

Understanding Why Lifespans Vary

For over one hundred years, women's lifespans have been longer than men's. From birth, women were expected to live longer than men, and once people made it to age 65, women still were expected to live more additional years than men were. Even as the average lifespan of male and female Americans has steadily increased, women are still the ones to join last call after the men have departed. Metaphorically speaking, of course. (Or not — we've heard those assisted living facilities have some pretty wild parties.)

There are some primary culprits for men's premature deaths, with heart disease and cancer overwhelmingly leading the disease pack. Increasingly, researchers are learning how significantly hormone health plays into overall health and longevity, too. Balanced hormones, including insulin, cortisol, testosterone, and dopamine, interact smoothly and support mental clarity, energy, stable mood, fertility, and many other processes. But when your lifestyle creates an imbalance of hormones (you're eating too much sugar, having too many stressors or navigating them ineffectively, or getting too much dopamine caused by endless doom-scrolling, among other causes), then you suffer negative consequences, including being prone to becoming overweight (a risk factor for most of the diseases in Part 4), carrying too much *visceral fat* (that is, fat between your internal organs, which is a risk factor for heart disease in particular), and experiencing mental health disorders (which can contribute to suicide).

This chapter attempts to explain why men don't live as long as women, and how hormones play a bigger role in longevity than previously understood.

Measuring the Divide in Men's and Women's Lifespans

From the early twentieth century, the primary contributor to men's deaths was smoking — more men smoked than women did. This contributed to higher rates of cardiovascular disease that resulted in death, and was responsible for the shorter lifespans that men faced.

Fast forward to more recent times and the decade before the COVID-19 pandemic. In 2010, the average lifespan for men was 4.8 years less than for women — the smallest gap in recent history. The biggest contributors to men's deaths pre-pandemic were heart disease, unintentional injuries, diabetes, suicide, and homicide.

But then the COVID-19 pandemic hit, and during the years surrounding it (2019-2021) the gap widened substantially to 5.8 years, the highest gap in history. The causes that made a huge dent in men's lifespans compared to women's were twofold:

» COVID-19, where men died at much higher rates (more were in homeless shelters and encampments, and in prison, which made it difficult or impossible to socially distance, and more worked in jobs that required frequent public interaction)

» Unintentional injuries, primarily drug overdoses, which women also faced but not to as great a degree

TECHNICAL STUFF

In addition to the effects of the COVID virus, researchers found that lifespans for both men and women declined during the pandemic. They attribute part of this drop to *deaths of despair* — fatalities linked to drug use, suicide, and alcoholic liver disease. Although attributed to women as well, men experienced a substantially higher number of these deaths.

The good news is, following the COVID-19 pandemic and using 2023 data, we seem to be seeing a turnaround. The gap between men's and women's lifespans narrowed from 5.8 to 5.3 years ("a lot" by researcher standards). The main reason was because COVID deaths plummeted — COVID had been the third biggest contributor to men's deaths, and as the virus began to fade, COVID lost seven slots and moved to tenth place.

Understanding the Leading Causes of Men's Death

Here are the primary contributors to men's deaths, noting that some of the bottom five have swapped places from 2021 to 2022 and then 2023 (the most recent data available):

>> Heart disease

>> Cancer

>> COVID

>> Accidents (also known as unintentional injuries)

>> Stroke

>> Chronic lower respiratory diseases

>> Diabetes

>> Suicide

>> Alzheimer's

>> Chronic liver disease & cirrhosis

Most of these are also leading causes of women's deaths, but in many cases the number of men dying is disproportionate to women. Here are some reasons why:

>> Men tend to store more visceral fat, which increases heart disease and diabetes risk. (Check out Chapters 15 and 20 for information on heart disease and diabetes, respectively.)

>> Women get some pre-menopause protection from estrogen.

>> Women's immune responses are generally stronger (a double-edged sword, as women are more prone to autoimmune diseases).

>> Men have higher smoking rates than women. Smoking (which we cover in Chapter 9) is a significant contributor to heart disease, which continues to be the number one killer of men and women. Smoking is also a substantial contributor to lung cancer (see Chapter 16) and chronic lower respiratory diseases (Chapter 19 has more on these).

>> Men drink more alcohol than women do. Excessive alcohol (which we cover in Chapter 9) is increasingly viewed as a contributor to a number of diseases on the list, and is a primary contributor to chronic liver disease and cirrhosis.

>> Men engage in riskier behavior. Whether the way they drive, the jobs they work, or the violence they're involved with, men are more at risk for fatal accidents (covered in Chapter 17).

>> Men are less likely to seek mental health help for depression (with more information in Chapter 7), and they're significantly more likely to commit suicide (accounting for eight of ten suicides in the United States).

>> Men go to the doctor less often and are less likely to get regular health screenings, which reduces their chances of identifying problems earlier, when they're easier to treat. (Chapter 10 has pointers on regular checkups so you can stay on top of things.)

Discovering How Hormones Underpin Your Health

Everyone has a miraculous, self-governing endocrine (hormone) system focused 24 hours a day and 365 days a year on helping your body function properly. The endocrine system produces and releases over 50 different *hormones* — the body's chemical messengers. Each hormone has a unique role and works to keep you feeling mentally, emotionally, and physically balanced. From insulin managing your blood sugar levels, to cortisol helping the body respond to stress (physical or psychological), hormones are at the core of our health, energy, and resilience daily.

REMEMBER

Emerging research highlights the vital role hormones play in our overall health and longevity. Advances in testing have allowed us to measure and monitor hormone levels with greater accuracy and autonomy than ever before. This collective effort has fundamentally begun reshaping our understanding of hormone health.

Our hormonal apparatus evolved to suit a world far different from the one we live in today. While our ancestors faced physical exertion, intermittent food availability, and natural stressors, modern life presents an entirely new set of challenges: processed foods, sedentary lifestyles, a loneliness epidemic, chronic stress, and environmental toxins. Our hormones are simply ill equipped to handle this new state of affairs.

The consequences of the imbalance between our biology and modern environment are staggering. Chronic hormone-related diseases such as type 2 diabetes (covered in Chapter 20), heart disease (covered in Chapter 15), and obesity (which is a risk for most of the diseases found in Part 4 and which is introduced in Chapter 4) are now leading causes of death globally.

WARNING

According to the World Health Organization (WHO, www.who.in), heart disease alone claims the lives of around 18 million people each year, while type 2 diabetes affects over 537 million adults worldwide and is responsible for nearly 2 million deaths annually. Both conditions often stem from *metabolic dysfunction* (when your body doesn't use fats, proteins, and carbohydrates as designed, and your blood sugar and insulin levels get out of whack) caused by modern dietary habits and lifestyles. We've come to learn that our hormones are alarm bells, warning us through uncomfortable symptoms that our current way of living isn't really working for us.

Speculating about the increase in hormone imbalances

At the heart of the rise in hormone imbalances lies a fundamental issue: Our minds and bodies are under unprecedented levels of strain, and we have become disconnected from the signals our symptoms are trying to convey. Despite the substantial body of research, Western medicine has often fallen short in addressing hormone imbalances through a biopsychosocial lens — one that recognizes the intricate interplay between biological, psychological, and social factors. The approach to treating hormone-related conditions remains fragmented, treating isolated symptoms individually, often with medication. Healthcare professionals tend to overlook the broader, interconnected systems at work, missing opportunities to address the root causes of hormonal imbalances and to view the body as a holistic, integrated entity.

TECHNICAL
STUFF

For instance, while stress is widely recognized as a key factor in hormone-related conditions like low testosterone and insulin resistance, conventional treatments often focus on short-term solutions such as medication or supplements. These approaches typically target the symptoms but fail to address the deeper, underlying causes of the stress. This is where the *biopsychosocial model* offers a more comprehensive perspective, emphasizing the need to tackle not just the biological symptoms, but also the psychological and social drivers of hormonal imbalances for a truly holistic approach to healing.

Diseases and conditions linked to hormones

REMEMBER

Maintaining healthy hormone levels requires constant care and attention, just like a garden needs ongoing maintenance. There will always be weeds that threaten to disrupt your hormonal harmony. The key is learning how to tend to your hormones throughout all stages of life, ensuring they remain resilient and adaptable to whatever comes your way to reduce the risk of developing more severe diseases and conditions linked to hormonal dysfunction in the future. Here are just a few brief examples:

» **Cardiovascular disease:** Hormones such as cortisol and insulin affect heart health; imbalances increase the risk of high blood pressure and heart disease.

» **Digestive disorders:** Cortisol and insulin play a critical role in gut health, influencing conditions such irritable bowel syndrome (IBS) and leaky gut (which itself can worsen heart disease).

» **Autoimmune diseases:** Fluctuations in hormones such as cortisol can trigger or worsen conditions like Hashimoto's, rheumatoid arthritis, and lupus.

» **Chronic fatigue:** Imbalances in cortisol, a key regulator of energy, often underlie persistent fatigue.

Overcoming Modern-Day Hormone Disruptors

REMEMBER

Modern *Homo sapiens* (that's us!) have thrived for thousands of years through movement, connection, and balancing short-term needs and long-term rewards. We hunted, gathered, and formed communities, and our bodies and brains evolved over time to function optimally when we have high levels of activity, close social bonds, and a natural rhythm between work and rest.

When you compare the way we live now to the lives of our ancient ancestors, it's clear these patterns have drastically shifted. We no longer need to chase or work hard for our meals or operate in tight-knit communities to make it through each day. Instead, we spend our time glued to screens, moving less, socializing virtually, and satisfying our every need with just a few taps of a device. While convenient, this way of life is making it harder for our ancient hormones to function at their best.

Moving your body and making technology work for you

We have long understood the connection between physical activity and overall health. In the modern world, most of us live far closer to a leisurely style of living than a physical one. In fact, the average adult in the United States now spends more than 10 hours a day sitting; only 23 percent of adults meet the recommended guidelines for both aerobic and muscle-strengthening activities.

Globally, the situation is similar, with WHO reporting that one in four adults worldwide are not physically active enough. In countries like the U.K., approximately 75 percent of workers spend nearly six hours sitting each workday, the consequences of which go beyond just physical fitness or aesthetics. Regular inactivity disrupts essential biological functions that regulate your hormones, including the release of *myokines* — a fascinating class of signaling molecules released by the muscles during physical activity. These "messengers" play a vital role in regulating two crucial hormones: insulin and cortisol, both of which are central to metabolic and stress-related processes in the body.

TECHNICAL STUFF

But how did this shift to moving less come about? Understanding the broader societal changes that have contributed to the decline in physical activity will help you start identifying practical strategies to overcome these barriers and reintegrate movement into your daily routine:

>> **Sedentary work environments:** Sedentary jobs in the United States have increased by 83 percent since 1950. Most modern jobs now involve little to no physical exertion, but that doesn't have to be a barrier to incorporating movement into your day. Taking short, frequent breaks to stand up, stretch, or walk around can break up long periods of sitting and help combat the effects of a sedentary job.

>> **Technological distractions:** The average American adult spends more than 7 hours a day consuming digital media, whether it's scrolling through social platforms, gaming, watching the news online, or binge-watching shows. However, instead of throwing your devices into a drawer and fighting against the use of technology, you can actually use them to your advantage. There are countless fitness apps, online exercise classes, and activity trackers designed to integrate movement in your life.

>> **Urbanization:** It's easy to see how urban sprawl, car dependency, and lack of green spaces can make incorporating physical activity a little trickier than it used to be, so you might have to get creative! Walking more during your commute (even parking farther away or getting off public transport a stop earlier) or seeking out local parks during weekends can make movement

more accessible and enjoyable. Even short bursts of physical activity — 10 to 15 minutes at a time — can add up to big health benefits, so choose to climb stairs rather than getting the elevator, walk up escalators rather than riding them, walk in place or around the office while on calls, or stretch during TV breaks.

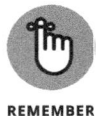

REMEMBER

>> **Time constraints:** Effective time management starts with setting clear boundaries. If you constantly feel overwhelmed or stretched too thin, you need to reevaluate how you're protecting your time to make room for the things that truly matter. Prioritizing exercise not only boosts your energy and improves hormone balance but makes you more efficient and productive in the other areas of your life. Shift your mindset to see exercise as investing in your future self rather than as time-consuming.

Overcoming disruption to traditional workplace models

REMEMBER

The workforce was once dominated by manufacturing, manual labor, and fixed office environments, but it's shifted toward knowledge-based, service-driven roles that are predominantly desk-bound, giving way to more flexible but less structured work environments that require people to have much greater self-awareness than was necessary for previous generations to manage our health effectively.

By being conscious of these modern challenges and making deliberate choices to prioritize your hormone health, you can transform your reality and thrive in this ever-evolving landscape. In the following sections, we outline the biggest hormone offenders so you can take steps to counteract them.

Reassessing exposure to artificial light

Widespread use of artificial light, particularly during winter months in the Northern Hemisphere when the sun may set as early as 3:00 p.m., can disrupt natural *circadian rhythms* (your internal biological clock). Among artificial light sources, blue light wavelengths are particularly problematic after sunset because they suppress the production of *melatonin* — your sleep hormone — delaying its release and making it harder to fall asleep and achieve restful sleep. Over time, poor sleep contributes to increased stress and worsens mood disorders, highlighting the need to minimize blue light exposure in the evening, such as from screens and LED lighting.

The health risks of prolonged artificial light exposure are evident in research on night-shift workers, who face increased risks of metabolic disorders such as type 2 diabetes and obesity. These effects are largely attributed to disrupted circadian rhythms and suppressed melatonin production.

Here are a few steps you can take:

>> Put phones and other digital devices away at least an hour before bedtime so you can fall asleep faster.

>> Get outside for even a 15-minute walk most days to get some natural light.

>> Install a light therapy lamp in your bedroom to help you wake up in the morning and stay synchronized with the sun.

Embracing the evolution of work for better health

Remote work seems here to stay, which demands a new mindset about how you engage with your work environment and care for yourself in this evolving landscape.

The following list looks at how you can approach this shift strategically, taking steps to ensure that while your work changes, your health remains a priority:

>> **Incorporate movement into your day:** Physical activity doesn't need to happen all at once, so make time for short bursts that can have a cumulative effect on improving your energy levels, boosting productivity, and balancing hormones.

>> **Prioritize work-life boundaries:** Set specific work hours, and when the workday is done, focus on activities that nourish your mind and body. This clear structure will not only improve your mental health and reduce stress but also allow your body to find its natural rhythm again.

>> **Spend time in nature:** Spending at least 120 minutes per week in nature has been shown to significantly improve mental, emotional, and physical health, according to a study published in the aptly named journal *Nature*. Those who spend time near blue spaces (bodies of water) report even greater benefits, including reduced stress and enhanced mental clarity.

>> **Use technology to your advantage:** Just as technology has disrupted traditional work models, it can also be used to improve your health. If you're feeling stretched for time or struggle to remember to implement your healthy habits at first, technology is there to help you.

Recognizing social media dopamine addiction

Dopamine is a neurotransmitter that plays a key role in how people experience pleasure, motivation, and reward. Whenever you experience something pleasurable, dopamine is released in your brain. This reinforces the behavior, making you want to repeat it for another hit of satisfaction.

Dopamine motivates us to seek out experiences that trigger its release, driving many of our day-to-day actions that cultivate or disrupt hormone balance such as what we eat, how much we exercise and how much stress our body experiences.

You can become addicted to the activities or substances that cause the dopamine spikes, which then creates a cycle of craving that pleasure again and again. It's important to take back control of your dopamine feedback loop because over time, excessive stimulation can actually decrease the number of dopamine receptors in your brain.

TIP

Here are some ways you can break the cycle:

>> **Limit screen time:** Reducing your time on social platforms by small increments to work toward a goal of only 1 to 2 hours per day. Most smartphones offer screen time trackers to help with this.

>> **Establish phone-free zones:** Create boundaries around your social media use by designating specific times or places where your phone is completely off-limits — in the bedroom, during meals, while exercising or working.

>> **Take regular digital detoxes:** Consider going on short *digital detoxes* where you take a break from social media entirely for a few days or a weekend to help reset your brain's dopamine response.

Experiencing short-term versus long-term gratification

The ability to deny yourself immediate pleasure for the sake of a greater long-term reward is strong predictor of your ability to achieve your goals. The reason so many of us struggle with this is not because we're "weak" or "undisciplined." Rather, it's due to the fact that we've been biologically hardwired to prioritize short-term gratification. For our ancient ancestors, rewards such as finding food or shelter were essential for survival, so our brains release dopamine when we experience these short-term rewards, reinforcing behaviors that lead to quick payoffs.

The modern challenge for us is that our *prefrontal cortex* — the part of the brain responsible for decision-making and long-term planning — has to work harder than ever to override our impulses for short-term rewards. In a world of convenience and instant gratification, everything is so easily accessible that it's become increasingly more challenging to prioritize long-term benefits over momentary satisfaction. This task becomes even more difficult when we're stressed, tired, or overwhelmed, which weakens the ability to delay gratification. This is why so many people struggle to make choices that support their long-term health.

REMEMBER

Developing the ability to zoom out and make decisions that will benefit future you is the secret weapon to managing your hormone health. Opting for immediate pleasures — such as sugary foods — may feel rewarding in the moment, but over time, it can lead to weight gain, insulin resistance, and type 2 diabetes. Additionally, constantly chasing quick dopamine hits can raise cortisol levels, contributing to chronic stress and anxiety that can diminish your motivation and focus over time, making it harder to engage in activities that require sustained effort.

Chapter **3**

Starting Smart: Making Changes that Last

Whether you want to improve your diet, add regular workouts to your weekly routine, cut down on drinking, or make other changes that'll help you feel better and navigate the world more easily, having a game plan will help you achieve your goals. A goal without a plan is just a wish!

In this chapter, we explain how to set up the solid, unshakable foundation you need to create (and most importantly, execute!) a personalized health plan. This chapter is all about designing a new lifestyle and mindset that works for you and supports your journey to better health and a longer life. So whether you need to develop awareness about your current routines, set achievable goals, figure out how to create new habits that stick, or find a supportive accountability buddy, this chapter lays the groundwork for real, tangible results.

Getting into the Mindset of Making Changes

REMEMBER

The human body possesses a remarkable ability to regenerate itself, which is a powerful asset when it comes to making changes to how you eat, move, manage stress, sleep, and engage in other new, healthier habits. If you haven't been taking optimal care of your body (and your spirit), then you may be facing some health concerns (like constant fatigue, excess weight, or mild depression) or even diseases. Although not all diseases or more serious conditions can be entirely reversed, some can, and any changes you make as you seek to live a better-quality life will certainly help alleviate symptoms and optimize the health you have. And similarly, such changes will positively improve how you feel and how your body acts, which may help you live longer and better enjoy the life you're living.

Riding the self-improvement roller coaster

REMEMBER

The process for achieving a healthier body and mind, like most changes, is far from linear. Working towards goals, like life, often feels like being strapped into a roller coaster: exhilarating highs where you can see your progress and feel amazing, and frustrating lows of setbacks or no evidence of any tangible changes despite your hard and consistent effort.

Humans are wired to seek stability and familiarity over discomfort. However, healing requires temporary discomfort for future gains. An essential part of this journey is creating new habits that stop you from seeking safety in habits you're familiar with, especially if those patterns are contributing to your less healthy life in the first place.

Being kind to yourself outside your comfort zone

If something doesn't challenge you, it doesn't change you, and remember that you certainly aren't going to get it "right" every day. You'll make mistakes and revert to old habits as you proceed on your path to improvement. Be kind to yourself rather than beating yourself up for every perceived failure or slip-up. Your willingness to show up for yourself, even when things get tough, is the most important thing. Your progress might look squiggly, like the line in Figure 3-1, or it might even feel like you're going backward, but over time you will trend upward.

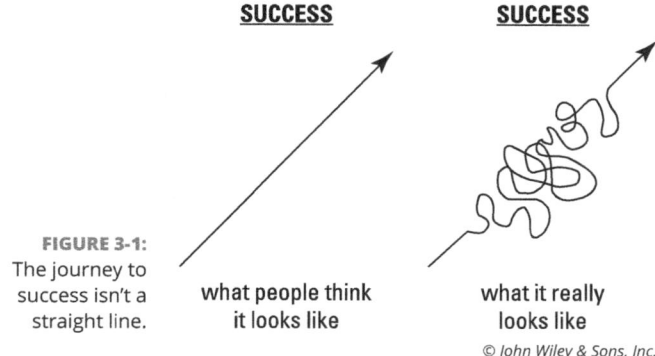

SUCCESS   SUCCESS

FIGURE 3-1:
The journey to
success isn't a
straight line.

what people think
it looks like

what it really
looks like

© *John Wiley & Sons, Inc.*

Building Your Game Plan for Health

So you've got big plans for retirement and need plenty of time to fulfill your dreams. Or you found your love later in life and want to do what you can to extend the time you have together. Or you're sick and tired of being sick and tired, and you're ready to make some changes to feel better now.

Whatever your motivation for learning about your health and making some improvements to live your best life, change starts with an action plan. Your action plan is the blueprint for a new lifestyle you can stick to for the long term. This is partly about ticking off tasks on a to-do list — who doesn't get satisfaction from that? It's also about aligning your daily habits and choices with your long-term goals how you want to live and how you want to feel.

REMEMBER

Developing an action plan involves four steps; we cover these throughout the rest of the chapter:

1. **Develop awareness.** Becoming aware of how things are now helps you determine what changes you want to make, and allows you to effectively define where you want to go and how you want to get there.

2. **Set long- and short-term goals.** You can't get from here to there if you don't know where "there" is — this is what you aspire to achieve. And the way to achieve a big goal is to break it up into smaller pieces that are easier to accomplish and that give you a chance to feel and celebrate progress.

3. **Create effective habits.** *Habits* are the behaviors that support you day to day in achieving your short- and long-term goals.

4. **Find an accountability buddy.** Every road trip is better with someone riding shotgun — you can support and motivate each other, celebrate successes and navigate setbacks together, and keep each other awake. I'll take a Twizzler.

Developing awareness

Awareness is the foundation for any meaningful change. To get to where you want to go, you need to understand where you're starting from, what got you there, and what roadblocks you need to overcome to move forward. Awareness also means paying closer attention to your physical, mental, and emotional symptoms and identifying the messages your body is sending you.

TIP

As you prepare to make your game plan, think about answers to the following questions:

>> What physical symptoms have you been experiencing regularly? For example, do you experience fatigue, digestive issues, muscle aches, low libido, or sleep disturbances?

>> When do these symptoms tend to flare up? Are there specific triggers, such as when you're stressed or when you eat particular items?

>> Do you need to follow up on your symptoms and get any testing done?

>> What behaviors do you engage in that may be hindering your progress to a better you? Are there certain people, environments, or situations that lead you to make unhealthy choices?

>> What habits do you want to change but find difficult to let go of? For example, do you procrastinate or engage in late-night scrolling, snacking, or negative self-talk? Do you overwork, stay busy, and avoid emotions?

>> What thoughts or beliefs tend to arise when you feel stuck in a rut or over-whelmed by challenges? Are these thoughts supportive or limiting? How might they be affecting your actions and decisions?

>> What are signs that indicate you're making progress, even if they feel small?

Setting long-term and short-term goals

The second step to making a game plan is to shift your focus toward the future by envisioning your healthiest, happiest self. You need to set intentional, clear goals that will serve as your "North Stars" to guide you over the bridge between where you are now and where you want to be.

TIP

Refer to your answers from the questions in the preceding section and use them to set both and long- and short-term goals. Focus on one goal at a time, and apply the SMART method (read more about SMART goals in the next section). This helps you create goals that challenge you while still being realistic and manageable.

Start with your big vision for the long term and break it down into actionable, short-term steps that will set you on the path to success.

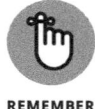

REMEMBER

We want to share an important point: Many people make the mistake of setting goals that are either too vague or too grandiose, so they set themselves up for failure. For instance, a goal such as "I want to feel better" lacks specificity and direction, whereas a goal along the lines of "I want to lose 50 pounds in a month" is unrealistic and unsustainable. What's much more effective is setting SMART goals, which challenge you but are achievable enough to foster momentum and keep you motivated.

Setting SMART goals

TIP

The *SMART method* is a well-established framework for effective goal setting. Each aspect of SMART — specific, measurable, attainable, relevant, and time-bound — ensures that goals are both actionable and realistic, paving the way for consistent, meaningful progress.

>> **Specific:** Make sure your goals are clear and well-defined. Rather than saying, "I want to be less stressed," be specific: "I want to lower my stress levels at work by practicing mindfulness meditation for 10 minutes every morning and going for a lunchtime walk."

>> **Measurable:** Make sure you have a way to track your progress. Instead of setting a vague goal such as "I want to have more energy and sleep better," you might say, "I want to increase my overall sleep levels by going to bed every night by 11:00 pm, putting all electronics in the kitchen by 10:00 pm, and reading for 30 minutes before lights out."

>> **Attainable:** Your goals should be realistic and manageable. They should stretch you but not so far that they feel impossible. For instance, setting a goal to reduce sugar intake by 50 percent within the next month is more attainable than trying to cut out all sugar overnight.

WARNING

Drastic changes, especially with things you crave, can backfire. Your brain often responds to restriction with an even stronger desire for the thing you're trying to avoid, which leads to more intense cravings.

>> **Relevant:** Make sure your goals align with your long-term objectives and values. Ask yourself, "Is this goal going to get me closer to the person I want to become?"

>> **Time-bound:** Give yourself a deadline to work toward. A time frame gives your goal structure and prevents you from procrastinating. One example is "I will meditate for 10 minutes before bed for the next 30 days."

Setting long-term goals

Long-term goals paint a picture of where you want to be in the months and years ahead and require sustained effort and commitment over the long term, so you first decide what your ultimate goal is. Once you have it established, you can then break it down into smaller, actionable, achievable steps so you don't get overwhelmed.

To set your long-term goals, consider what the happiest and healthiest version of you looks and feels like. What would your daily routine be? What environments would you spend time in? What people do you surround yourself with?

Your goals will be specific to you, but here are some examples:

>> Wake up feeling energized, excited, and optimistic

>> Exercise every day within a supportive gym community and look forward to it

>> Feel confident in my body's abilities that allow me to keep up with my energetic kids

>> Enjoy life as a non-smoker who's able to savor all flavors of a meal

Setting short-term goals

Once you have your big vision down, you can create stepping stones to help you get there. They can be actions or changes that you're able to realistically achieve within a few days or weeks. They're meant to give you quick wins. Some examples include joining a gym and committing to workouts by adding them to your calendar. If necessary, you may also want to set the goal of having a comprehensive physical exam and related vaccinations and recommended tests based on your age.

Creating effective habits

REMEMBER

This step is where real transformation begins. In his bestselling book, *Atomic Habits* (Avery, 2018), continuous-improvement expert James Clear explains that small, consistent behaviors compound to create significant, lasting change when repeated regularly. The key, Clear emphasizes, is not solely to fixate on the goals you want to achieve, but rather to focus on building the systems and structures that support those goals. While goals define the desired outcome, it's the habits — the daily processes and actions — that drive you toward those outcomes.

TIP

Read through the rest of this section to familiarize yourself with the frameworks for successfully building and breaking habits. Then consider which health-supportive habits you need to implement and use the habit loop framework to help you craft your new habit and adding it to the tracking log we provide later in this chapter. You can also apply this framework to breaking your current habits that are misaligned with your goals.

You don't have to overhaul your entire lifestyle at once; instead, start small and focus on incremental changes. Choose one or two habits that feel most accessible for you and begin with them. Once you've established consistency with those, you can gradually layer in more habits so they build over time. This way, you create sustainable change that supports your goals without feeling overwhelmed. Remember, the goal is progress and consistency, not perfection.

Creating new habits

Forming lasting habits requires more than just willpower; it involves understanding the cues, cravings, and rewards that drive your behavior. By designing habits that align with your lifestyle and making them enjoyable and easy to integrate, you're more likely to stick with them in the long term. In this section, we walk you through the steps of making habits stick:

1. **Make it obvious (cue).**

Identify the cue or trigger that initiates the habit loop. A time of day, a location, or even an emotional state could all be cues. For example, if your goal is to engage in regular physical activity, you could set a cue by placing your workout clothes in a visible spot the night before. The idea is to remove barriers between you and the habit, making the desired action as seamless as possible.

TIP

One technique to use is *habit stacking,* which means you attach your new habit to an existing one that's already firmly established. For example, you could pair your morning dog walk with a mindfulness podcast. This way, you're pairing a new behavior with something you already do automatically, creating a natural flow.

2. **Make it attractive (craving).**

If a habit feels like a chore then it's unlikely to last without a motivator. It's helpful to find ways to make your new habit something you look forward to. James Clear suggests using *temptation bundling* — linking something you want to do with something you need to do. For example, if you enjoy listening to podcasts but struggle to make time for daily workouts, you can bundle them together. This pairs an attractive reward with the behavior you want to reinforce.

3. **Make it easy (response).**

The easier a habit is, the more likely you are to stick with it. This means scaling down behaviors to something manageable, such as doing one push-up or meditating for one minute. By removing the friction, you create momentum. Once you get started, it becomes easier to do more.

4. **Make it satisfying (reward).**

To effectively reinforce habits, your brain requires a sense of immediate gratification, which enables you to tap into the *dopamine-reward loop* (where something you do generates pleasure, which makes you want to do it more, so you generate more pleasure, and loop-de-loop we go). One way to do this is by tracking your habits. Create a visual cue, such as marking an X on a calendar each time you complete your habit. Doing this creates a sense of accomplishment and taps into the very human desire not to break the streak.

Breaking old habits

REMEMBER

Certain habits, such as skipping exercise to sleep in or picking up a ready-made meal on the way home rather than using the healthy food you have in the fridge to make a quick meal, undermine your progress. You can take the following steps to combat that tendency and break existing habits you want to change:

1. **Make it invisible (remove the cue).**

Remove the triggers that initiate the behavior. (Go back to the questions in the section "Developing awareness" to help with this.) Bad habits thrive on cues, just as good habits do. To eliminate bad habits, distance yourself from the cues that spark them.

TIP

For example, if you tend to overindulge on carbohydrate-heavy or processed snacks while watching football with your family on Sundays, start by removing these snacks from your home and replacing them with healthier (yet still delicious) alternatives. Or try substituting a different activity during commercial breaks, such as a brief walk or stretching. The goal here is to make it more difficult to indulge in the behavior by removing its triggers from your environment and replacing them with more supportive cues for healthier choices.

2. **Make it unattractive (reframe the craving).**

Habits usually persist because you associate them with some level of reward, even if the reward is fleeting or damaging in the long run. To break a habit, reframe the behavior and make it unattractive. One great way to do this is by focusing on the negative long-term consequences of the habit.

TIP

For instance, if you find yourself reaching for a few beers to relax, reframe that craving by visualizing how it could be affecting your health. Imagine the long-term effects, such as gaining weight, disrupting your sleep cycles, or increased inflammation. Associating the habit with these undesirable outcomes can make the habit feel less rewarding and help you resist it more easily.

3. **Make it difficult (increase friction).**

   The more difficult you make a habit, the less likely you are to follow through with it. For example, if you check your phone the moment you wake up each day, make it harder to do that by leaving your phone in another room or in the hallway overnight.

4. **Make it unsatisfying (create accountability).**

TIP

   One of the most powerful tools for breaking a habit is *accountability.* When your actions have consequences beyond yourself, it becomes much harder to justify continuing the behavior. One way to harness this is by setting up a system where there's a real consequence for your actions. For example, if you're trying to cut down on smoking, you could commit to donating a significant amount of money to a cause you *don't* support every time you smoke a cigarette.

The power of identity in breaking habits

REMEMBER

Breaking habits is about so much more than willpower or discipline. Every time you resist the urge to engage in a bad habit, you're casting a vote for the person you want to become. You're not simply trying to stop a behavior; you're focusing on aligning with your new identity, which it much more powerful.

For instance, instead of saying, "I'm trying to stop overeating," shift your mindset to, "I'm someone who respects their body's fullness cues and nourishes themselves with healthy, balanced meals." This mental shift toward seeing yourself as someone who naturally makes decisions that align with their goals and values is transformative.

Finding an accountability buddy

Humans are inherently social creatures, and the ability to create meaningful, lasting change is magnified when we're supported and surrounded by others. As the famous African proverb says, "If you want to go fast, go alone; if you want to go far, go together." Therefore, the last step of your action plan is to find an accountability buddy.

Understanding the importance of norms and expectations

REMEMBER

The company we keep matters for our health, because we humans are deeply influenced by social norms. What's considered "normal" behavior within a particular social circle or community tends to set a baseline for how the people in those groups behave as individuals. So if you're surrounded by a group that drinks, smokes, or eats processed foods, it can become more difficult to resist those behaviors yourself. Conversely, in a group that prioritizes fitness, sobriety, healthy diets, or mindfulness, those behaviors become part of the expected routine, which subtly encourages everyone to align with the group's norms.

Powering up with accountability

One of the key psychological theories behind accountability is the concept of *commitment devices.* These are external motivators or agreements that encourage you to stick to your goals because you feel a greater sense of responsibility. For example, signing up for a charity run to motivate yourself to exercise works because you've made an external commitment to a cause. When you share your intentions and progress with someone else, you're far less likely to let things slip through the cracks. In fact, you get to harness the positive energy and momentum that comes from knowing someone else is invested in your growth and cheering you on.

REMEMBER

Having someone who understands your journey and regularly checks in on your progress can help alleviate the loneliness that often accompanies personal transformation. Change isn't easy — especially when it requires sacrificing short-term comforts, summoning grit, and drawing on determination. An accountability buddy can provide the extra push you need when your motivation slips (or your old patterns and behaviors creep back in). This person can also offer fresh perspectives when inevitable challenges arise and celebrate your wins with you. They may help you see progress you might otherwise overlook. Plus, by supporting each other, you create a positive feedback loop of encouragement, pushing each other to new heights.

Building your support network

REMEMBER

It's important to acknowledge that not everyone around you may fully understand the health improvements you're seeking to make or why you're trying to make them.

Identify at least one person in your life who could be your accountability buddy. If no one immediately comes to mind, explore options in online communities or consider enlisting a professional, such as a personal trainer, nutritionist, or therapist. When you've found your person (or people), initiate a conversation with them about your mutual goals and how you can keep each other on track. Then, plan your first check-in within the next week to set your accountability system in motion!

2
Longevity Isn't Luck — It's Lifestyle

IN THIS PART . . .

Start eating clean and navigate early hurdles to get a good mix of healthy foods.

Decide how much and how intense your physical activity should be, and pick some activities that keep you engaged.

Understand weights, reps, and sets so you can create — and get started on — a training plan.

Recognize and combat stress, make connections to limit loneliness, and fortify your mental health.

Figure out what makes for good sleep and make changes based on your current habits.

Reassess the roles that smoking and drinking play in your life and make changes to put your health first.

Find the right primary care provider, prepare for an annual physical, and get the recommended vaccines for your age.

Chapter **4**

Eating Better Now So You Can Live Longer Later

O nce upon a time, people simply sat down to dinner, eating to fill an empty stomach or just for the pleasure of it. Nobody said, "Wow, that cream soup is loaded with calories," or asked whether the bread was a high-fiber loaf, or fretted about the chicken being served with the skin still on. No longer. Today, the dinner table can be a battleground — with yourself or others — between health and pleasure. Maybe you or a loved one plan your meals with the precision of a major general moving their troops into the front lines, or maybe you get a lot of take-outs or meals from the freezer section of the grocery store. For a lot of guys who try to eat mindfully, choosing what's good for you over what just tastes good can feel like a lifelong battle.

This chapter aims to end the war between your need for good nutrition and your equally compelling need for tasty meals. Living a better and hopefully longer life is a great goal, but it's less compelling if you feel you're not allowed to enjoy what you consume when getting your three squares.

Figuring Out Food

Why did we evolve with such complicated digestive systems when other organisms can simply absorb nutrients from their surrounding environment? Read on to find out.

Fueling up with food

The human body is amazing — it can do all sorts of work, like replacing a roof, moving couches up two flights of stairs, running a six-minute mile, analyzing pages of data to create a two-sentence synopsis, and doing the Dougie. To do all this work, your body needs *energy*, and the fuel for energy is the food you eat. The amount of energy in food is measured in *calories,* the amount of heat produced when food is burned (*metabolized*) in your body cells. Without enough food — fuel — you don't have enough energy to run your body. No surprise there.

Categorizing macronutrients and micronutrients

REMEMBER

Food is more than just fuel. It's also the source of essential building blocks that your body and brain need to grow, repair, and age. Nutrients can be broadly categorized into two groups: macronutrients and micronutrients.

Macronutrients

Macronutrients are the nutrients your body needs in larger amounts. They are the primary sources of energy and the building blocks for various cellular processes. A healthy diet is comprised of a mix of the following:

» **Carbohydrates** provide glucose, the main energy source for your body and fuel for neurons. Examples of carbs include fruits, vegetables, grains (like rice, pasta, breads, and cereals), and some legumes (like peas) and beans (like chickpeas).

» **Protein** supplies essential amino acids to build and repair tissues, and synthesize hormones and neurotransmitters. Examples include chicken, fish, eggs, pork, and beef; milk and other dairy products; some beans (like black beans) and legumes (like lentils).

» **Fat** provides essential fatty acids, energy, and helps absorb vitamins while forming 60 percent of your brain's structure. Examples of fats include oils (such as olive, vegetable, coconut), nuts (like walnuts and almonds), and seeds (including sunflower, pumpkin, and chia).

REMEMBER

Some foods cross over and can be counted in more than one category. Examples include lentils and black beans (high in protein but also high in carbs), some nuts and seeds (high in fat but also relatively rich in protein), and some fruits or vegetables (avocado is technically a fruit but is so high in fat that it's often categorized as a fat). The free versions of apps such as MyFitnessPal and Chronometer provide nutrition data on thousands of foods. You can also find nutrition info at fdc.nal.usda.gov (look in the section called Foundation Foods).

TIP

Lean proteins such as chicken and fish are better for your body than higher fat proteins (for example, beef and bacon). Whole grains (like brown rice, whole wheat bread, and oats) are better for you than refined grains (such as white flour, white rice). Take a look at Chapter 15 for information on making heart-healthy nutrition choices.

Micronutrients

Micronutrients include vitamins and minerals, are needed in microscopic amounts, but are still very important. Vitamins are *organic*, meaning they're made by living organisms such as plants. Minerals are *inorganic*, meaning they come from the soil or water. Together vitamins and minerals support a wide range of your physiological and cellular needs. Examples include:

>> Key brain vitamins include B vitamins for energy and neurotransmitter synthesis, vitamin C for antioxidant protection, and vitamin E for cell membrane health.

>> Essential minerals such as magnesium aid synapse transmission, zinc supports brain function, and iron is vital for oxygen transport and energy metabolism.

Making Food Choices Based on Their Nutrition

A healthful diet provides sufficient amounts of all the nutrients that your body needs. You need some carbs, some protein, and some fats every day to keep your body humming. The question is, how much is enough, and how do you monitor that you're getting what you need?

Different sets of recommendations help you determine how much is enough, and each one comes with its own virtues and deficiencies. The recommendation you're most likely familiar with, and the one this chapter covers, are the *RDA* guidelines (short for *Recommended Dietary Allowance*).

Understanding RDAs to keep your nutrition on point

The Recommended Dietary Allowances (RDAs) originally were designed to make planning several days' meals in advance easy for you. The *D* in RDA stands for *dietary*, not daily, because the RDAs are an average. You may get more of a nutrient one day and less the next, but the idea is to hit an average over several days.

RDAs offer recommendations for protein and 18 essential vitamins and minerals. What nutrients are missing from the RDA list of essentials? Carbohydrates, fiber, fat, and alcohol.

The thinking is, if your diet provides enough protein, vitamins, and minerals, it's almost certain to provide enough carbohydrates and probably more than enough fat. But being forewarned is being forearmed, so here are some pointers for determining reasonable amounts of calories, carbohydrates, dietary fiber, fats, protein, and alcohol:

» **Balance what you eat with how much you move.** See the section "Determining how many calories you need" for specifics on how many calories a person of your weight, height, and level of activity needs to consume each day.

» **Make foods with complex carbohydrates and dietary fiber the base of your total daily calories.** These should make up to 900 to 1,300 calories and up to 25 grams dietary fiber on a 2,000 calorie per day diet.

» **Concentrate on unsaturated fats.** Not all fats are created equal — some are healthier for your body than others. Unsaturated fats are better for you, and include plant-based foods such as vegetable oils, nuts, and seeds.

» **Drink alcohol only in moderation.** That means a maximum of two drinks per day for a man. For more on alcohol consumption, see Chapter 9.

Deciphering RDAs on nutrition labels

All prepackaged foods now include a nutrition label so you can easily understand how well (or poorly) a particular food delivers nutrients to help you fuel up. Fresh foods may not all come with labels, but you can get nutrient information from popular apps such as My Fitness Pal and Cronometer and websites such as `MyPlate.gov`.

TECHNICAL STUFF

Nutrient listings use the metric system. RDAs for protein are listed in grams. RDAs for vitamins and minerals are shown in milligrams (mg) and micrograms (mcg). Here are the units you'll see on the nutrition labels of your favorite foods:

>> g = gram

>> mg = milligram = 1/1,000 of a gram

>> mcg = microgram = 1/1,000,000 of a gram

>> IU = international unit

>> RE = retinol equivalent = the amount of "true" vitamin A in an IU

>> a-TE = alpha-tocopherol equivalent = the amount of alpha-tocopherol in a unit of vitamin E

Figuring out your RDAs based on your age

Table 4-1 shows the most recent RDAs for *vitamins* for healthy men; Table 4-2 shows RDAs for *minerals* for healthy men. Where no RDA is given, an AI is included. (*AI* stands for *adequate intake* and are used for eight nutrients that are considered necessary for good health, even though nobody really knows exactly how much your body needs. Not to worry: sooner or later, some smart nutrition researcher will come up with a hard number and move the nutrient to the RDA list.)

TABLE 4-1   **Vitamin RDAs for Healthy Male Adults**

Age (Years)	Vitamin A (RE/IU)†	Vitamin D (mcg/IU)‡*	Vitamin E (a-TE)	Vitamin K (mcg)*	Vitamin C (mg)
Males					
19–30	900/2,970	15/600	15	120	90
31–50	900/2,970	15/600	15	120	90
51–70	900/2,970	15/600	15	120	90
71 and older	900/2,970	20/800	15	120	90

*Adequate Intake (AI)

†The "official" RDA for vitamin A is still 1,000 RE/5,000 IU for a male; the lower numbers listed on this chart are the currently recommended levels for adults.

‡The current recommendations are the amounts required to prevent vitamin D deficiency disease; recent studies suggest that the optimal levels for overall health may actually be higher, in the range of 800–1,000 IU a day.

TABLE 4-2   # Mineral RDAs for Healthy Male Adults

Age (years)	Calcium (mg)*	Phosphorus (mg)	Magnesium (mg)	Iron (mg)	Zinc (mg)	Copper (mcg)
19–30	1,000	700	400	8	11	900
31–50	1,000	700	420	8	11	900
51–70	1,200	700	420	8	11	900
71 and older	1,200	700	420	8	11	900

Adequate Intake (AI)

Age (years)	Thiamin (Vitamin B1) (mg)	Riboflavin (Vitamin B2) (mg)	Niacin (NE)	Pantothenic acid (mg)*	Vitamin B6 (mg)	Folate (mcg)	Vitamin B12 (mcg)	Biotin (mcg)*
19–30	1.2	1.3	16	5	1.3	400	2.4	30
31–50	1.2	1.3	16	5	1.3	400	2.4	30
50–70	1.2	1.3	16	5	1.7	400	2.4	30
71 and older	1.2	1.1	16	5	1.7	400	2.4	30

Adequate Intake (AI)

Age (years)	Iodine (mcg)	Selenium (mcg)	Molybdenum (mcg)	Manganese (mg)*	Fluoride (mg)*	Chromium (mcg)*	Choline (mg)*
19–30	150	55	45	2.3	4	36	550
31–50	150	55	45	2.3	4	36	550
51–70	150	55	45	2.3	4	30	550
71 and older	150	55	45	2.3	4	30	550

Adequate Intake (AI)

Adapted with permission from Recommended Dietary Allowances (Washington D.C.: National Academy Press, 1989), and DRI panel reports, 1997–2004.

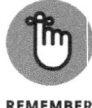

REMEMBER

The slogan "No Sale Ever Is Final," printed on the sales slips at one of our favorite clothing stores, definitely applies to nutritional numbers. RDAs and AIs should always be regarded as works in progress, subject to revision at the first sign of a new study. In other words, in an ever-changing world, here's one thing of which you can be *absolutely* certain: The numbers in this chapter will change. Sorry about that.

DO I NEED SUPPLEMENTS?

Many people take one or more dietary or nutritional supplements either every day or occasionally. Today's dietary supplements include vitamins, minerals, herbals and botanicals, amino acids, enzymes, and many other products. Dietary supplements may come in the form of tablets, capsules, powders, energy bars, and drinks. Common dietary supplements include vitamins C, D, and E; minerals like calcium, magnesium, and iron; herbs such as echinacea and garlic; and specialty products like glucosamine, probiotics, and fish oils.

When you select a dietary supplement, you'll notice the Supplement Facts panel on the packaging that lists the contents, amount of active ingredients per serving, and other added ingredients (like fillers, binders, and flavorings). Serving size is often suggested by the manufacturer, but your doctor may recommend a different amount that's appropriate for you.

Dietary supplements should *not* take the place of the variety of foods that are necessary for a healthy diet. Supplements are meant to be just that — supplements. Dietary supplements can be an addition to a healthy diet that will help you get essential nutrients, but mustn't be used as a substitute or replacement.

Some supplements may interact with certain medications, so if you're taking medications to manage any health conditions, talk to your doctor before starting to take supplements.

Firing Up the Body with Calories

Automobiles burn gasoline to get the energy they need to move. Your body burns (*metabolizes*) food to produce energy in the form of heat that keeps you warm and (as energy) powers your every move and thought.

The amount of heat produced by metabolizing food is measured in a unit called the *kilocalorie* — the amount of energy it takes to raise the temperature of 1 kilogram of water 1 degree on a Centigrade (Celsius) thermometer at sea level.

TECHNICAL STUFF

Nutritionists commonly substitute the word *calorie* for *kilocalorie*. Strictly speaking, a true calorie is just 1/1,000 of a kilocalorie, but the word *calorie* is easier to say and easier to remember, so that's what you see when you read about the energy in food.

Understanding calories — because a doughnut ain't a salad

When someone says that a serving of food — say, one banana — has 105 calories, that means your metabolizing the banana produces 105 calories of energy your body can use for work.

Different foods have different amounts of calories depending on their nutritional components. For example, high-fat foods have more calories than low-fat foods because a gram of fat has more calories than a gram of carbs or protein or alcohol:

>> Fat has 9 calories per gram.

>> Carbohydrates have 4 calories per gram.

>> Protein has 4 calories per gram.

>> Alcohol has 7 calories per gram.

In other words, ounce for ounce, proteins and carbohydrates give you fewer than half as many calories as fat. That's why — again, ounce for ounce — high-fat foods, such as cream cheese and doughnuts, are calorie-rich, while low-fat foods, such as fruits and vegetables, are not.

WARNING

Sometimes foods that seem like they should be equally low calorie really aren't. You have to watch all the angles, paying attention to fat in addition to protein and carbohydrates. Here's a good example: A skinless chicken breast and a hamburger are both high-protein foods. So you think both should have the same number of calories per ounce. But because the chicken is skinless, it contains very little fat, while the hamburger has a lot. So a 3-ounce serving of skinless chicken gives you 140 calories, while a similarly sized 3-ounce burger yields 230 to 245 calories, depending on the cut of the meat and its fat content. (This is where apps such as Chronometer and MyFitnessPal come in handy — it's hard to remember all these nutrition nuances.)

Determining how many calories you need

Think of your energy requirements as a bank account. You make deposits when you consume calories. You make withdrawals when your body spends energy on work. Nutritionists divide the amount of energy you withdraw each day into two parts:

>> **The energy you need when your body is at rest** (called *resting energy expenditure,* or REE), which accounts for 60 to 70 percent of all the energy you need each day.

>> **The energy you need to do your daily "work,"** which includes everything from brushing your teeth in the morning to walking the dog before dinner or working out in the gym.

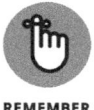

REMEMBER

To keep your energy account in balance, you need to take in enough each day to cover your withdrawals. Figuring out exactly how many calories you need each day can be a consuming task. Luckily, Table 4-3 shows the calorie recommendations as estimated by the U.S. Department of Agriculture and Health and Human Services.

Note: In this context, *sedentary* means a lifestyle with only the light physical activity associated with daily living; *moderately active* means a lifestyle that adds physical activity equal to a daily 1.5-to-3-mile walk at a speed of 3 to 4 miles per hour; *active* means adding physical activity equal to walking 3 miles a day at the 3 to 4 miles per hour clip.

TABLE 4-3 **Daily Calorie Needs for Healthy Men Based on Activity Level**

Age (years)	Sedentary	Moderately Active	Active
19–30	2,400	2,600–2,800	3,000
31–50	2,200	2,400–2,600	2,800–3,000
51–60	2,200	2,200–2,400	2,400–2,800
61–65	2,000	2,400	2,800
66–75	2,000	2,200	2,600
76+	2,000	2,200	2,400

Source: https://www.webmd.com/diet/features/estimated-calorie-requirement.

EATING A MEDITERRANEAN STYLE DIET

The MedDiet, rich in fruits, vegetables, whole grains, legumes, nuts, olive oil, and fish (plus a little red wine), has been linked to numerous health benefits like lower risks of heart disease, diabetes, obesity, dementia, and improved mental health. Its anti-inflammatory, antioxidant properties make it ideal for reducing obesity and, with its plant-based focus, it has a low environmental impact, offering both health and sustainability benefits.

(continued)

(continued)

Rather than being a strict optimization protocol, the MedDiet is like a set of guiding principles that influence how you select, prepare, eat, and enjoy food. Here's a quick summary of what you should eat on a Mediterranean-style diet:

- **Veggies and fruits:** Load up on a variety of colorful vegetables and fruits.
- **Extra virgin olive oil:** Use this as your main source of fat — it's both tasty and healthy!
- **Whole-grain breads and cereals:** Think whole-grain goodness such as whole wheat bread and hearty cereals.
- **Legumes and beans:** Chickpeas, kidney beans, lentils — these are your new best friends.
- **Nuts and seeds:** Snack on a handful of nuts or sprinkle seeds over your meals.
- **Fish and seafood:** Treat yourself to fish and seafood regularly.
- **Herbs and spices:** Flavor your dishes with onion, garlic, and a variety of herbs and spices such as oregano, coriander, and cumin.

Wondering about meat and dairy? No worries! You can definitely include:

- **Yogurt, cheese, and milk:** Enjoy these in moderation.
- **Lean proteins:** Chicken, turkey, and eggs are all great choices.
- **Red meat and sweets:** Keep these to small amounts and occasional treats.
- **Processed meats and packaged foods:** Try to limit these to rare occasions.

And what about alcohol? If you enjoy a drink, wine (especially red wine) is a traditional part of this diet. Just remember, it's all about moderation and enjoying it with meals.

Eating Clean to Power Your Present and Protect Your Future

Awareness of clean eating has increased in recent years, with magazines, books, websites, and other media dedicated to advancing this concept. But what does it mean to eat clean? And how does it line up with your goal of avoiding heart disease, cancer, and the other big health risks guys face? All great questions that we answer in this section.

First, a definition: *eating clean* is simply another way to say "eating healthy." The principal goal is to base your diet on consuming whole, unprocessed foods as much as possible. These foods don't need to be organic, although you can certainly choose organic foods if you can afford them and feel you'd derive additional benefits from them.

REMEMBER

Clean eating comes with big perks. For starters, sticking to foods lower on the food chain loads you up with cancer-fighting nutrients your body actually knows what to do with. You're also cutting empty calories from refined sugar and unhealthy fats, helping you maintain a healthy weight (reducing a risk factor for heart disease and other health conditions) and avoid additives tied to health risks.

Applying clean eating principles

TIP

Eating better can feel confusing at first — calories, macros, fiber, protein . . . it's a lot to think about. But clean eating keeps it simple, using commonsense rules you can actually stick to. Here are some points to keep in mind as you move toward a clean diet:

>> **Focus on eating nutrient-dense foods as close to their natural state as possible.** This means avoiding processed food (anything in a box, can, or container that has a long shelf life and contains a bunch of unpronounceable ingredients) whenever you can and favoring nutrient-dense foods, such as fresh produce, whole grains, legumes, and lean meats (chicken, turkey, fish) and dairy.

>> **Expand your palate by eating a wide variety of wholesome foods.** Variety is the spice of life, and eating a broad range of foods helps keep food boredom at bay. Plus, you're more likely to get a great mix of nutrients without having to make too many decisions about what to eat when.

>> **Plan on eating five or six times daily.** Eating small, frequent meals is healthier than gorging yourself with large meals. Spreading out your meals helps keep your blood glucose levels stable, provides a steady stream of energy, and helps ward off the negative effects of eating big meals, like indigestion and sleepiness.

>> **Use the New American Plate to guide your meal ratios.** This method, created by American Institute for Cancer Research, comprises a plate made up of two-thirds (or more) of vegetables, fruits, and whole grains or beans and one-third (or less) of an animal protein. If you're a vegetarian, substitute a plant-based source of protein, such as beans or tofu, for the meat. Alternatively, you can use a whole grain that's high in protein, like quinoa. Find an example of the New American Plate here: www.aicr.org/cancer-prevention/healthy-eating/new-american-plate.

>> **Strive for *more* than five fruits and vegetables, and get colorful!** Fruits and vegetables are the healthiest foods on Earth. A considerable amount of disease-fighting power is contained in the very compounds that give produce its pigment. By varying the color of the produce you eat, you'll get a wider array of nutrients. Plus, you'll be creating a beautiful plate — and, as they say, you eat with your eyes first.

Avoiding "dirty" foods (most of the time)

Certain foods just aren't clean, often because they contain large quantities of compounds that aren't healthy. Because clean eating isn't meant to be a restrictive diet (it's a lifestyle, man!), don't beat yourself up if you occasionally eat any of the items we outline here. As long as you avoid them most of the time, you're good.

TIP

Many people find the 80–20 rule works well for them: Try to focus on eating clean 80 percent of the time if you can, which means 20 percent of your choices can be a little more relaxed.

Here are foods and other items to avoid whenever possible:

>> **Artificial sweeteners** are synthetic sugar substitutes that are often significantly sweeter than sugar. They don't provide any nutritive benefits, and they may cause greater weight gain than sugar (and obesity is a known risk factor for heart disease and cancer). You're better off adding a little honey, Sucanat, or other natural sweetener to your food or simply going without. The more sweets you cut out of your diet, the less you'll crave them.

>> **Fast foods** like burgers, pizza, and fries are most certainly unhealthy and can contribute to weight gain if eaten frequently. They're also highly processed to make them last longer and taste better. But many of today's fast-food restaurants offer healthier options like salads, plain baked potatoes, grilled chicken sandwiches, and fruit smoothies, so next time you need to consider a drive-thru, order one of the healthier options.

>> **Processed foods**, also called *convenience foods,* have been altered from their natural states and have a long shelf life, lots of additives (such as artificial colors and flavors), and little nutritive value. You know, like those boxed dinners that line the middle aisles of the grocery store, or the hot dogs and other nitrate-preserved meats.

TIP

When you need to consider convenience foods, take the time to read labels — two seemingly similar items may have very different nutrient stats. And if you do end up indulging in a boxed dinner or having hot dogs, eating foods that are high in vitamin C may help counteract any potential ill effects.

Vitamin C can combat the inflammation triggered by certain additives, and some evidence suggests that vitamin C–rich foods can prevent nitrates from being transformed into cancer-causing compounds.

>> **Refined sugar, sodium, and saturated and trans fats** have little nutritive value and can cause ill health effects when eaten consistently or in larger quantities. Eating lots of refined sugar gives you nothing but empty calories and can lead to weight gain and diabetes; excess sodium intake can lead to fluid retention and high blood pressure; and saturated and trans fats can clog blood vessels, leading to heart disease.

Deciding to take it slow or jump right into clean eating

Because eating clean is a lifestyle, you have the flexibility to ease into it or to dive in headfirst. To avoid pronounced cravings for unhealthy food you no longer eat and to reduce feelings of deprivation — both of which place you at higher risk of reverting back to your old eating habits — we recommend you start slowly. Simply start replacing some of your unhealthy staples with clean substitutes. For example, have unsweetened iced green tea in place of soda, carrot sticks instead of potato chips, or low-fat plain yogurt with some berries instead of pudding. As you get comfortable with your initial replacements, simply keep making more replacements until you're at your goal clean eating level.

Managing cravings

Food cravings aren't a sign of weakness, but they may be a sign of addiction, particularly if your diet has largely consisted of processed foods. When you nourish your body with nutrient-dense foods, that double-chocolate fudge cake you enjoyed so much before may be entirely too sweet for you now. Until you get to this point, you may crave those unwholesome eats and go through a withdrawal period.

TIP

Try these tips to tackle any cravings you experience:

>> Keep unwholesome foods out of the house.

>> Distract yourself with a 20-minute activity like taking a walk, pulling weeds, or shooting some hoops.

>> Have a healthy snack that mimics your craving.

Handling feelings of deprivation

It's normal to feel a sense of deprivation as you remove foods from your diet that you're accustomed to, or that have brought you comfort, or that are associated with happy memories. But in some cases, the deprivation may be spurred on by factors you can control and remedy without straying from your clean eating plan.

TIP

If you starting feeling deprived, ask yourself these questions:

>> **Are you eating too bland?** Make sure you're seasoning your food well with spices, herbs, and a variety of condiments.

>> **Are you getting enough calories?** Don't restrict calories; just make sure you're getting your calories from nutrient-dense sources so you reap the greatest health benefits.

>> **Are you being too strict or taking it too quickly?** The goal is to *eventually* be eating mostly clean (like the 80-20 rule we mention earlier in this chapter). If you suddenly switched completely away from a diet high in processed foods, take a step back and slow your transition so your body can better adjust to your new way of eating.

>> **Are you failing to reward yourself in other ways?** If you often treated food as a reward and clean foods aren't yet fitting that bill, you may need to set up more non-food rewards for yourself.

Discovering nature's flavor enhancers

As you adjust to eating clean foods, you may think they taste bland or unappealing compared with the foods you've been consuming. This isn't because clean foods aren't flavorful; it's because food manufacturers pump processed foods with sugar, sodium, and additives to ramp up their flavor. During the transition, you're simply noticing that absence.

Your palate will eventually come to appreciate the unique flavors of clean foods, which often have many more subtle notes than any food manufacturer can achieve.

But while you make the adjustment (and even once you have), you don't have to eat whole foods just as they are to keep them clean. Give some of these natural and minimally processed flavor enhancers a try:

>> **Lemon and citrus juices:** These acidic juices can perk up the flavor of everything from chicken and fish, to produce and whole grains. They can also keep foods like avocados and bananas from turning brown, making them

more palatable when added to certain recipes, like guacamole and fruit salad. As a bonus, you get a healthy dose of vitamin C.

» **Fresh herbs:** Herbs are like little flavor bombs, and they're packed with phytochemicals. They can be used in any dish.

» **Hot peppers:** Hot peppers such as jalapenos or habaneros can add a kick to your foods, whether you're adding them directly to a recipe or you get industrious and make your own hot sauce.

» **Spices:** If you peruse the baking aisle in any grocery store, you'll see there are a vast number of spices, which can be used to flavor everything from sweet treats to savory dishes.

» **Salt:** Don't feel bad about sprinkling on a little salt, particularly if your diet now includes very few processed foods. Just be sure to limit your total sodium intake to less than 2,300 mg daily or to no more than 1,500 mg if you're older than age 51 or have high blood pressure, diabetes, or chronic kidney disease. That's less than ¼ teaspoon of salt daily.

» **Condiments:** Mustard reigns supreme in its ability to impart flavor. Other condiments include salsa, guacamole, mayonnaise, and naturally brewed low-sodium soy sauce. Avoid condiments made with artificial flavors and colors, such as prepared barbecue sauces.

Chapter **5**

Breaking a Sweat Five Days a Week

E xercise is one of your greatest tools for helping you feel better, look better, and potentially live a longer, happier life. Luckily, exercise can be fun and healthfully addictive, as well as having residual benefits on your mental and emotional health. Our bodies weren't designed to be sedentary, despite the way our lifestyles have changed over the years. Getting adequate physical activity helps you achieve your health goals, and if you choose a form of exercise you like, you'll even enjoy yourself in the process. The level of enjoyment that you experience will help you to heal and ward off other illness and complications as well.

WARNING

If you're already navigating a serious healthcare condition, such as diabetes, heart disease, prostate cancer, or other diagnoses, make sure to consult your primary-care physician before beginning specific exercise plans.

Getting Off the Couch: Why Exercise Is Essential

The benefits of exercise on overall physical health and well-being are hard to deny. The following is just a partial list of health benefits you can expect from frequent, consistent exercise. Specifically, exercise

>> Normalizes blood pressure

>> Improves overall cardiovascular health

>> Reduces some cancer risks and may prevent recurrences or the progression of prostate cancer

>> Decreases the risk of diabetes

>> Improves muscle and joint function

>> Reduces inflammation

>> Strengthens bones

>> Improves memory and brain functioning

Regular exercise also improves mental health. Frequent exercisers have less depression and anxiety. They also have better focus and handle stress more effectively. Find a drug that can do all that for both mental and physical health, and you'll become rich and famous!

TIP

Evidence has shown that not only is exercise necessary to good health, but that spending too much time on sedentary activities is bad for your health. So as you change up some of your lifestyle habits, make sure to limit sedentary time. Get up every 30 minutes and move around. If you spend much of your day sitting at a desk, you can also try out a standing desk and alternate standing with sitting on a stability ball.

Determining How Much You Should Exercise

Unless you have a specific physical restriction, you have no limitation on what kind of exercise or how much you can do. You should select one or more activities that you enjoy and will continue to perform. If you're new to exercise, it's a good idea to build exercise slowly (find out more in the later section of this chapter, "Easing in, not opting out").

Dialing in the right effort for you

TIP

In the past, exercise physiologists wanted you to monitor your exercise intensity by periodically checking your heart rate. Your exercise heart rate was supposed to be based on your age. The usual formula to figure this out is to take the number 220, subtract your age, and multiply that number by 60 to 75 percent to get the recommended heart rate zone for aerobic exercise.

Now studies have shown that people can sustain aerobic exercise at higher heart rates. Perhaps the best way to know whether you're meeting your exercise goals is to use the perceived exertion scale described in the sidebar "Checking the Value of Your Exercise."

The younger you are, the faster your exercise heart rate may be. Your exercise heart rate is an individual number. If you're a world-class athlete training for your ninth marathon, your exercise heart rate may be higher. If you have some heart disease, your exercise heart rate may be significantly lower.

Deciding how often to exercise

The amount of physical activity you should aim for has fluctuated in the past, based on evolving research. Experts now recommend that you should get at least 150 minutes of moderate-intensity physical activity per week (plus strength training twice per week) to get the best benefit for your body. Or if you like an intense workout, you can get the same benefits with 75 minutes per week of vigorous-intensity activity, or some combo of the two. And you can split up these 150 minutes however you want. Exercise for 30 minutes five days a week, or 45 minutes three days per week. The 150 minutes (or more) is what matters.

REMEMBER

What happens when you take a break? Maybe you're swamped with life and pause making time for physical activity, or you get injured, or you just lose motivation? How long can you stop exercising before you start to decondition? It takes only about two to three weeks to lose some of the fitness your exercise has provided. Then it takes up to six weeks to get back to your current level, assuming that your holiday from exercise doesn't go on too long. So when you're struggling to fit in exercise, even one or two sessions in a week is better for you than none; you can pick back up as soon as you're able.

CHECKING THE VALUE OF YOUR EXERCISE

Use the perceived exertion scale to easily assess how hard you're exercising. Exercise is given a descriptive value ranging from *extremely light* to *extremely hard* based on how hard it is to perform. You want to exercise to a level of *somewhat hard* — you'll be at your target heart rate in most cases. As you get into shape, the amount of exertion that corresponds to *somewhat hard* will increase.

Here's a description of these various levels of exercise:

- **Extremely light exercise** is very easy to do and requires little or no exertion.
- **Very light exercise** is like walking slowly for several minutes.
- **Light exercise** is like walking faster but at a pace you can continue without effort.
- **Somewhat hard exercise** is getting a little difficult but still feels okay to continue.
- **Very hard exercise** is difficult to continue. You have to push yourself, and you're very tired. At this level, you have trouble talking. The very hard level of exercise is most beneficial, but it isn't for everyone. Be sure to check with your doctor before engaging in very hard exercise to make sure that it's safe for you.
- **Extremely hard exercise** is the most difficult exercise you've ever done.

You should be able to talk or sing comfortably while doing aerobic exercise. If you can't, you're probably in the *very hard* (or even *extremely hard*) zone.

Warning: Don't continue exercising if you have tightness in your chest, chest pain, severe shortness of breath, or dizziness.

Choosing What Moves You to Get Moving

In order to hit your 150 minutes of moderate physical activity weekly, you first need to understand what we mean by "moderate." *Moderate exercise* has a moving definition. If you're out of shape, moderate exercise for you may be slow walking. If you're in good shape, moderate exercise may be jogging or cross-country skiing. Moderate exercise is simply something you can do without getting out of breath.

The following factors can help you determine your choice(s) of activity:

>> Do you like to exercise alone or with company? Pick a competitive or team sport or a group fitness class if you prefer company.

>> Do you like to compete against others or just yourself? Running or walking are activities you can do alone.

>> Do you prefer vigorous or less-vigorous activity? Less-vigorous activity over a longer period is just as effective as more-vigorous activity.

>> Do you live where you can do activities outside year-round, or do you need to go inside a lot of the year? Find a sports club if weather prevents year-round outside activity.

>> Do you need special equipment or just a pair of running shoes?

>> What benefits are you looking for in your exercise — cardiovascular, strength, endurance, flexibility, or body fat control? You should probably look for all these benefits, but you may have to combine activities to get them all in.

>> Do you have any balance problems? If so, swimming and water aerobics are great choices for you.

Sizing up the benefits before you break a sweat

TIP

A good starting point in your activity selection is to focus on the benefits. Table 5-1 gives you some ideas.

TABLE 5-1   **Match Your Activity to the Results You Want**

If You Want to . . .	Then Consider . . .
Build up cardiovascular condition	Vigorous basketball, pickle ball, squash, cross-country skiing, handball, swimming, aerobics, dancing
Strengthen your body	Low-weight high-repetition weight lifting, gymnastics, swimming, mountain climbing, cross-country skiing, biking, Pilates, Tai chi
Build up muscular endurance	Gymnastics, rowing, cross-country skiing, vigorous basketball, Pilates, resistance training
Increase flexibility	Gymnastics, yoga, judo, karate, soccer, surfing
Control body fat	Handball, pickle ball, squash, cross-country skiing, vigorous basketball, singles tennis

TIP

Hundreds of fitness videos are available for free online that you can even do while seated in a chair. You can swim, bike, row, or do armchair exercises where you move your upper body vigorously.

Cross-training, where you do several different activities throughout the week, is a good idea. Cross-training reduces the boredom that may accompany doing one thing day after day. It also permits you to exercise regardless of the weather because you can do some things indoors and some outside. So don't feel limited to choosing just one activity from the previous list.

REMEMBER

As you consider the activity (or activities) you want to pursue, remember that the social benefits of exercise are very important, too. You're together with people who are concerned with health and appearance. These people usually share many of your interests. People who like to jog often like to hike and climb and camp, too. Many lifetime partnerships begin on one side of a tennis court and on the dance floor.

Considering calories canceled

Table 5-2 lists a variety of activities, including some that don't exactly fit into the category of exercise or physical activity but are activities you may find yourself doing a fair bit. Next to each activity, we include the amount of kilocalories that a 125-pound person, a 175-pound person, and a 225-pound person burn in 20 minutes.

TABLE 5-2 **Calories Burned in 20 Minutes at Different Body Weights**

Activity	Kilocalories Burned (125 pounds)	Kilocalories Burned (175 pounds)	Kilocalories Burned (225 pounds)
Standing	24	32	43
Walking, 4 mph	104	144	199
Running, 7 mph	236	328	456
Gardening	60	84	118
Writing	30	42	59
Typing	38	54	77
Carpentry	64	88	121
House painting	58	80	110
Playing baseball	78	108	149
Dancing	70	96	132
Playing football	138	192	267
Golfing	66	96	139

Activity	Kilocalories Burned (125 pounds)	Kilocalories Burned (175 pounds)	Kilocalories Burned (225 pounds)
Swimming	80	112	157
Skiing, downhill	160	224	314
Skiing, cross-country	196	276	389
Playing tennis	112	160	229
Hatha yoga	76	105	145

Everything you do burns calories. Even sleeping and watching television use 20 kilocalories in 20 minutes if you weigh 125 pounds.

TECHNICAL STUFF

Here's an interesting tidbit. There's a sweet spot when you're planning a running fitness regime. A study published in the *Journal of the American College of Cardiology* in February 2015, which followed joggers for a total of 12 years, showed that 1 to 2.4 hours of light jogging per week is the healthiest form of running. Over the 12-year period, strenuous joggers were as likely to die as sedentary non-joggers. So don't feel like you need to train for a marathon in order to get the benefits of running.

Easing in, not opting out

Men can have very different overall levels of health. Some men are generally physically strong and fit, while others haven't exercised much in years, spending a lot of their time behind a desk, watching tv, or playing video games.

How long and how intensely you exercise depends on how active you are. Active men can generally exercise far more vigorously, and for longer periods of time, than sedentary men can. But it's important to keep in mind that engaging in physical activity is good for your body no matter how long or hard you're moving. So, if you've been leading a pretty low-key and inactive life, you shouldn't jump right into your new exercise program by running the Boston Marathon or climbing Mount Everest. You need to build up slowly with exercise, as your own doctor can tell you. In fact, it's very important to check your exercise plan with your doctor first.

If you're new to exercise, it's a good idea to build exercise slowly by increasing the amount of exercise you get by an additional 10 percent per week in order to prevent injury and excess fatigue. Once you top out at 150 minutes weekly, you've met the recommended minimum for overall health benefits. We said recommended *minimum* — exercising more than 150 minutes per week is beneficial for your body, so keep increasing by 10 percent (up to 300 minutes per week) if you want to support your body's health even more.

Walking into Wellness, One Step at a Time

TIP

The special needs of some of the activities we talk about earlier in this chapter may turn you off exercising. If so, then we have good news for you — the best exercise that you can sustain for life is right at your feet. A brisk daily walk improves heart function, adds to muscular endurance, and helps control body fat. Walking is an excellent exercise for most men, regardless of physical fitness or any existing health conditions. Other good exercises are bicycling, swimming, and jogging.

The federal government cooked up a walking plan that's easy to follow (see Table 5-3). It helps you start slow and build up without burning out. Use the program as-is, or tweak it to fit your pace.

TABLE 5-3   **Your Get-Going Walking Program**

Week	Warm-up	Exercise (Walking)	Cool-down	Total Time
1	5 min.	5 min.	5 min.	15 min.
2	5 min.	7 min.	5 min.	17 min.
3	5 min.	9 min.	5 min.	19 min.
4	5 min.	11 min.	5 min.	21 min.
5	5 min.	13 min.	5 min.	23 min.
6	5 min.	15 min.	5 min.	25 min.
7	5 min.	18 min.	5 min.	28 min.
8	5 min.	20 min.	5 min.	30 min.
9	5 min.	23 min.	5 min.	33 min.
10	5 min.	26 min.	5 min.	36 min.
11	5 min.	28 min.	5 min.	38 min.
12	5 min.	30 min.	5 min.	40 min.

During the warm-up portion of the walking program, walk at a comfortable pace and then work up to a brisker pace for the exercise portion. When you're ready for the cool-down phase, start walking slower so that you can get your heart rate down.

After you complete Week 12, you can stick with this 30 min (exercise portion) plan and do it five times per week to meet your 150 minutes, or you can keep increasing your exercise walking time if you plan to have fewer than five exercise sessions each week or want to aim for something higher than 150 weekly minutes.

TIP

Don't have very much time to exercise? Walking doesn't take a lot of time; almost everyone can budget a short period of time for walking on most days. Eliminate a few mindless TV programs, and there you have it — enough time. Take your partner or child with you on your walk for some quality time together. Or break your walking across two or three short sessions in a day. What's most important is the 150 minutes of moderate activity, not how you choose to get there.

Chapter **6**

Weight Training for Life

Modern living provides every convenience except one: a lot of natural physical activity. From young to old, we ride in cars, use remote controls, step into elevators, play on smartphones, and shop online. Many activities that required us to get up out of the chair and use our muscles no longer exist. The result: We need to add weight training to our lives to stimulate our bodies and our brains to keep us healthy and strong.

Men of all ages benefit from weight training. The risks of doing nothing are greater than the risks of injury from exercise — even for the frail and elderly. Whether you're a beginner who wants to get started safely or you're already fit and you want to improve your performance, weight training improves your current condition (whatever that is) and helps you achieve your goals of feeling stronger and better about yourself.

Goal-Setting for Success

TIP

Many men set weight-training goals. Many of them even set realistic ones. But too often, guys don't fulfill their ambitions — for many reasons. Follow the pointers in the following to be more successful in achieving your goals.

>> **Identify why your goals are important.** You're much more likely to stick to a plan of action if you remind yourself often why it's important to you.

>> **Use S.M.A.R.T. goals** — specific, measurable, achievable, reasonable, and timed.

>> **Seek to stick to your plan for at least eight weeks.** Fifty percent of people typically drop out of a new exercise program within the first six weeks, according to research evidence. Studies also tell us that it takes about eight weeks of doing a new behavior to create a new habit. Know that after you've passed the first eight weeks of consistent training, you're well on your way to successfully achieving your goals and maintaining a lifetime of fitness.

REMEMBER

Life happens. If you fall off track, don't waste precious time beating yourself up with negative thoughts. Simply assess what interfered with your regular training, benefit from the experience, and get right back into your program.

Figuring Out Your Reps and Sets

Repetitions, often shortened to *reps,* refer to a single rendition of an exercise. For example, pressing two dumbbells straight above your head and then lowering them back down to your shoulders constitutes one complete repetition of the dumbbell shoulder press. A *set* is a group of consecutive reps that you perform without resting. When you've done 12 repetitions of the dumbbell shoulder press and then put the weights down, you've completed one set. If you rest for a minute and then perform 12 more repetitions, you've done two sets.

Beginners should start with one set for each of the major muscle groups listed under "Knowing Weight-Routine Essentials," later in this chapter. That's roughly 11 sets per workout. The American College of Sports Medicine recommends one-set training because most of your gains occur from that first set. Of course, you'll gain more strength and faster results with more sets, but your program takes more time. After a month or two, you may want to increase the number of sets. But then again, you may not. If your goal is to gain moderate amounts of strength and maintain your health, one set may be as much as you ever need to do.

TIP

Based on how long you've been weight training and your fitness goals (and we're not talking about fittin' a whole cheeseburger into your mouth), we recommend the following:

>> To focus on increasing **muscular endurance,** do at least 12 reps or more, but only two to three sets.

For older adults, we recommend doing between 10–15 reps using light weights.

TIP

>> To **increase muscle size,** do 6 to 12 reps, but more sets — anywhere from three to six.

>> To **increase muscular strength,** do fewer reps, no more than six, and anywhere from two to six sets each.

Knowing Weight-Routine Essentials

If an orchestra were to play Vivaldi's *Four Seasons* minus the string section, the piece would lack a certain vitality and depth. Likewise, if you leave out a key element of your weight workout, you may end up with disappointing results. So, follow these guidelines:

>> **Focus on major muscle groups.** Be sure that your routines include at least one exercise for each of the following muscle groups:

  • **Lower body:** Butt or buttocks (glutes), front thighs (quadriceps), rear thighs (hamstrings), calves, shins

  • **Upper body:** Chest (pecs), back, shoulders (delts), front of upper arms (biceps), rear of upper arms (triceps)

  • **Middle body:** Abdominals (abs)

>> **Do exercises in the right order (sequence).** In general, work your large muscles before your small muscles (follow the order in the preceding bullet). This practice ensures that your larger muscles — such as your butt, back, and chest — are challenged sufficiently. Save your abs for last so they can help stabilize you throughout your training session.

>> **Appreciate the value of rest and recovery.** When you train, you stress or overload your muscles. Microscopic tears occur in the muscle fibers. When you rest, your body repairs these tears and your muscles become stronger. So remember that rest and good nutrition are just as important to your training as your workouts.

>> **When life gets busy, don't stop training completely.** You may find it difficult to do your full routine when your schedule is very full, so remember that something is always better than nothing. Even training one day a week, especially if performed at a higher intensity, can be very valuable to prevent a loss of strength over time.

Building a Training Plan that Meets You Where You Are

When it comes to weight training, one size doesn't fit all. In order to create a program that best meets your needs, you need to know what your conditioning level is, what you want to achieve with your training, and how to set goals and monitor your progress for success.

REMEMBER

Half of all people who begin a new training program quit before they're really even started — within the first six to eight weeks. Why? Most people say that the reason for quitting is that they don't have enough time. A research study of prison inmates, who had all the time in the world for their exercise program, showed the same dropout rate. Leading behavioral scientists have concluded that the real reason people don't stick to new exercise programs isn't lack of time — it's because changing your habits for something new is difficult, especially if motivation is lacking.

Identifying your fitness level

Before you begin weight-training exercises, start by getting a sense of your fitness level. Here are some key questions to ask yourself:

>> **When was the last time you did a sit-up?** Have you been consistently exercising for the past 6 to 12 months, or can you not remember the last time you worked out?

If you answered not at all or not consistently in the past 6 months, even if you were an athlete in high school, you're a beginner. If you've been working out three to five times a week for six months, you're in the intermediate category. And if you've been working out consistently, lifting weights three to five times a week, and your progress has slowed or come to a halt, you're in the advanced category.

>> **How much cardio do you get?** Aerobic exercise is really important for good circulation and maintaining a healthy heart.

If you get winded walking upstairs, you're a beginner. If you can maintain your level of energy during aerobic activities, you're in the intermediate category. And if you play a team sport on a large field, you're in the advanced category.

>> **How would you rate your strength?** If you've never lifted weights or it's been a while (even if you were an athlete in high school), you're a beginner. If you're familiar with weight-training concepts and you currently lift light to moderate weights on a regular basis, you're in the intermediate category.

And if you can lift 100 pounds for eight to ten reps, you're in the advanced category.

>> **How flexible are you?** If you do plenty of strength training and cardio, but you don't do any stretching, you're creating an imbalance in your body. Flexibility plays a big part in overall fitness.

If you're sedentary and you can't touch your toes, you're a beginner. If you stretch major muscle groups two to three times a week, you're in the intermediate category. And if you can progress through an advanced level of yoga poses or variable stretches, you're in the advanced category.

WARNING

Having answered these four questions, you should have a general sense of whether you're a beginner, advanced, or in between. If you're in doubt, err on the side of taking it easier in the beginning — you can always work up to a more advanced level, but if you push too hard in the beginning, you may injure yourself.

Creating your first weight-training plan

TIP

Here's what each of these categories means in terms of the weight-training exercises in this chapter:

>> **Beginner:** If you're at the beginner level, start out doing one set of ten repetitions per exercise. You can always add another set of ten reps when you feel you've mastered the proper form. Also, plan on weight training twice a week, alongside your 150 minutes of cardio physical activity.

Listen to your body and don't move forward until you feel you're ready.

REMEMBER

>> **Intermediate:** If you're at the intermediate level, do one set of 15 repetitions of each exercise. If you feel confident that you're using proper form and one set is too easy, you can add another set of 15 reps. Otherwise, complete two weeks of training before adding a second set of 15 reps to each exercise.

>> **Advanced:** If you're at the advanced level, start out with two sets of 20 repetitions. Using a high amount of reps leads to increased muscle endurance rather than strength and size.

Getting a Great Lower-Body Workout

Your butt and legs are the largest muscle groups in your body, and these muscles carry you everywhere you go. Having strong lower-body muscles is key to living independently into old age. Being able to stand up from chairs, pick yourself up off the floor, climb stairs, step out of cars, and even get off the toilet are key factors to enjoying life on your own. Your lower body muscles, therefore, deserve plenty of attention.

This section covers just two exercises — squats and lunges. Both work your butt and your legs simultaneously, so you get a lot of bang for your buck with each.

Working out your butt and legs: Squat

In addition to strengthening your butt muscles, the squat also does a good job of working your quadriceps and hamstrings.

If you have hip, knee, or lower-back problems, you may want to try the modified version.

Getting set

Hold your arms straight out in front of you or hold a dumbbell in each hand for more of a challenge. Stand with your feet as wide as your hips and with your weight slightly back on your heels. Pull your abdominals in and stand up tall with square shoulders (see Figure 6-1a).

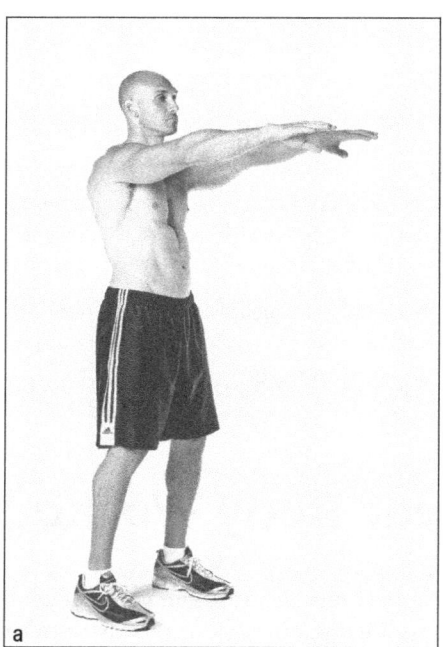
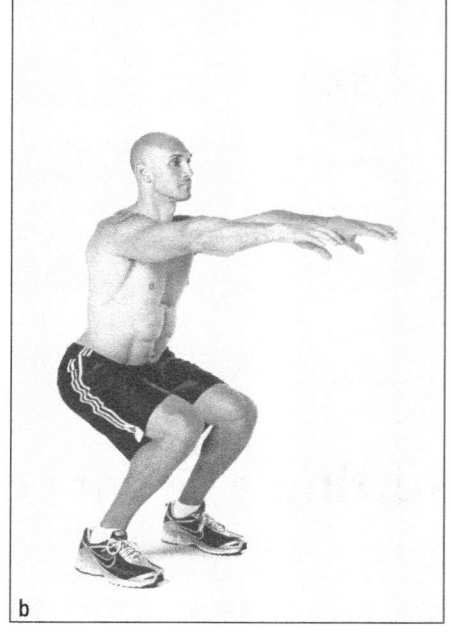

FIGURE 6-1:
Squat.

a

b

Photo by Nick Horne

The exercise

Sit back and down, as if you're sitting into a chair (see Figure 6-1b). Lower as far as you can without leaning your upper body more than a few inches forward. Don't lower any farther than the point at which your thighs are parallel to the floor, and don't allow your knees to shoot out in front of your toes. When you feel your upper body fold forward over your thighs, straighten your legs and stand back up. Take care not to lock your knees at the top of the movement.

Do's and don'ts

- » DON'T allow your knees to travel beyond your toes. We know we said this before, but it bears repeating.

- » DON'T look down. Your body tends to follow your eyes. So if you're staring at the ground, you're more likely to fall forward. Instead, keep your head up and your eyes focused on an object directly in front of you.

- » DON'T shift your body weight forward so your heels lift up off the floor. When you push back up to the standing position, concentrate on pushing through your heels.

- » DON'T arch your back as you stand back up.

Working out your butt and legs: Lunge

The lunge is a great overall lower-body exercise: It strengthens your butt, quadriceps, hamstrings, and calves.

WARNING

If you feel pain in your hips, knees, or lower back when you do this exercise, try using a chair to touch your butt to — it'll keep you from sitting too far down toward the floor.

Getting set

Stand with your feet as wide as your hips and your weight back a little on your heels, and place your hands on your hips. Pull your abdominals in and stand up tall with square shoulders.

The exercise

Lift your right toe slightly and, leading with your heel, step your right foot forward an elongated stride's length, as if you're trying to step over a crack on the sidewalk. As your foot touches the floor, bend both knees until your right thigh is parallel to the floor and your left knee is perpendicular to the floor. Your left heel will lift off the floor (see Figure 6-2). Press off the ball of your foot and step back to the standing position.

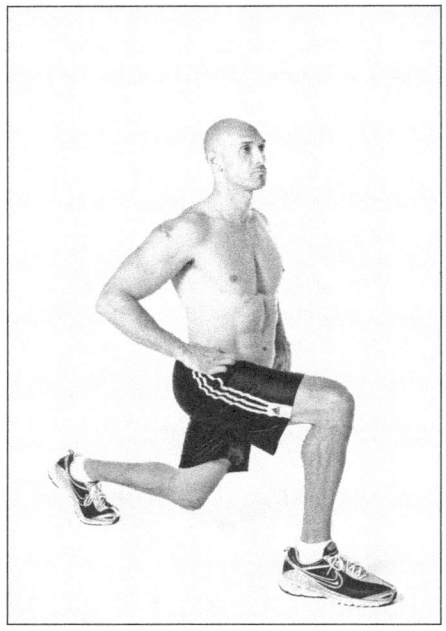

Photo by Nick Horne

FIGURE 6-2:
Lunge.

Do's and don'ts

» DO keep your eyes focused ahead; when you look down, you tend to fall forward.

» DON'T step too far forward or you'll have trouble balancing.

» DON'T lean forward or allow your front knee to travel past your toes.

Getting Started with an Upper-Body Workout

Your upper body muscles are essential for everyday living. For example, when you move your arms in virtually any direction — up, down, backward, forward, side-ways, diagonally, or in circles — your shoulders are in charge or at least involved. Regular training makes your upper-body strong and keeps it that way.

Working out your chest: Push-ups

Push-ups target your chest muscles along with the abdominal muscles and butt to give good core strength and allover toning.

Getting set

Straighten your arms and lift your body in push-up position so that you're balanced equally on your palms (see Figure 6-3a). Tuck your chin a few inches toward your chest so that your forehead faces the floor.

The exercise

Lower your body toward the floor, bending your elbows out to the side (see Figure 6-3b). Straighten your arms pressing against the floor to return to starting position. Complete ten repetitions.

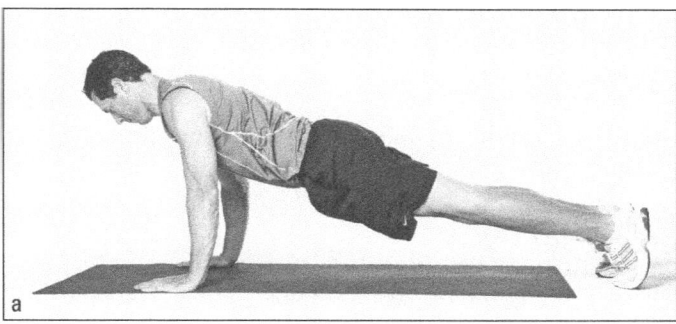

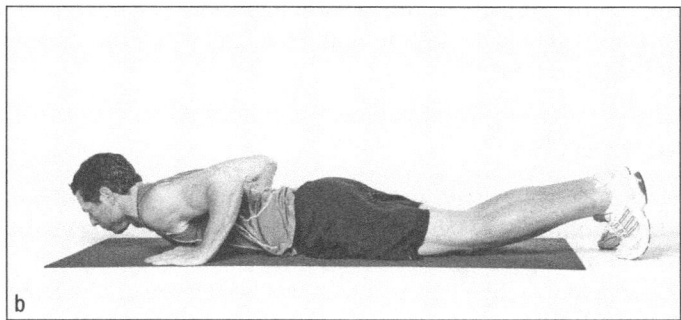

FIGURE 6-3:
Push-up.

Photo by Nick Horne

Do's and don'ts

>> DO keep your abdominal muscles tight to help you maintain your balance.

>> DO use proper breathing, inhaling as you lower and exhaling as you press back up.

>> DON'T arch your back. Keep it straight and in line with your head and the rest of your body.

Working out your back: Band lat pull-down

The band lat pull-down, which uses an exercise band, works your upper-back muscles (your *latissimus dorsi* or "lats") with some emphasis on your shoulders and biceps.

TIP

Bands are particularly helpful if you want to keep up your strength and work out when you travel. Make sure that you use a band designed for exercising. In general, the shorter and/or the thicker the band, the harder it is to pull and the more resistance it provides.

WARNING

Be especially careful to follow the form guidelines if you're prone to neck discomfort.

Getting set

Sit in a chair or stand with your feet hip-width apart and hold an end of the exercise band in each hand. Raise your arms over your head with your left palm facing in and your right palm facing forward just above shoulder level (see Figure 6-4a). Your elbows should be slightly bent. Stand tall with your abdominals pulled in and your knees relaxed.

The exercise

Keep your left arm still. Bend your right elbow down and out to the side, as if you're shooting an arrow straight up into the air. Keeping your wrist straight, pull the band until your right hand is to the side of your right shoulder, the band is tight, and your right elbow points down (see Figure 6-4b). Slowly straighten your arm. Switch sides, alternating arms as you complete the set.

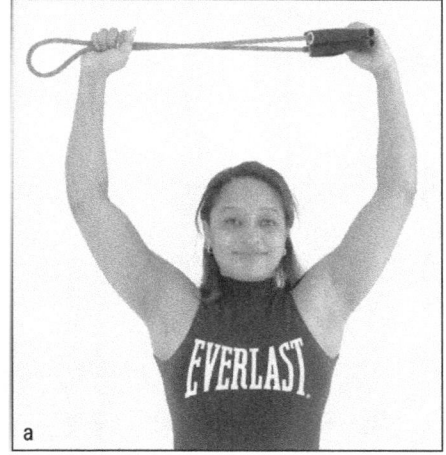
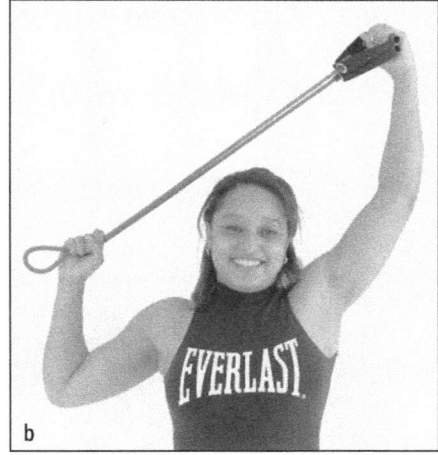

FIGURE 6-4:
Band lat
pull-down.

Photo by Zoran Popovic

Do's and don'ts

>> DO make sure that the band is securely in place before each set.

>> DO be especially careful to follow the form guidelines if you're prone to neck discomfort.

>> DON'T allow your shoulders to hunch up.

Working out your back: One-arm dumbbell row

The one-arm dumbbell row targets your back, but also emphasizes your biceps and shoulders.

WARNING

Be careful with this exercise if you have lower-back problems.

Getting set

Stand in a lunge position, left foot forward, making sure your knee doesn't jut out past your toes. Hold a dumbbell in your right hand with your palm facing in. Let your right arm hang down underneath your right shoulder. Tilt your chin toward your chest so your neck is in line with the rest of your spine (see Figure 6-5a).

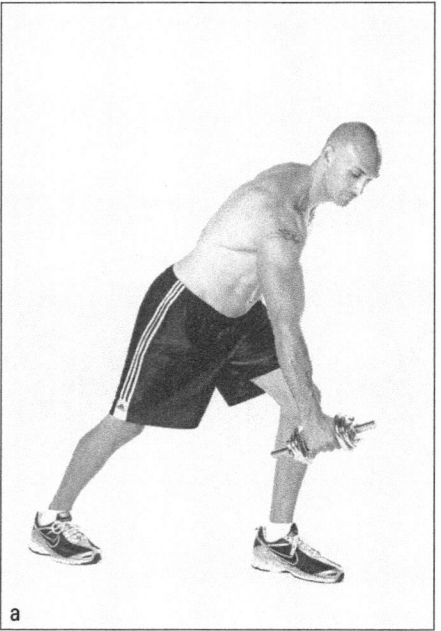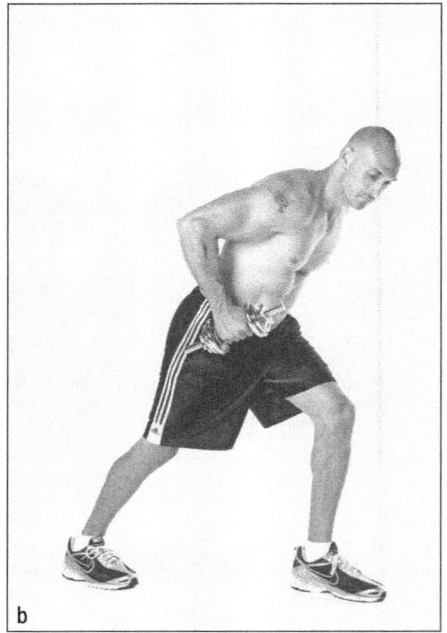

Photo by Nick Horne

FIGURE 6-5:
One-arm
dumbbell row.

The exercise

Pull your right arm up, keeping it in line with your shoulder and parallel to the ceiling (see Figure 6-5b). Lift your arm until your hand brushes against your waist. Lower the weight slowly back down.

Do's and don'ts

» DO remember that, although your arm is moving, this is a back exercise. Concentrate on pulling from your back muscles (right behind and below your shoulder) rather than just moving your arm up and down.

» DO keep your abs pulled in tight throughout the motion.

» DON'T allow your back to sag toward the floor or your shoulders to hunch up.

» DON'T jerk the weight upward.

Working out your shoulders: Dumbbell shoulder press

The dumbbell shoulder press targets the top and center of your shoulder muscles. This exercise also works your upper back and triceps.

Use caution if you have lower-back, neck, or elbow problems.

Getting set

Hold a dumbbell in each hand and sit on a bench with back support. Plant your feet firmly on the floor about hip-width apart. Bend your elbows and raise your upper arms to shoulder height so the dumbbells are at ear level. Pull your abdominals in so there's a slight gap between the small of your back and the bench. Place the back of your head against the pad (see Figure 6-6a).

The exercise

Push the dumbbells up and in until the ends of the dumbbells are nearly touching directly over your head (see Figure 6-6b) and then lower the dumbbells back to ear level.

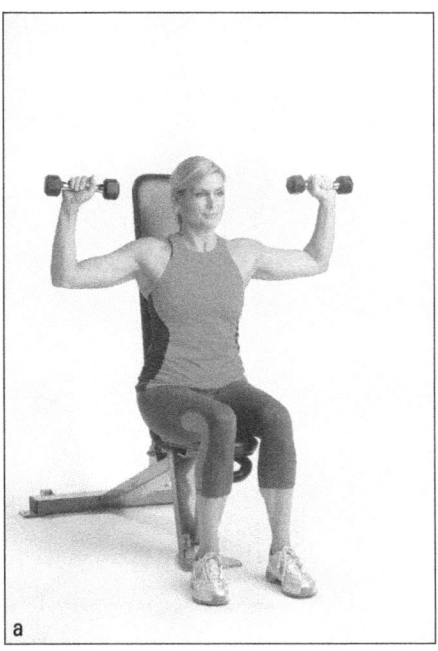
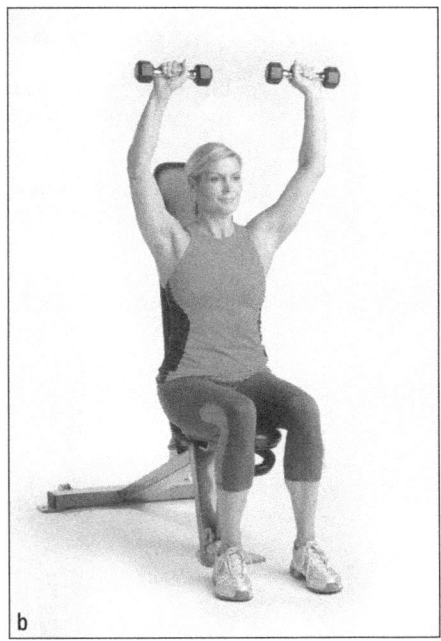

FIGURE 6-6:
Dumbbell
shoulder press.

Photo by Nick Horne

Do's and don'ts

➤➤ DO keep your elbows relaxed at the top instead of locking them.

➤➤ DO stop lowering the dumbbells when your elbows are at or slightly below shoulder level.

» DON'T let your back arch a great degree off the back support.

» DON'T wiggle or squirm around in an effort to press the weights up.

Working out your shoulders: Lateral raise

The lateral raise works the center of your shoulder muscles. Make sure that you use stellar technique if you have neck or lower-back problems.

Getting set

Hold a dumbbell in each hand and stand up tall with your feet as wide as your hips. Bend your elbows a little, turn your palms toward each other, and bring the dumbbells together in front of the tops of your thighs (see Figure 6-7a). Pull your abdominals in.

The exercise

Lift your arms up and out to the side until the dumbbells are just below shoulder height (see Figure 6-7b). Slowly lower the weights back down.

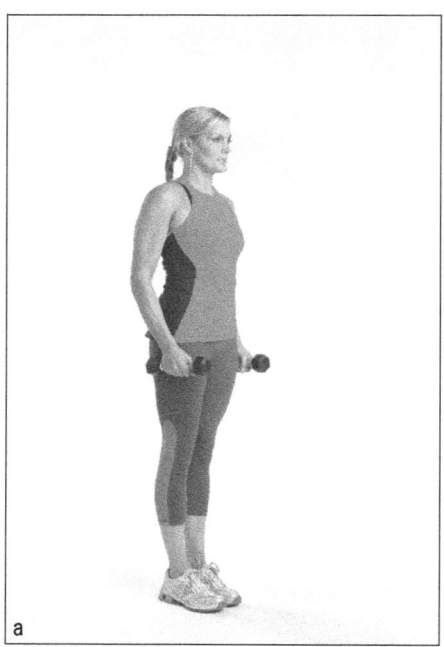 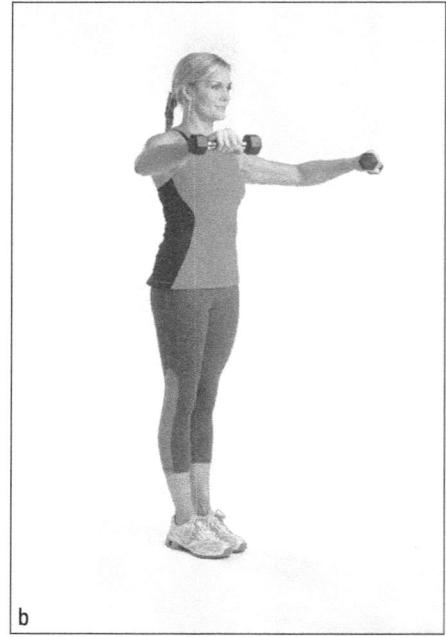

FIGURE 6-7: Lateral raise.

a

b

Photo by Nick Horne

TIP

It may help to imagine that you're pouring two pitchers of lemonade on the floor in front of you.

Do's and don'ts

» DO lift from the shoulders; in other words, keep your elbows stationary.

» DON'T arch your back, lean backward, or rock back and forth to lift the weights.

» DON'T raise the weights above shoulder height.

Working out your biceps: Barbell biceps curl

The barbell biceps curl targets your biceps.

WARNING

Be especially careful if you have elbow problems. Whenever you add weight and bend a joint, it increases the stress to that joint. Therefore, if you have a weakened joint, you need to exercise extreme care not to overdo it and cause an injury. If you have lower-back problems, you may want to choose a seated biceps exercise instead.

Getting set

Hold a barbell with an underhand grip and your hands about shoulder-width apart. Stand with your feet as wide as your hips, and let your arms hang down so the bar is in front of your thighs (see Figure 6-8a). Stand up tall with your abdominals pulled in and knees relaxed.

The exercise

Bend your arms to curl the bar almost up to your shoulders (see Figure 6-8b), and then slowly lower the bar *almost* to the starting position.

Do's and don'ts

» DON'T swing your elbows out wide as you bend your arm to raise the weight. Keep your elbows close to your body *without* supporting them on the sides of your stomach for leverage.

» DON'T just let the weight fall back to the starting position. Lower it slowly and with control.

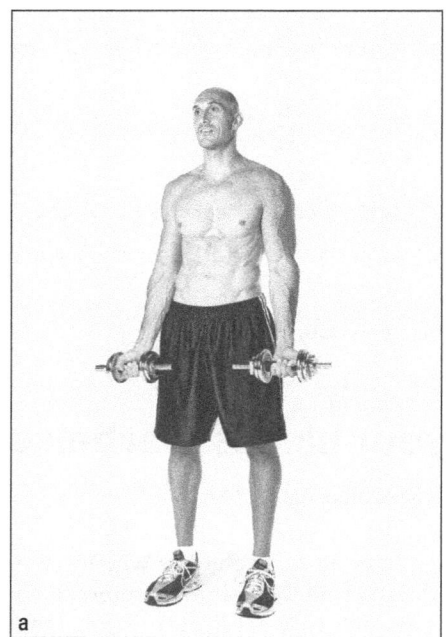
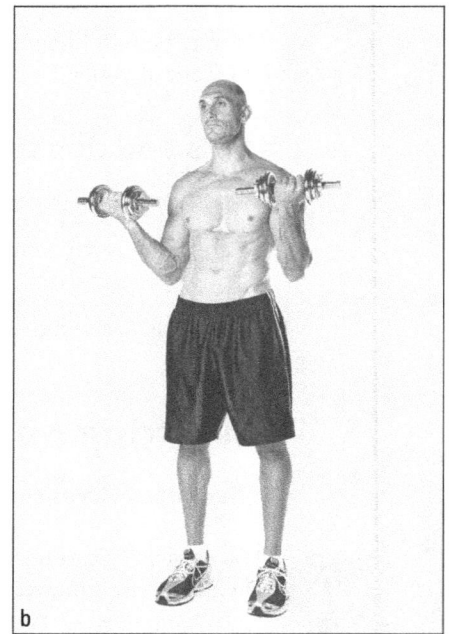

Photo by Nick Horne

FIGURE 6-8:
Barbell
biceps curl.

Working out your triceps: Triceps kickback

The triceps kickback works your triceps.

WARNING

Use caution if you have elbow or lower-back problems.

Getting set

Hold a dumbbell in your right hand, and stand in a lunge position. Lean forward at the hips until your upper body is at a 45-degree angle to the floor. Bend your right elbow so your upper arm is parallel to the floor, your forearm is perpendicular to the floor, and your palm faces in (see Figure 6-9a). Keep your elbow close to your waist. Pull your abdominals in and relax your knees.

The exercise

Keeping your upper arm still, straighten your arm behind you until the end of the dumbbell is pointing down (see Figure 6-9b). Slowly bend your arm to lower the weight. When you've completed the set, repeat the exercise with your left arm.

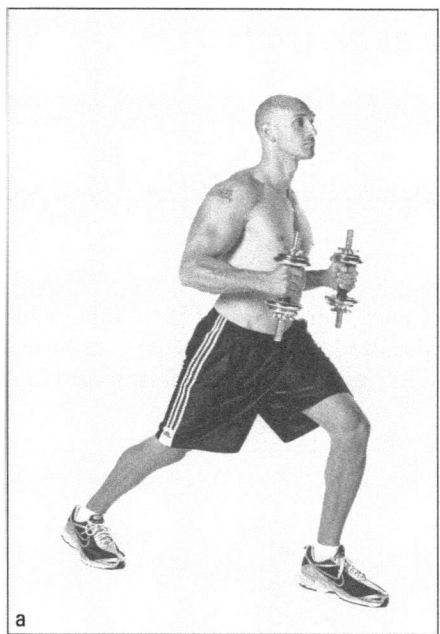
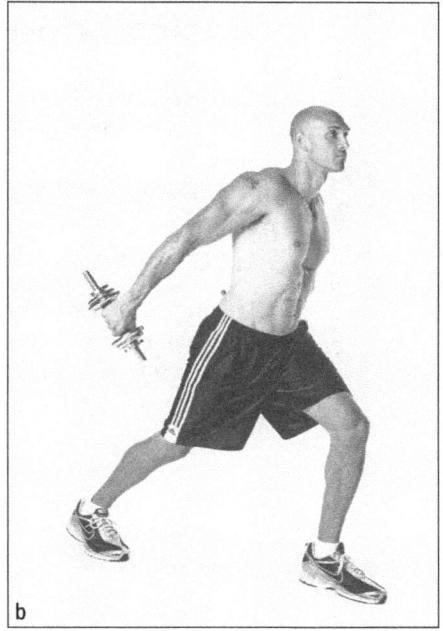

FIGURE 6-9:
Triceps kickback.

a b

Photo by Nick Horne

Do's and don'ts

>> DO keep your abdominals pulled in and your knees relaxed to protect your lower back.

>> DON'T lock your elbow at the top of the movement; do straighten your arm but keep your elbow relaxed.

>> DON'T allow your upper arm to move or your shoulder to drop below waist level.

Working Out Your Abdominals

Sitting, driving, and slouching lead to weak abdominal muscles. And with weak abdominals comes a weak lower back. Strengthening the abs or abdominals works wonders for your entire body. Better posture, better balance, and feeling more stable with all your movements are the results you can expect from building strong abdominals.

Basic abdominal crunch

The basic abdominal crunch is the fundamental abdominal exercise that works all your abdominal muscles.

Pay special attention to your form if you have lower-back or neck problems.

Getting set

Lie on your back with your knees bent and feet flat on the floor hip-width apart. Place your hands behind your head for support. Keep your head upright and don't press it into your chest. Gently pull your abdominals inward (see Figure 6-10a).

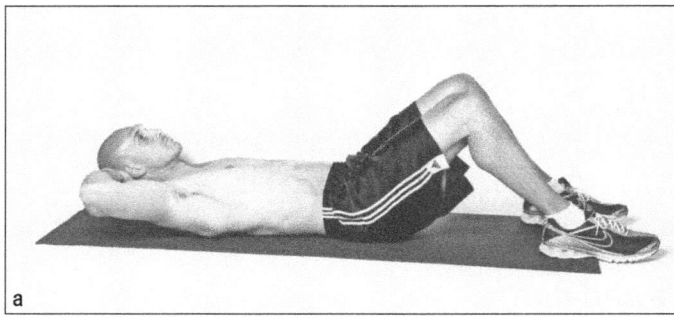

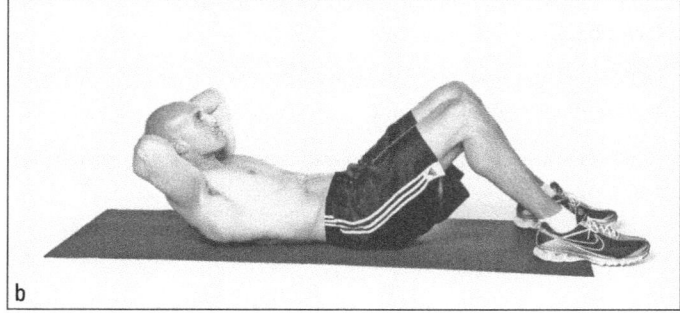

FIGURE 6-10: Basic abdominal crunch.

Photo by Nick Horne

The exercise

Curl up and forward so your head, neck, and shoulder blades lift off the floor (see Figure 6-10b). Hold for a moment at the top of the movement and then lower slowly back down.

Do's and don'ts

>> DO keep your abdominals pulled in so you feel more tension in your abs and so you don't overarch your lower back.

>> DO curl as well as lift.

>> DON'T pull on your legs with your hands.

Reverse crunch

The reverse crunch emphasizes the lower portion of your main abdominal muscles (the *rectus abdominis*).

Use caution if you're prone to lower-back discomfort.

Getting set

Lie on your back with your legs up, knees slightly bent, and feet in air. Rest your arms on the floor and place your fingertips behind your head. Rest your head on your hands, relax your shoulders, and pull in your abdominals (see Figure 6-11a).

The exercise

Lift your butt 1 or 2 inches off the floor so your legs lift up and a few inches backward (see Figure 6-11b). Hold the position for a moment, and then lower slowly.

Do's and don'ts

>> DO keep your shoulders relaxed and down.

>> DO keep the crunch movement small and precise; you don't have to lift very high to feel this exercise working.

>> DO use a minimum of leg movement.

>> DON'T thrust or jerk your hips.

>> DON'T involve your upper body at all.

>> DON'T cross your feet at the ankles.

>> DON'T roll your hips so your buttocks and back come way off the floor. This type of movement involves your front hip muscles more than your abdominals.

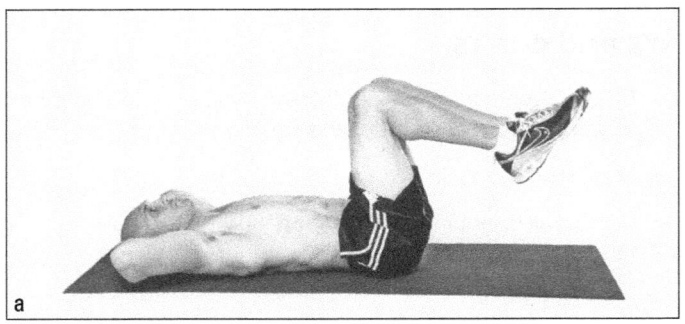

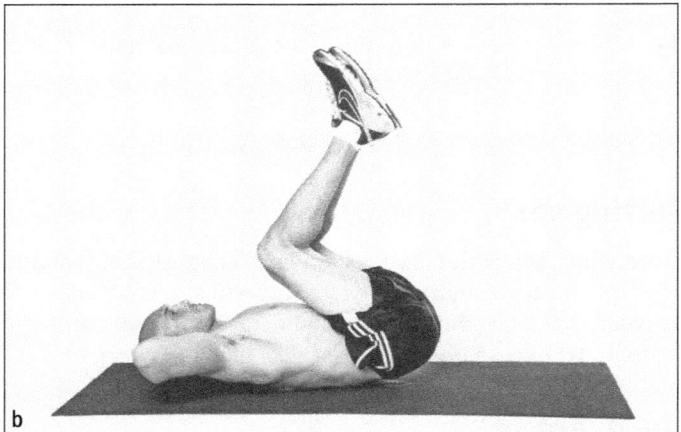

FIGURE 6-11:
Reverse crunch.

Photo by Nick Horne

Chapter **7**

Getting Real about Stress, Loneliness, and Mental Health

Stress, loneliness, anxiety, depression — they're the heavy hitters quietly wearing down men's health and happiness. Stress is your body's built-in alarm system, meant to help you handle challenges, but when it's always blaring, it can wreck your mind and body. Loneliness, meanwhile, can quickly erode happiness, self-worth, and even physical health. Left unchecked, both can open the door to anxiety and depression — conditions that are more than just "worrying too much" or "feeling down."

This chapter cuts through the noise to explain what stress really is, why you feel it, and how to get the upper hand before it takes a toll. You'll also find out why building and maintaining connections — at home, with friends, and in your community — are just as vital to your health as exercise and diet. And we'll break down anxiety and depression in plain language, with a quick look at proven treatment options.

REMEMBER

Your mental health isn't separate from your physical health — it's the foundation.

Sizing Up Stress

Despite literally hundreds of studies about stress, a precise definition is frustratingly difficult to come up with. Perhaps the best simple definition came from Canadian scientist Hans Selye, who in 1956 defined *stress* as "the nonspecific response of the body to any demands made on it" in his pioneering book *The Stress of Life* (McGraw Hill, 1978).

The *demand* (the thing that stresses you out, be it a traffic jam, power outage, or deadline) and the *response* (your internal reaction to, say, a $2,000 car-repair bill or any other demand) are the key components of stress. No doubt you're faced with many demands (stressors) every day. How you respond is up to you, but remember that the way you respond can contribute either to improved cardiac health or to increased cardiac risk.

Realizing stress can be good as well as bad

Your stress-response systems enable you to respond to threats, challenges, or opportunities. Without a response, you'd be unable to manage or adapt to changing situations.

Many people don't realize that having positive stress is possible. A certain amount of stress may be necessary for you to reach your optimal performance. Low stress leads to boredom and poor performance. However, when stress becomes excessive or when your response to the stress becomes negative, your health in general, and your cardiac health in particular, may be harmed.

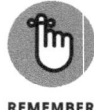

REMEMBER

Stress can be characterized in two ways:

>> **Positive (*eustress*):** Motivates and promotes learning; enhances performance and builds resilience; often seen in positive challenges (such as preparing for sports competition).

>> **Negative (*distress*):** Stress from perceived threats, leading to anxiety, poor performance, and physical/emotional symptoms; often tied to chronic stress.

Understanding the balance of stress can help you optimize your performance and manage your stress levels effectively. By recognizing your optimal stress level, you can aim to maintain it for better productivity and well-being.

Unpacking stress's whole-body beatdown

Stress profoundly affects, among other systems, the hormonal (*endocrine*) system, the immune system, and the digestive system.

Stress first impacts the hormonal system, causing visible changes in the adrenal glands — your body's stress hormone factories. Then it weakens the immune system and wreaks havoc on the digestive system, damaging the intestinal lining and disrupting gut health.

TECHNICAL STUFF

Over time, the continuous flood of cortisol begins to affect every tissue in your body. The overstimulation of your adrenal glands leads to exhaustion and adrenal fatigue, disrupting the production of essential hormones like estrogen, testosterone, and progesterone, which results in menstrual irregularities, infertility, sexual dysfunction, and a decreased libido. The constant release of cortisol also dampens your immune system, leaving you more susceptible to illness, and weakens your digestive system, contributing to issues like leaky gut and irritable bowel syndrome (IBS).

REMEMBER

Chronic stress further disrupts your body's natural balance (*homeostasis*) by slowing metabolism, altering thyroid function, and increasing the risk of metabolic disorders such as insulin resistance and type 2 diabetes. Mental health also takes a hit, creating a vicious cycle where stress and hormonal imbalances feed off each other, damaging both mind and body.

Understanding Your Stress Response System

There's more to your stress-response system than just the simple "fight or flight" response.

TECHNICAL STUFF

The *hypothalamus-pituitary-adrenal* (HPA) axis, which is your body's main stress-response system that helps you react and adapt to situations, is closely intertwined with the nervous system. When the nervous system detects a perceived threat or something unfamiliar, it signals the hypothalamus to activate the HPA axis. This triggers a cascade of hormonal responses, including the release of cortisol and adrenaline, which prepare the body to respond to the challenge by heightening alertness, increasing heart rate, and mobilizing energy — ultimately helping to ensure your safety.

The following sections go into a little more detail.

Assessing the influencers

One of our favorite academic articles, published in *Nature Reviews Neuroscience* in 2009, coined the term "neuro-symphony of stress," emphasizing how your brain runs a whole orchestra of mediators — neurotransmitters, neuropeptides, and hormones — to help you deal with stress. Some kick in within seconds, others stick around for weeks, all working together so you can handle both immediate and prolonged challenges.

REMEMBER

Many factors influence how you perceive and respond to stress, which is why your brain and body need a complex repertoire. Some factors include:

>> Duration of the stressor, which can last from seconds to years (acute versus chronic)

>> Type of stressor (physical versus psychological)

>> Context (such as the time of day)

>> Your age, sex, and genetic background play a role

>> Your stages of life, from childhood to old age

Your "stress neuro-symphony" ensures that your brain and body can handle anything from a sudden scare, such as a spider jumping on you, to prolonged stress, such as caring for a dying relative. By understanding how these different mediators work together, you can better manage feeling "stressed" and experience resilience and thrive when you're challenged.

Figuring out your dual stress response system

Imagine your brain and body working together in a finely tuned neuro symphony to handle the challenges, or stressors you face every day. Two major systems play leading roles:

>> Hypothalamic-Pituitary-Adrenal (HPA) axis

>> Autonomic Nervous System (ANS)

When you face an immediate stressor, such as a hairy spider or loud noise at night, your ANS kicks in with a neurally mediated quick-fire response, providing a burst of energy and alertness through the rapid release of adrenaline and neural activation of tissues such as blood vessels and your pupils.

The swift ANS response is often followed by the slower, hormone-mediated HPA axis activation, which sustains your response if the stressor persists by releasing cortisol to maintain energy supply and modulate bodily functions.

Layering in stress hormones

Adrenaline, noradrenaline, and cortisol are three key signaling molecules that orchestrate your brain and body's response to threats, challenges, and opportunities. Here's what you need to know:

>> **Noradrenaline** (known as *norepinephrine* in the United States) increases heart rate, blood flow, and regulates blood vessel constriction, as well as increases arousal, alertness, vigilance, and memory formation.

>> **Adrenaline** (known as *epinephrine* in the United States) quickly increases heart rate, breathing, dilates pupils, and releases glucose.

>> **Cortisol** is what your body releases when you encounter a threat or challenge, and it helps you respond and adapt to stressors by:

- Promoting glucose release for quick energy

- Regulating metabolism of fats, proteins, and carbs

- Enhancing alertness, focus, and memory

REMEMBER

Adrenaline, noradrenaline, and cortisol are not simply switched on or off in response to threats. Instead, their levels each adjust like a volume dial, turning up or down as needed.

HIGH AND LOW CORTISOL: WHAT IT MEANS FOR YOUR BODY

Cortisol is not a villain. You need it to help appropriately respond to stress and regulate your energy, metabolism, sexual arousal, and immune responses. But when it remains elevated for too long, you begin experiencing symptoms such as

- Anxiety, irritability, and restlessness

- Weight gain, especially around the abdomen

(continued)

(continued)

- High blood pressure and blood sugar spikes

- Sleep disturbances, like difficulty falling or staying asleep

On the flip side, when the adrenal glands (which regulate cortisol levels) become overworked, cortisol production eventually drops to protect the body, which leaves you feeling

- Fatigued, no matter how much sleep you get

- Mentally foggy and struggling to concentrate

- Weak, with low stamina and motivation

- Emotionally depleted, leading to feelings of depression or apathy

Low cortisol levels are essentially your body's way of signaling that it can no longer keep up with the constant demands placed upon it. Essentially, the body has shifted into survival mode, and energy is conserved by shutting down nonessential functions, leaving you exhausted and burnt out.

Deciding how to act: Fight, flight, freeze, and fawn

The concepts of fight, flight, freeze, and fawn (sometimes called befriend) are useful metaphors to describe how humans and other animals respond to threats. Responses vary greatly depending on the individual and the specific threat.

>> The *freeze* response, often the initial reaction to a threat, lets you "stop, look, and listen." This hypervigilant state helps you assess the situation. By remaining still, prey can avoid detection by predators that primarily see movement. This response is associated with heightened alertness and caution.

>> Following the freeze response, you may be lucky enough to *flee* (take *flight*) from danger. If an escape route isn't possible, all that's left for you to do is *fight*. But this sequence — flight then fight — doesn't always play out. For example, someone trained in martial arts may be more likely to fight an attacker in a dark car park than someone with no training.

>> The *tend and befriend* or *fawn* response is the idea that humans often seek social support when we're stressed. When you face a threat, you may tend to your children for their protection or call your Mum or Dad for mutual support and comfort.

Recognizing the Risks of Stress

Everyone responds to stress differently. Australians may befriend hairy huntsman spiders, whereas visitors may see them as deadly threats. This reminds us that stress responses aren't inherently good or bad; they vary widely and depend on context. It's prolonged or excessive stress that leads to wear and tear on the body and brain.

Stress — like diet exercise, genes, sleep, relationships — is an important risk factor for disease ranging from cardiovascular diseases to dementia. Too much stress for too long can throw your body out of balance and raise your risk of illness and burnout.

WARNING

Here's a list of well-established health consequences of toxic or chronic stress.

>> **Burnout:** A state of exhaustion caused by long-term stress, often related to work or caregiving, leaving you feeling drained and unmotivated.

>> **Anxiety:** Chronic stress keeps your body and brain on high alert, leading to constant worry and tension, which can develop into anxiety disorders.

>> **Depression:** Chronic stress can lead to biochemical changes in the brain, causing mood regulation issues and potentially leading to depression.

>> **Poor cardiovascular health:** Chronic stress produces cortisol and adrenaline, which can damage your heart and blood vessels over time, increasing the risk of heart disease.

>> **Metabolic issues:** Stress can alter your metabolism, leading to weight gain and raising the risk of diabetes and other metabolic problems.

>> **Weakened immune system:** Chronic stress weakens your immune system, making you more prone to infections and illnesses.

>> **Sleep problems:** Stress often disrupts sleep, leading to a vicious cycle that worsens brain, body, and mental health.

Keeping Stress and Anger at Bay

Do you get bent out of shape when the weather ruins your plans? When a driver cuts you off? When a last-minute project keeps you late at work? If you do, you're risking serious damage to your heart, which can stand up to only so much stress and anger. Reducing these risk factors is up to you, and it's not as hard as you may think.

TIP

Stress may be dangerous for the heart (and many other bodily systems), but fortunately some simple strategies may significantly lower stress and thereby improve your health. Here are four ways to lower the stress in your life and, in doing so, reduce your risk of developing diseases that contribute to men's premature deaths:

» **Modify or eliminate circumstances that contribute to stress.** People often don't realize that daily habits can compound problems with stress. Cutting back on coffee, tea, energy drinks, and other caffeinated beverages, for example, may make a substantial difference in your stress levels. Fatigue and insomnia may also contribute to stress, so be sure to get plenty of sleep whenever you're experiencing symptoms of stress. And avoid using alcohol as a way to relax. Although it may seem to offer a temporary release from stress, it usually leads to greater problems.

» **Live in the present.** It may sound simple, but many people spend an inordinate amount of time either regretting the past or fearing the future. Strategies such as *biofeedback* (where you can learn to train your body's automatic functions through real-time biological monitoring), visualization, and medications can help you live in the present and substantially lower stress levels.

» **Get out of your own way.** Many people compound the inevitable stresses of their daily lives by layering on negative feelings concerning these stresses. Recognizing that no one can live a life that is completely free of stress is as important as trying not to compound the problem by allowing feelings of negativity or low self-worth to make stress worse.

» **Develop a personal plan for stress.** Developing a personal plan to alleviate stress is one of the most effective ways to handle it on an ongoing basis, instead of allowing it to become free-floating anxiety. Daily exercise, meditation, and taking timeouts (either alone or with family) are effective ways of controlling the stresses that crop up every day.

TIP

TEN-MINUTE TIMEOUTS AGAINST STRESS

"Step away for ten a day": Short, calming breaks from your daily routine can lower your stress dramatically. Try one of these techniques:

Go outside. The right short break outside can ease the tension. Do stroll, clear your mind, smell the flowers, and people watch. Don't think about your schedule, outline that memo, or pick at a worry.

Tune into calm. You can also get away right in your office or easy chair. Simply find a quiet, comfortable spot. Allow no interruptions. Sit quietly and focus on becoming calm. Consciously clear your mind, gently pushing away any intruding thoughts of work or problems. Listening to quiet music, visualizing peaceful scenes, or focusing on deep, slow breathing may help. A luxurious stretch at the end of your ten minutes can be a nice transition back to activity.

Listen to your body. Using biofeedback techniques can help you foster a relaxed state. Our research found that people who take ten minutes each day to focus on relaxing were able to dramatically reduce their stress levels. They used the same techniques that we described earlier, but they also relied on a heart-rate monitor as their point of focus. Sitting quietly, focus on your heart rate and imagine it going lower. Using the other visualization techniques in combination with biofeedback can enhance your ten-minute timeout.

Meditate. Practicing any of several formal types of meditation can be useful to anyone who enjoys it. *Meditation For Dummies,* 4th Edition (John Wiley & Sons, Inc., 2016) can get you started.

Catnap. If you're one of those lucky souls who can drop instantly to sleep and wake refreshed in 10 or 15 minutes, you can experience the ten-minute timeout in one of its most satisfying forms (at least, so say its devotees).

Adding More Firepower to Your Destressing Tool Kit

You've probably heard it a million times: "Mindfulness is the key to managing stress." While this sentiment is well-intentioned, it can sometimes feel like trying to fit a square peg into a round hole.

Take a look at the following different strategies that you can mix and match, to create your personal tool kit for navigating life's challenging moments.

Breathing your way to calmness

Numerous positive health outcomes are measured in people practicing deep breathing. These include reduced heart rate, lower blood pressure, better lung capacity and function, reduced cortisol, enhanced mental focus, and improved emotional regulation.

TIP

Here are a few ways to use your breath to reduce stress:

>> **Physiological sigh:** Inhale deeply through the nose, followed by a second shorter inhale, then slowly exhale through your mouth (as if through a straw).

>> **Box breathing:** Inhale for four counts, hold for four, exhale for four, and pause for four before repeating. Navy SEALs use it to stay calm and focused.

>> **4-7-8 breathing:** Inhale for four seconds, hold for seven, and exhale for eight. A variation on box breathing with a different rhythm.

>> **Diaphragmatic breathing:** Breathe deeply into the diaphragm, not the chest, feeling your belly rise while keeping your chest still.

Using mind-body practices

TIP

Engage your mind and your body to help you navigate when life feels stressful:

>> Participate in cold water swimming or ice baths to release endorphins improving your mood.

>> Get regular exercise, which includes everything from walking to team sports to gym sessions.

>> Use relaxation techniques such as progressive muscle relaxation, visualization, or guided imagery to reduce physical tension.

>> Take up activities such as tai chi or qigong, which combine gentle physical movements with mindfulness.

Tweaking your lifestyle and habits

TIP

Make changes to your lifestyle to help deal with stress and minimize stressors in the first place:

>> Maintain a balanced diet of fruits, vegetables, lean proteins, and whole grains.

>> Ensure you get regular quality sleep every night.

>> Limit caffeine and alcohol.

>> Take regular breaks from screens and social media.

>> Keep a gratitude journal to focus on positive aspects of your life.

>> Learn to say no and set personal and professional boundaries to protect your time and reduce your risk of burnout.

>> Prioritize tasks, set realistic goals, and take breaks to manage your workload effectively.

Bringing more joy into your life

Making time for personal enjoyment and fun can also help you manage stress more effectively.

TIP

Check out the following ways to do so:

>> Indulge in the activities or hobbies you enjoy, such as reading, gardening, painting, or playing music, to relax and unwind.

>> Spend time outdoors in green or blue spaces.

>> Engage with your community by volunteering to create a sense of purpose and connection.

>> Write your thoughts and feelings down in a journal to process emotions and gain perspective.

>> Laugh! Watch a funny movie, read a good book, or spend time with people who make you laugh.

>> Use art, music, dance, or writing to relieve emotions and stress.

Limiting Loneliness by Making Connections

Guys who have trouble connecting with others and developing intimate relation-ships also may have a higher risk of developing heart disease and other conditions that contribute to shorter lifespans. The opposite also is true: Those who have strong relationships with others also have a healthier, better life.

Understanding the importance of connection

REMEMBER

The importance of human connection can't be overstated. Social isolation isn't just an emotional experience but a biological one because it triggers stress responses that can harm the body over time. Research continues to link loneliness and a lack of close relationships to increased inflammation, which, when chronic, is associated with a wide range of serious health issues, including those covered in this book.

Also, when people feel isolated or disconnected, they often turn to unhealthy coping behaviors to manage those feelings, such as excessive alcohol consumption, binge eating, lack of exercise, social withdrawal, or even using social media as an emotional crutch. All these activities are linked to dysregulation in tier 1 hormones cortisol and insulin, compounding stress on the body and creating a vicious feedback loop that becomes tough to break. (Check out "Understanding Your Stress Response System" earlier in this chapter for more on how hormones and stress are related.)

Friendships, on the other hand, activate the release of endorphins and other feel-good hormones, such as dopamine and oxytocin, which in turn stimulate your immune system's natural killer cells that target diseases and viruses. Studies also show that those with fewer or no close connections are more susceptible to psychological conditions like depression and are less equipped to fend off illness.

Research consistently shows that partnered individuals tend to eat better, exercise more, and are less likely to engage in harmful behaviors such as smoking or excessive drinking, all contributing to a protective effect on overall health and longevity. Studies on long-term, cohabiting, and married couples indicate that they live longer than their single counterparts on average.

REMEMBER

The research might make it sound like long-term partnership is the magic bullet, but remember that it's not about whether you're single or partnered; it's about the quality of the connections you have. Whether you're spending time with a close friend, family member, or even a beloved pet, moments of genuine connection are nourishing for your nervous system, which doesn't care about your relationship status. Your nervous system just wants you to feel safe and supported, like you belong, and surrounded by love, in whatever form that comes.

Suffering the lonely heart

Technology has made our world intensely hyperconnected. The paradox is that our constant connectivity has us feeling more isolated than ever and increasingly disconnected from meaningful human interactions. The World Health Organization

(WHO, www.who.int) now recognizes loneliness as a serious public health problem that's comparable in its health risks to smoking 15 cigarettes a day and obesity.

Here are some additional research findings that show that individuals who feel isolated and alone are much more likely to experience health problems, including heart disease and cancer:

>> The prestigious *New England Journal of Medicine* published a study of more than 2,300 men who had survived a heart attack. The risk of death for participants who were classified as socially isolated and having a high degree of stress was more than four times that of participants with low levels of stress and isolation. These relationships held up even when the study was controlled for other cardiac risk factors, such as smoking, diet, exercise, and weight.

>> In a Duke University study of 1,400 men and women who had blockage of at least one coronary artery (determined by coronary angiography), study participants who weren't married and didn't have at least one close confidant were more than three times more likely to have died at follow-up than participants who were married and/or had a confidant.

>> In a third study, participants who suffered a recent heart attack and lived alone experienced twice the risk of dying after a heart attack when compared with participants who lived with one or more other individuals and described their relationships as close.

TECHNICAL STUFF

In many other studies conducted in diverse cultures, social isolation has been found to increase the risk of heart disease, sudden death, and cancer. In response, countries such as Japan and the U.K. have appointed "ministers of loneliness" who are tasked with developing strategies to combat the rising rates of loneliness and social isolation, particularly among younger citizens, older populations, and men.

Linking loneliness and pornography

One underrecognized contributor to the growing loneliness crisis is pornography consumption. A study from the Institute for Family Studies (https://ifstudies.org) revealed that daily pornography use among young adults is strongly linked to higher rates of depression and loneliness, underscoring the need for a broader conversation about how people interact with digital content, and more importantly, how people prioritize and cultivate meaningful human connections in an era where digital consumption often takes precedence over real-world intimacy.

Distinguishing loneliness from aloneness

Being alone doesn't always mean being lonely. In fact, solitude gives you wonderful opportunities for reflection, emotional processing, creativity, and mental restoration. Loneliness, in contrast, occurs when isolation is not a choice, or when there's a disconnect between how much social interaction you're craving or desiring and what is available for you.

REMEMBER

It's not just about physical isolation; you can feel lonely, disconnected, or unseen even when you're surrounded by other people. This happens when the social interactions you're having lack depth or meaning, when you don't feel emotionally connected to the people around you or you don't feel like you can be your true, authentic self. Loneliness is a deeply subjective experience. So for some, being physically alone doesn't result in loneliness at all, whereas others may feel profoundly lonely even though they have a huge family and social circle. The quality of your interactions matters far more than the quantity. People with closer friendships and higher-quality relationships built on empathy and intimacy that allows them to feel seen and heard experience more life satisfaction and less loneliness and depression.

Reconnecting Authentically with Others and Yourself

If you feel lonely, don't feel ashamed for feeling that way; you have the power to seek out and prioritize deeper, more meaningful relationships where you can express your whole self, flaws and all, without fear of rejection or ridicule.

TIP

Taking steps to reconnect with your authentic self through creative outlets, nature, and mindfulness can have a profound impact on your health. Activities such as painting, drawing, journaling, or even walking in nature reduce cortisol levels and increase feel-good hormones such as dopamine, endorphins, and oxytocin. They also enhance your resilience, giving you the emotional energy and capacity needed to put yourself out there and form genuine relationships.

Additionally, oxytocin — your bonding hormone — is released when you engage in real-world, meaningful interactions, even something small, like a friendly chat with your local barista. They don't need to be lengthy or profound conversations to positively impact your hormone levels. They just need to be genuine.

TIP

If you feel isolated or lonely, here are some additional suggestions for making some connections:

>> Invest time and thought in friends and/or family as seriously as you do in your work.

>> Join an interest or hobby group. From chess clubs to gardening clubs, book clubs to folkdance societies, running clubs to writing classes, an activity-related group that matches your interests is out there for you to benefit from.

>> Find a third place. Beyond home and work, people long have benefited from a close connection to a *third place* in their communities. For many it's their church, synagogue, mosque, or temple. For others, it's a social group, community organization, or other activity or group that is meaningful to them. The identity of your third place isn't as important as the fact that you have one.

Fortifying Your Body through Mental Wellness

In 2023, the White House acknowledged that the nation faced "a mental health crisis," with 40 percent of U.S. adults experiencing depression or anxiety in 2021. Gallup estimated that 22 percent of Americans had symptoms severe enough to disrupt their daily lives for two weeks or longer. One-third of U.S. teens had anxiety disorders, and nearly one in five faced a major depressive episode in 2023. This concerning trend isn't limited to the United States. Globally, WHO reports that nearly 1 billion people are now living with a mental health disorder, with depression and anxiety leading the way.

If you think you might be facing anxiety or depression, take a look at the following sections.

Anxiety: Everybody's doing it

Stroll down the street and about one in four of the people you walk by has significant problems with anxiety. And almost half of the people you encounter will struggle with anxiety to one degree or another.

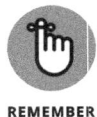

REMEMBER

Anxiety involves feelings of uneasiness, worry, apprehension, and/or fear, and it's the most common of all the emotional disorders. In other words, you definitely aren't alone if you have unwanted anxiety.

Life has always been menacing. But today people around the world are glued to screens watching, reading, or hearing about the latest horrors in real time. It can be difficult to get a break from all the bad news.

Anxiety results in all sorts of thoughts, behaviors, and feelings. When your anxiety begins to interfere with day-to-day life, you need to find ways to put your fears and worries at ease.

Recognizing the symptoms of anxiety

You may not know if you suffer from problematic anxiety. That's because anxiety involves a wide range of symptoms. Each person experiences a slightly different constellation of these symptoms.

Thinking anxiously

Folks with anxiety generally think in ways that differ from the ways that other people think. You're probably thinking anxiously if you experience:

>> **Approval addiction:** If you're an approval addict, you worry a great deal about what other people think about you.

>> **Living in the future and predicting the worst:** When you do this, you think about everything that lies ahead and assume the worst possible outcome.

>> **Dependency:** Some people believe they must have help from others and are unable to achieve on their own.

>> **Perfectionism:** If you're a perfectionist, you assume that any mistake means total failure.

>> **Poor concentration:** Anxious people routinely report that they struggle with focusing their thoughts. Short-term memory sometimes suffers as well.

>> **Racing thoughts:** Thoughts zip through your mind in a stream of almost uncontrollable worry and concern.

Behaving anxiously

We have three words to describe anxious behavior — avoidance, avoidance, and avoidance. Anxious people inevitably attempt to stay away from the things that make them anxious. Whether it's snakes, heights, crowds, freeways, parties, or paying bills, anxious people search for ways out.

In the short run, avoidance lowers anxiety. It makes you feel a little better. However, in the long run, avoidance actually maintains and heightens anxiety.

Finding anxiety in your body

Almost all people with severe anxiety experience a range of physical effects. These sensations don't simply occur in your head; they're as real as this book you're holding. The responses to anxiety vary considerably from person to person and include the following:

>> Accelerated heartbeat

>> Shallow, rapid breathing

>> A spike in blood pressure

>> Dizziness

>> Fatigue

>> Gastrointestinal upset

>> General aches and pains

>> Muscle tension or spasms

>> Sweating

WARNING

These are simply the temporary effects that anxiety exerts on your body. Chronic anxiety left untreated poses serious risks to your health as well.

Seeking help for your anxiety

Most people simply choose to live with anxiety rather than seek professional help. Some people worry that treatment won't work. Or they believe that the only effective treatment out there is medication, and they fear the possibility of side effects. Others fret about the costs of getting help. And still others have concerns that tackling their anxiety would cause their fears to increase so much that they wouldn't be able to stand it.

TIP

Stop adding worry to worry. You're reading this chapter, and that's a start. You can significantly reduce your anxiety through a variety of strategies. Many don't have to cost a single cent, and if one doesn't work, you can try another. Most people find that at least a couple of the approaches work for them.

Untreated anxiety may cause long-term health problems. It doesn't make sense to avoid doing something about your anxiety.

Matching symptoms and therapies

Anxiety symptoms appear in three different spheres. Treatment corresponds to each of these three areas.

>> **Thinking symptoms** pertain to the thoughts that run through your mind. One of the most effective treatments for a wide range of emotional problems, known as *cognitive therapy,* deals with the way you think about, perceive, and interpret everything that's important to you,

>> **Behaving symptoms** pertain to the things you do in response to anxiety. *Behavior therapy* deals with actions you can take and behaviors you can incorporate to alleviate your anxiety. Some actions are fairly straightforward, like getting more exercise and sleep and managing your responsibilities. *Exposure* can feel a little scary and involves breaking your fears down into small steps and facing them one at a time.

>> **Feeling symptoms** pertain to how your body reacts to anxiety. Anxiety sets off a storm of distressing physical symptoms, such as a racing heartbeat, upset stomach, muscle tension, sweating, dizziness, and so on. Making a few tweaks to your lifestyle such as increased exercise, better diet, and adequate sleep help a little. But our primary recommendation is to figure out how to approach distressing physical symptoms with an accepting attitude.

Some people, with the advice of their doctor, choose to take medications for their anxiety.

Helping yourself or calling in a pro

It's possible you can be your own best mental health helper. A number of studies support the idea that people can deal with important, difficult problems without seeking the services of a professional. People clearly benefit from self-help. They get better and stay better.

Then again, sometimes self-help efforts fall short, especially when anxiety is moderate to severe in intensity. Sometimes professional consultation is the most effective way to get the guidance and support you need.

Detecting depression

Everyone feels down from time to time. But depression is more than a normal reaction to unpleasant events and losses. Depression deepens and spreads well beyond sadness, disrupting both the mind and the body in serious, sometimes deadly ways.

Depression impacts every aspect of life. In fact, even though a number of types of depression exist, all types of depression affect people in four areas, although each individual may be affected in different ways. Take a look at the next sections for more information.

Dwelling on bleak thoughts

When you get depressed, your view of the world changes. The sun shines less brightly, the sky clouds over, people seem cold and distant, and the future looks dark. Your mind may fill with recurrent thoughts of worthlessness, self-loathing, and even death. Typically, depressed people complain of difficulty concentrating, remembering, and making decisions.

WARNING

If you're having serious suicidal thoughts, you need an immediate evaluation and treatment. If the thoughts include a plan that you believe you may actually carry out now or in the very near future, go to a hospital emergency room. They have trained personnel who can help. If you're not able to get yourself to an emergency room, call 911 for more rapid attention. The National Suicide Helpline is particularly useful and is staffed 24/7: Call 988 or 800-273-TALK (800-273-8255).

Dragging your feet: Depressed behavior

Not everyone who's depressed behaves in the same way. Some people speed up and others slow down. Some folks sleep more than ever, while others complain of a dreadful lack of sleep.

TIP

Although everyone is different, certain behaviors tend to go along with depression. Do your actions and behaviors concern you? Depressed people tend to either feel like they're walking in wet cement or running full speed on a treadmill.

Reflecting upon relationships and depression

Depression damages the way you relate to others. Withdrawal and avoidance are the most common responses to depression. Sometimes depressed people get irritable and critical with the very people they care most about.

When you're depressed, you turn away from the very people who may have the most support to offer you. Either you feel that they don't care about you, or perhaps you can't muster up positive feelings for them. You may avoid others or find yourself irritated and crabby.

Feeling funky: The physical signs of depression

Depression typically includes at least a few physical symptoms. These symptoms include changes in appetite, sleep, and energy. However, for some people, the experience of depression *primarily* consists of physical symptoms and doesn't necessarily include as many other symptoms such as sadness, withdrawal from people, lack of interests, and missed work.

TIP

Many folks who experience depression primarily in physical terms are very unaware of their emotional life. Sometimes, that's because they were taught that feelings are unimportant. In other cases, their parents scolded them for crying or showing other appropriate feelings such as excitement or sadness.

If your depression shows up primarily in physical terms, medications or some other physical remedy may seem like the best choice for you.

Finding help with psychotherapy

Psychotherapy involves work with a therapist using psychological techniques to alleviate emotional problems. And psychotherapy works well for treating depression. Incredibly, psychotherapy comes in literally hundreds of different forms and types; it's also practiced by a wide array of professionals. Take a look at the following for information about the types of psychotherapy that are known to work for treating depression.

REMEMBER

The following therapies have been proven to be effective for treating depressions and, for many, produce excellent results within a reasonable time frame:

>> **Cognitive therapy:** In brief, cognitive therapy operates on the assumption that the ways in which people think about, perceive, and interpret events plays a pivotal role in how they feel. For the treatment of depression, no psychotherapy has received as much support as cognitive therapy. Flat out, it works. It works at least as well as medication does for treating depression, and it appears to provide a degree of protection against relapse — something that medication can't do.

>> **Acceptance and Commitment Therapy (ACT):** ACT has many similarities to cognitive and behavior therapies. However, it places greater emphasis on accepting all feelings and emotions rather than trying to rid yourself of

them entirely. Accepting feelings, paradoxically, helps soften them. It also works on value clarification and commitment to living a life based on your personal values.

» **Behavior therapy:** Studies have found that changing your behavior can also improve the way you feel and alleviate depression. Behavior therapy focuses on helping you to change behaviors (such as increasing your pleasurable activities and teaching you ways to solve problems). Most practitioners of behavior therapy also include at least some cognitive techniques in their work. Many of these professionals call themselves cognitive-behavioral therapists.

» **Interpersonal therapy:** This type of therapy attempts to help people identify and modify problems in their relationships, both past and present. This approach has also been shown to alleviate depression about as well as medication. Sometimes this method of therapy delves into issues involving loss, grief, and major changes in a person's life, such as retirement or divorce.

Most people aren't aware that hundreds of different types of therapy exist. If you cast around, you may run into practitioners of psychoanalysis, hakomi therapy, eye movement desensitization reprocessing (popularly referred to as EMDR), client-centered therapy, transactional analysis, and Gestalt therapy, just to name a few. We believe that many of these therapies likely have value, and some may work for depression. However, the scientific literature is limited on these other types of therapy as applied to depression. We suggest that you start with therapies that have been fully established as effective.

Exploring the self-help option

Everyone who's dealing with depression can benefit from self-help. *Self-help* refers to efforts you make on your own, without professional assistance, to deal with your depression.

Choosing the right self-help approach depends in part on your personal preferences and style. The following list covers the most common self-help options.

» **Books:** Reading several different self-help books is a pretty good idea. Even though you may hear some suggestions more than once, repetition helps you remember, and all authors have slightly different ways of explaining concepts. Books can also provide you with a whole lot of information that would take a therapist many sessions to cover. And you can refer to the information as often as you need to. Finally, if you combine reading with therapy, it may just take you less time to get better.

REMEMBER

Make sure that the authors of any self-help book that you purchase have credentials and experience helping others deal with depression.

>> **Videos:** For folks who learn best by hearing or seeing, videos have merit. Look for the same author credentials and information on effective approaches that we note for books.

>> **Self-help groups:** People with common problems gather in these groups to share information and experiences. The members help themselves and each other by expressing feelings and solving problems together. The National Alliance for the Mentally Ill (www.nami.org) offers information about local support groups. In addition, your local chapter of United Way (an international network of local non-profits; www.unitedway.org) likely has a directory of community resources.

>> **Websites:** You can find a wide range of resources related to depression on the internet. Be cautious about unqualified, though well-meaning, individuals serving up advice, and especially beware of outright frauds.

WARNING

Numerous unscrupulous entrepreneurs hawk various types of books, herbs, videos, and other types of merchandise that promise prompt relief from depression with little or no effort. Buyers beware! No miracle cures exist for overcoming depression.

Chapter **8**

Getting Enough Zzz's

E very night, billions of people close their eyes, surrendering to a state that has puzzled and fascinated scientists, philosophers, and poets alike for centuries: sleep. For something so universal, sleep remains one of the most complex and poorly understood processes of the human body. Sleep is not just a nightly shutdown; it involves a complex dance of chemical messengers from the brain that interact with biological rhythms. Sleep is a vital activity that underpins all bodily processes — from memory to immunity.

Getting healthy sleep isn't just about how much time you spend in bed — it's about paying attention to your body, your lifestyle, and the many factors that affect your sleep. By making small changes to your daily habits — from diet and exercise to screen time and stress management — you can improve the quality of your sleep and feel more alert, rested, and energized throughout the day.

Moving From Dozing to Dreaming: The Mechanics of Sleep

Sleep may feel like a single continuous experience, but beneath the surface, sleep harbors an intricate symphony of biological activity. From the gentle transitions of light sleep to the vivid dreams of *REM sleep* (which is nothing to do with Peter Buck, it stands for rapid eye movement and refers to a sleep stage responsible for memory consolidation, emotional processing, and learning), every stage plays a unique role in restoring your body and mind.

Stages and states of sleep

A typical night's sleep follows a repeating cycle that lasts roughly 60–90 minutes (sometimes as long as 120 minutes) and moves through various stages of non-REM (NREM) and REM sleep.

TECHNICAL STUFF

NREM sleep forms the foundation of restorative sleep and dominates most of the sleep cycle. NREM sleep consists of stages N1 through N3, starting with light sleep (stage N1), progressing to slightly deeper sleep (stage N2), and ending with deep sleep (stage N3):

>> **Stage N1:** This is the gateway to sleep — a light, transitional stage marked by slower brain waves. Your muscles relax and eye movements slow down. People often don't realize they're asleep during this stage.

>> **Stage N2:** Often called *intermediate sleep*, this stage makes up 40 to 55 percent of your nightly rest. It features hallmark brain wave patterns that consolidate memories and suppress external stimuli.

>> **Stage N3:** Also known as *slow-wave sleep, delta sleep,* or *deep sleep*, this stage is essential for physical recovery. During the N3 stage, your body repairs tissues, clears brain toxins, and strengthens the immune system.

REM sleep occurs about 90 minutes after you fall asleep and recurs multiple times throughout the night. Each period of REM sleep grows longer. During REM, your brain activity mimics wakefulness, but your body remains in a state of temporary paralysis. REM is when the majority of your dreams occur, and experiencing it is critical for emotional regulation and memory consolidation.

If you have healthy sleep architecture, you cycle through these stages multiple times during the night, with the amount of deep sleep (N3) being higher earlier in the night and REM sleep increasing in the latter part of your night's sleep.

REMEMBER

But the sleep cycle doesn't always follow such a simple pattern because individuals can pass through sleep stages in a seemingly random order throughout the night. For example, some people can pass through the sleep stages in an order more like N1, N2, N1, REM, N2, and then N3.

Disruptions to sleep architecture — whether from stress, external noise, sleep or medical disorders, or lifestyle factors — can lead to fragmented sleep, which causes you to feel less refreshed even if you've spent sufficient time in bed.

Sleep components and characteristics

During sleep, your conscious mind takes a break, but your body and brain perform critical maintenance that supports your health and well-being. Sleep is marked by distinct neurophysiological and physical changes, all of which help restore your energy and optimize your body's functions. Here's a quick glance at them:

» **Circadian system:** Your sleep-wake cycle is largely controlled by your sleep drive and by your circadian sleep-wake rhythm, which follows a roughly 24-hour cycle (see later in this chapter). One of the strongest influences on this rhythm is light. Exposure to light in the morning can allow you to wake up earlier, and evening light can delay the onset of sleep.

» **Dreams:** Most dreaming occurs during REM sleep, when the brain is highly active, particularly in the limbic system, which governs emotions. Dreams play a role in emotional processing, learning, and even simulating waking-life scenarios. Dreams also reflect the activity in regions of the brain associated with vision and emotion, which can make dreams richly sensory and often emotionally intense. Interestingly, dream recall happens primarily when you briefly wake during or after REM sleep, which is a natural part of nightly cycles.

» **Effects on body systems:** During the transition from wakefulness to light sleep, your breathing changes as it switches from conscious control to an autonomic mechanism, and during REM sleep, your breathing becomes shallower and irregular. Similarly, other body systems react, including

- *Your heart rate and blood pressure* can fluctuate during REM sleep.

- *Your digestive system* undergoes a change, with gastric acid secretion peaking in the early morning hours, and during REM sleep, your digestion is generally more active.

- *Growth hormone secretion* surges during deep NREM sleep, promoting repair and growth of tissues.

- *Body temperature* varies during sleep and, during REM sleep, your body can't regulate temperature as efficiently, leading to unpredictable swings in temperature.

» **Differences due to sex:** Women tend to sleep longer than men, and differences in *EEG activity* (electrical signals in your brain) between women and men occur during the sleep stages. Additionally, sleep disturbances are common during pregnancy, postpartum, and menopause.

» **Neurotransmitters:** These chemical messengers play a role in regulating NREM and REM sleep. For example, GABA (gamma-aminobutyric acid) is an inhibitory neurotransmitter that slows down brain activity and helps induce sleep, and orexin (hypocretin) stabilizes wakefulness and prevents transitions to sleep.

>> **Racial and ethnic differences:** Racial minorities are more likely to experience sleep disruptions and shorter sleep durations, and cultural practices vary among ethnic groups with respect to co-sleeping and napping.

>> **Wake-sleep and sleep-stage regulation:** A group of nuclei in the brainstem plays a major role in the promotion of sleep and wakefulness, and also in alternating NREM and REM sleep. If the balance of the neurotransmitters in the brainstem is off, you can experience disorders of excessive sleep (such as narcolepsy) or too little sleep (such as insomnia).

Changes in sleep, movement, and behavior during the night

Your body undergoes a dynamic array of changes as it transitions between sleep stages and cycles. These changes in heart rate, brain activity, and even physical movements are critical to your body's restorative processes:

>> **Body movements:** While you may shift positions or adjust your blanket during lighter stages of sleep (like N1 and N2), your body becomes more relaxed as you transition into deeper stages. This relaxation conserves energy and promotes recovery. On the other hand, disorders such as restless legs syndrome (RLS) or REM sleep behavior disorder (RBD) disrupt this stillness and can lead to excessive or even dangerous movements during the night.

>> **Brain activity and dreaming:** Your brain stays busy while you sleep. Deep sleep (N3) is a time for synchronized delta waves, which help your brain strengthen memories and recover from the day's demands. As the night progresses and REM sleep takes over, dreaming is more likely to occur, and activity ramps up in brain areas tied to emotions and creativity.

>> **Heart rate and breathing:** Your cardiovascular and respiratory systems respond to the demands of each sleep stage. In deep sleep (N3), your heart rate and breathing slow and become regular (when compared to the wake state), creating the perfect conditions for physical repair.

>> **Hormonal shifts:** Hormones work behind the scenes to keep your body in balance while you sleep. Growth hormone peaks during deep sleep, repairing tissues and supporting muscle recovery, while *cortisol* — your primary stress hormone — dips to its lowest levels early in the night. This delicate hormonal choreography prepares you for both physical restoration and the challenges of the next day.

>> **Temperature regulation:** Sleep also impacts how your body handles its internal temperature. During NREM sleep, your core temperature naturally drops, which helps you stay comfortable and enter deeper stages of rest.

TIP

During REM sleep, however, your body's temperature regulation turns off, leaving you more vulnerable to external factors like a hot or chilly room. A bedroom set to a cool 60–67 degrees F can help you maintain comfort throughout the night.

If you wake up frequently feeling overheated, try adjusting your room's temperature or swapping out heavy blankets for breathable, lightweight options. Small changes to your environment can make a big difference.

These nightly changes are part of the body's intricate design to promote health and restoration, but disruptions may throw these processes off balance, leaving you feeling groggy and unfocused the next day.

REMEMBER

If you experience repeated disruptions to sleep cycles — whether because of lifestyle factors or medical conditions — you may see long-term impacts on your physical and mental health. If you experience persistent sleep difficulties, consult a healthcare professional for personalized advice and solutions.

Figuring Out if You're Rested or Just Used to Being Tired

Getting enough sleep isn't just about the number of hours in bed. Quality, consistency, and how you feel during the day are all critical factors that define whether your sleep is adequate. Doctors generally recommend that adults aim for about seven to nine hours of sleep each night, but individual people's needs vary based on factors such as age, lifestyle, and overall health.

How much sleep do you really need?

Your sleep requirement is as personal as your fingerprint. Some people naturally function well with less than seven hours of sleep, and others may need closer to nine hours. The goal is to figure out what amount of sleep works best for you. Just because your partner or friend thrives on less sleep doesn't mean that your body will do the same.

To make attaining your sleep goal a bit more interesting, the amount of sleep you need also changes as you age. Here are some typical age-related sleep ranges:

>> **Newborns:** 14–17 hours per day

>> **Children:** 9–12 hours per night

>> **Adolescents:** 8–10 hours per night

>> **Adults:** 7–9 hours per night

>> **Elderly:** 7–8 hours per night

But what happens if the amount of sleep you get regularly falls outside of these typical ranges? The distinction between short sleep and long sleep becomes important in this discussion. While sleep patterns can vary, consistently getting too little or too much sleep may be a red flag signaling possible sleep disorders or other health issues.

To break down the distinction:

>> **Short sleep (six hours or less):** Research shows that consistently sleeping less than six hours per night increases your risk of serious health conditions, such as coronary heart disease, stroke, obesity, diabetes, mental health issues, and even *all-cause mortality* (the total number of deaths from any cause). This relationship between short sleep and serious health conditions can go both ways. Short sleep can contribute to the onset of these health problems, but existing medical conditions — such as chronic pain or anxiety — can also lead to shorter sleep.

>> **Long sleep (nine hours or more):** Regularly sleeping more than nine hours is also linked to poor health outcomes, including diabetes, hypertension and other cardiovascular conditions, obesity, and cognitive decline. People who report long sleep durations often experience underlying health conditions such as depression or sleep apnea, which can extend the overall time they spend asleep.

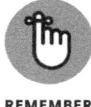

REMEMBER

Both short and long sleep often connect to underlying issues, rather than being causes for atypical sleep duration by themselves. If you find that you regularly sleep less than six hours or more than nine hours and feel tired, checking in with a healthcare provider to find out whether an underlying medical condition could be affecting your sleep is worthwhile.

Clues that you're not getting enough sleep

If you're waking up tired despite getting enough hours of sleep, you should evaluate your sleep environment, nighttime habits, and overall sleep quality. Are you waking up refreshed, or do you feel groggy and tired throughout the day? Some people may function well on the lower end of the typical range of sleep hours, while others need more sleep to feel their best. Even though feeling tired is a pretty common occurrence, don't shrug it off, especially if the feeling is persistent.

Chronic sleep deprivation can lead to serious long-term effects, including a higher risk for heart disease, diabetes, and depression.

The best way to know if you're getting enough sleep is by paying careful attention to how you feel during the day after a night's sleep. Here are some clues:

>> **Cognitive impairment:** Poor attention, memory issues, or difficulty concentrating may be signs that you need more sleep. Lack of sleep affects vigilance, learning, and higher-order cognitive functions, such as driving a car or making complex decisions at work.

>> **Daytime sleepiness:** You shouldn't feel excessively sleepy during the day if you're getting enough sleep. Falling asleep during meetings, while driving, or while reading can be a major sign of sleep deprivation.

>> **Near accidents or microsleeps:** If you've experienced near misses or accidents due to momentary lapses into sleep (*microsleep* is the technical term for the situation in which your brain shifts from wake to sleep for a few seconds), this could be a strong sign that you need to improve your sleep duration or quality.

If you experience a microsleep and close your eyes while driving — even for a few seconds — the result could be a fatal accident. Officers typically use information from accident scenes to determine the causes of accidents. For example, finding no skid marks shows that the driver wasn't applying the brakes, and the conclusion might be that they likely experienced a lapse of consciousness — such as a microsleep.

>> **Mood changes:** If you notice that you're more irritable, moody, depressed, or anxious, you may not be getting sufficient sleep.

>> **Physical signs:** Sudden weight gain or increased hunger could indicate that your sleep quality is poor. Sleep affects your appetite-regulating hormones (such as ghrelin and leptin), and your appetite may increase.

If you experience any of the sleep-deprivation clues noted in this section, try increasing your sleep by 15-minute increments each week. For example, if you currently sleep 7 hours but still feel sleepy, try going to bed 15 minutes earlier and maintaining your usual wake time for a week. Continue this process (of increasing sleep time by 15 minutes for a week, while maintaining wakeup time as the anchor) until you no longer feel sleepy during the day. If adding segments to your sleep time doesn't work to improve daytime sleepiness, you may need to consider that your issue isn't the quantity of sleep, but the quality of sleep instead.

Understanding and Maintaining Healthy Sleep

Healthy sleep isn't just about how long you sleep (the quantity), but it's also about the quality. Sleep that restores your body and mind has specific characteristics, and understanding these can help you assess whether you're truly getting both the quantity and the quality of sleep you need. While everyone's sleep needs vary slightly, some universal markers of healthy sleep apply across all ages. Healthy sleep has three main components that together create the foundation for feeling refreshed and alert during the day:

>> **Continuity:** Having enough sleep is important, but so is having uninterrupted sleep. Healthy sleep should occur in one consolidated block, without frequent awakenings. Fragmented sleep — even if the total hours add up to a sufficient amount — reduces your time in restorative stages such as deep sleep and REM.

>> **Depth:** The intensity of sleep, particularly during deep sleep, is critical for physical recovery and memory consolidation. While you may not be able to measure sleep depth directly at home, you can assess it by how refreshed you feel upon waking. People who regularly experience shallow or disrupted sleep often wake up groggy, with lingering fatigue.

>> **Duration:** The National Sleep Foundation (www.thensf.org) recommends seven to nine hours of sleep per night for adults, with slight variations depending on individual needs. Children and teens require more because their developing bodies and brains rely heavily on restorative rest. Sleeping consistently within your recommended range is one of the most important steps toward maintaining overall health.

The role of circadian rhythms

TIP

Healthy sleep is deeply tied to your *circadian rhythms* — the internal biologic clock that regulates your sleep-wake cycle. These rhythms are influenced by natural light and darkness, which signal your body to release sleep-promoting hormones such as melatonin. Aligning your schedule with these rhythms can improve the quality of your life.

>> **Evening habits:** Dim the lights in your home as bedtime approaches, and avoid blue light from screens. These behaviors may impact melatonin signals to your body that it's time to wind down.

>> **Morning routines:** Expose yourself to natural light within the first hour of waking. This practice helps regulate your circadian rhythms and promotes alertness during the day.

For those who struggle with circadian misalignment — such as shift workers or frequent travelers (who cross time zones) — establishing consistent sleep routines and using tools such as light therapy devices can help reset your internal clock.

TIP

Struggling to make changes? Start small. Focus on one aspect of your sleep, such as your bedtime routine, and gradually build from there. Consistency is more important than perfection.

Nutrition, exercise, and sleep

TIP

Getting good nutrition and regular exercise are essential for maintaining healthy sleep. Here are some general guidelines regarding eating and drinking:

>> **Eat foods rich in unsaturated fats and high in fiber** to help promote deeper, more restorative sleep.

>> **Avoid refined sugars, processed foods, and large amounts of carbohydrates,** which might leave you feeling groggy and less alert.

>> **Start the day with a balanced breakfast** to improve not only sleep quality, but also motivation during morning routines.

>> **If you're a shift worker, steer clear of heavy meals during night shifts** to avoid disrupting your sleep later.

>> **Avoid alcohol and caffeine in the evening** to keep them from interfering with your ability to fall asleep or stay asleep.

Regular exercise can improve sleep quality and total sleep time (quantity). Sleep research shows that exercise can improve the symptoms and sleep quality in individuals who have sleep disorders such as insomnia, obstructive sleep apnea (OSA), restless legs syndrome (RLS), and periodic limb movements during sleep (PLMS).

Getting Better Sleep Based on Your Life Stage

Sleep needs change as people age, and what works for one age group may not be as effective for another. Tailoring sleep habits to different life stages ensures that you get the most restful, restorative sleep possible for all stages. (And although some teenagers may consider themselves men, we're providing guidance here for guys older than their teens.)

Sleep needs for young men and guys in their prime

Adults often struggle to balance sleep with work, family, and social responsibilities. Many fall short of the recommended seven to nine hours of sleep, which can lead to chronic sleep debt. Adults cycle through NREM and REM sleep throughout the night. However, factors such as stress, poor diet, and lifestyle choices (such as alcohol or caffeine consumption at inappropriate times) can often disrupt sleep. And chronic stress can lead to insomnia, in which individuals struggle to fall asleep, or wake frequently during the night. Cortisol, the stress hormone, stays elevated and prevents relaxation.

TIP

Prioritize stress management techniques such as meditation, deep breathing, or yoga to improve sleep. Reduce alcohol and caffeine intake, especially in the evening. Also maintain a consistent sleep schedule, create a relaxing bedtime routine, and ensure that your sleep environment is comfortable.

Characteristics of men's sleep

When you examine sleep throughout adulthood, you find that total sleep time progressively declines. You also find a corresponding increase in wakefulness after sleep onset, which results in lower *sleep efficiency* (proportion of time someone is asleep while they're in bed).

Here are some specifics related to the sleep experience in adults:

>> **Adult sleep is lighter:** They experience a decrease in deep slow-wave (N3) sleep, an increase in lighter stages of sleep (N1 and N2), and REM sleep tends to hover at around 25 percent of total sleep time from the mid-20s on. As adults age, their circadian sleep-wake system gradually becomes less robust with poorer quality of sleep at night and more drowsiness during the day. Adults also have a decreased ability to rebound from nights of either partial or total sleep loss compared to when they were younger.

>> **Sleep (and other) disorders become more prevalent and disruptive to sleep:** Disorders such as OSA, RLS, and chronic insomnia occur more frequently in adults.

Other medical disorders can also arise and take the form of hypertension, heart disease, thyroid disease, chronic obstructive pulmonary disease (COPD), gastroesophageal reflux disease (GERD), chronic pain, type 2 diabetes, and cancer. Also, mental conditions such as depression and anxiety can disrupt sleep during adulthood.

>> **Many medications prescribed for adults to treat any of these sleep, medical, or psychiatric disorders may potentially worsen sleep:** For example, stimulants prescribed for the daytime sleepiness of narcolepsy, bronchodilator medications for asthma, and some antidepressants can negatively affect sleep.

Dos and don'ts for healthy adult sleep

Check out Table 8-1 for some important do's and don'ts for healthy sleep as an adult.

TABLE 8-1 **Sleep-Related Do's and Don'ts for Adults**

What to Do	How to Do It
Do	
Maintain a healthy lifestyle	A healthy diet and regular exercise regimen promote sleep and stable circadian sleep-wake rhythms.
Establish a regular sleep-wake schedule	Go to bed near the same time each night and awaken near the same time each day for all days of the week. Keeping wakeup time constant is especially critical.
Allow adequate sleep time	Make time for at least 7 hours of sleep per night.
Set up a conducive sleep space	Make sure that your bedroom matches your preferences for temperature, noise level, mattress and pillow firmness, and light exposure.
Use light to synchronize your body's sleep-wake cycle	Within 5 minutes of awakening, go outside (into the sunlight) or stay in an indoor area that receives significant sunlight for 30 minutes to align your sleep-wake cycle with your desired awakening time. If you typically awaken before dawn, applying a UV-filtered light box (10,000 lux and 18" from eyes) is an acceptable substitute for sunlight. Conversely, avoid bright light for a few hours before bedtime to prevent it from delaying your sleep onset.
Establish a regular relaxing pattern before sleep	Meditation, yoga, or a warm bath can help to promote sleep.
Create and manage a *worry list*	A few hours before bedtime, write down all the items that are bothering you to serve as a *placeholder* for the worries. (You don't have to deal with them immediately, but don't forget to address them.) This practice can lessen the chance that these worries flood your mind the moment your head hits the pillow. For more on managing stress, take a look at Chapter 7.

(continued)

TABLE 8-1 *(continued)*

What to Do	How to Do It
Don't	
Engage with stimulating substances and activities close to bedtime	Avoid exercise, caffeine, nicotine, alcohol, heavy meals, or heavy liquid intake for at least two hours before bedtime.
Take OTC medications that you haven't vetted	Discuss any other-the-counter (OTC) medication with your healthcare provider. *Note:* An exception would be melatonin; a 0.3 mg dose of melatonin may help those who have symptoms of insomnia.
Watch TV or read in bed	Avoid these activities unless they definitely make you drowsy.
Work in bed	Avoid activities that require mental effort or may cause stress — such as working. Also, avoid using a smartphone, tablet, or computer (even with blue-blocking software) at least 30 minutes before bedtime.
Nap during the day	Power through the day without naps so that you avoid affecting your night's sleep. You may take a short nap (10 to 20 minutes) to avoid driving when drowsy, and taking a nap at the same time of day for a set amount of time is okay because your body will become used to taking this daily nap. Enhance the benefits of this short nap by taking caffeine just prior to the nap, which allows the caffeine to enter your system and help with alertness.
Linger in bed longer than 20 minutes if you can't fall asleep (or back to sleep)	Get up and go to another room, do something that makes you drowsy (meditation, for example), and then go back to bed when you feel drowsy. This is important for reconditioning your body to associate the bedroom as a place to sleep.

Sleep needs for silver foxes

The good news for older adults is that the decline in total sleep time (as well as N3 and REM sleep) and the ability to fall and stay asleep appears to plateau at about the age of 60 years. The bad news is that wakefulness after sleep onset increases and the ability to fall asleep continues to decrease with advanced age.

Older adults typically need around seven to eight hours of sleep, although as people age, sleep efficiency declines, and older adults experience more fragmented sleep. Older adults often feel sleepy earlier in the evening and wake up earlier in the morning; this *advanced sleep phase* represents a normal shift in the timing of their circadian sleep–wake rhythm.

WARNING

Although older adults appear to be more resilient to the effects of sleep loss than younger adults, older adults who regularly sleep less than six hours have increased risk of cognitive dysfunction and mortality. Additionally, an association between excessive daytime sleepiness in the elderly and subsequent cognitive decline and dementia is suggested.

Sleep interference, from medical to mental

As people age, they're more likely to develop medical issues (such as musculo-skeletal pain) and mental health conditions (such as anxiety or depression) that interfere with sleep quality and duration. And like younger adults, older adults often face sleep disorders such as OSA, RLS, and chronic insomnia, which make getting restorative sleep harder to do. Managing these conditions with medication can also affect your sleep. Here are some aspects that relate to using medications to treat the conditions that older people might develop:

>> **Discuss with your doctor about using the lowest possible dose** of medication that still works effectively but minimizes side effects.

>> **Ask about medications that are more sedating (rather than alerting)** if you need to take them near bedtime

>> **Avoid medications that increase nighttime bathroom visits** so that they are less likely to cause frequent urination at night.

>> **Review the half-life of any medication** that could cause daytime drowsiness with your doctor.

Sleeping like a younger man

To optimize your sleep if you're an older adult, you can look to the recommendations for younger adults. Specifically, older adults should

>> **Maintain a consistent sleep schedule** even though retirement may eliminate the pressure to go to bed and wake up at specific times — no alarm clock needed!

>> **Address sleep-disrupting conditions like OSA** to minimize fragmentation of sleep.

>> **Practice relaxation techniques** to reduce night-time wakefulness.

>> **Possibly introduce short, strategic naps (those that last no longer than 30 minutes),** which can improve alertness and mood without disrupting nighttime sleep.

Long or frequent naps may worsen insomnia and can disturb your normal sleep-wake rhythm.

Be sure to get your mental health regularly assessed, especially if you've lost some of your social support system due to death of loved ones. Compared to younger adults, maintaining regular physical activity and exercise (for example, walking or stretching), and light exposure during the day, are even more important for older adults because of the alterations in sleep and circadian rhythms that accompany normal aging. Regular physical and social activity can improve sleep quantity and quality in older adults, including those who are residing in nursing homes.

Seeing the Signs of Sleep Gone Sideways

Sleep deprivation is more than an occasional restless night — it's a state that affects your body, mind, and daily life. Whether caused by external factors, lifestyle habits, or underlying sleep disorders, the consequences of insufficient sleep can be profound. Recognizing the signs of sleep deprivation early is key to addressing the problem and restoring balance to your sleep-wake cycle.

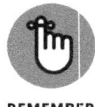

Avoid *sleep debt* — the accumulation of lost sleep over time — to prevent frequent *microsleeps*. These uncontrollable episodes of sleep can occur during the day and lead to life-threatening situations, especially when you're driving or operating hazardous machinery.

COMMON SLEEP DISORDERS

Not all sleep problems are caused by poor habits or external factors — many stem from underlying disorders that require targeted treatment. Some of the most common sleep disorders include

- **Insomnia:** A condition in which you have difficulty falling asleep, staying asleep, or getting enough rest. This sleep disorder is one of the most common; it affects about one in six Americans. Stress, anxiety, and medical conditions are common triggers.

- **Hypersomnias:** A group of disorders that cause symptoms such as excessive daytime sleepiness and sometimes sudden sleep attacks. *Narcolepsy* is a well-known hypersomnia that also features symptoms such as hallucinations when falling asleep or waking up that are frequently accompanied by temporary paralysis of voluntary muscles, and *cataplexy* (a sudden muscle weakness often triggered by strong emotions).

- **Obstructive sleep apnea (OSA):** A common sleep-related breathing disorder that affects about 24 percent of men between the ages of 30 and 60. OSA is marked by pauses or decreases in your breathing during sleep.

- **Restless legs syndrome (RLS):** A common condition that involves an uncontrollable urge to move the legs, especially at night, disrupting both falling asleep and staying asleep. You may also have unpleasant sensations (for example, feeling like bugs are crawling on your skin) or also experience periodic limb movements during sleep (PLMS), in which your legs kick or twitch during the night and wake you up (or, more commonly, wake up your bedpartner).

- **Sleepwalking:** Sleepwalking happens when you get up and walk around during deep sleep, even though you're not fully awake. If you've ever seen someone sleepwalking, they might seem alert, but they won't remember it the next morning.

- **Delayed sleep-wake phase disorder:** One of several circadian rhythm sleep disorders in which you struggle to fall asleep and wake up at the times you want. You might find yourself staying up late and having a hard time getting up early in the morning.

Recognizing the symptoms and signs of sleep disorders is the first step toward effective treatment.

Types of sleep deprivation

Specific types of sleep deprivation can affect your sleep in various ways that curtail the amount of restful sleep you experience on a nightly basis.

>> **Acute sleep deprivation:** Not sleeping for one or more nights, either missing total or partial sleep during these nights. This may be caused, for example, by work deadlines, illness, or family situations.

>> **Chronic sleep loss and fragmentation:** Getting less sleep consistently over an extended time frame either by a reduction in your total sleep time (voluntarily or involuntarily) or by fragmentation of your sleep.

>> **Partial and sleep-stage deprivation:** For partial sleep deprivation, your total sleep time is reduced so that you get less sleep than usual. In the case of sleep-stage deprivation, you may have a medical condition or be taking medications that reduce certain stages of sleep.

Warning signs of sleep deprivation

Sleep deprivation can manifest in many ways, some more subtle than others:

>> **Cognitive impairments:** Difficulty concentrating, memory lapses, or slower decision-making. Sleep is essential for processing and retaining information, so even one night of poor rest can leave you feeling foggy.

>> **Emotional changes:** Increased irritability, anxiety, or mood swings. Without enough REM sleep, your brain struggles to regulate emotions effectively, and may result in or exacerbate anxiety and mood disorders, such as depression.

>> **Psychosocial changes:** Overreaction to minor annoyances, impaired social judgment, loneliness/social isolation, strained family and intimate relationships, and struggles in the workplace may be challenging effects of poor sleep.

>> **Physical symptoms:** Persistent fatigue, weakened immune function, or changes in appetite. Chronic sleep deprivation is linked to a higher risk of conditions like diabetes, heart disease, and obesity.

>> **Unintended sleep episodes:** Falling asleep during the day, even in inappropriate settings like meetings or while driving. This is a clear sign that your body is desperately trying to recover lost rest.

WARNING

If you notice any of these signs, take them seriously. Chronic sleep deprivation can have far-reaching consequences for your health and safety.

Long-term impacts of sleep loss

Prolonged sleep loss goes beyond day-to-day symptoms and increases the risk of severe health issues over time. Research shows that insufficient sleep disrupts nearly every system in the body:

>> **Cardiovascular disease:** Sleep deprivation raises blood pressure and increases inflammation, both of which contribute to heart disease and stroke.

>> **Endocrine effects:** Increased levels of cortisol and stress hormones may lead to a range of mental and physical issues.

>> **Gastrointestinal issues:** Research studies demonstrate that sleep disruption can affect the gut microbiome and lead to gastrointestinal issues such as bloating and constipation.

>> **Impaired mental health:** Chronic sleep loss is closely linked to conditions such as depression and anxiety, as well as reduced emotional resilience.

MEDICAL DISORDERS AND MEDICATIONS

Sleep disorders aren't the only causes of sleep loss. Many common medical disorders and medications — both prescription and over-the-counter (OTC) — frequently disrupt sleep. Conditions such as asthma, chronic obstructive pulmonary disease (COPD), diabetes, thyroid disease, and gastroesophageal reflux disease (GERD) can significantly impact both the quantity and quality of your sleep. Pain (physical, emotional, or psychological) is also a common cause of sleep loss.

Certain medications, including steroids, decongestants, cardiovascular drugs, and stimulants, can interfere with your ability to sleep at night. Additionally, substance abuse — particularly involving alcohol and nicotine — can severely disrupt sleep patterns.

>> **Metabolic changes:** Lack of sleep disrupts the hormones that regulate hunger, leading to overeating and weight gain.

>> **Musculoskeletal effects:** Sleep loss can hamper muscle repair and growth, as well as bone density — all factors that can lead to slow recovery from injuries.

>> **Reproductive problems:** Sleep deprivation can reduce testosterone levels in men.

>> **Respiratory disorders:** Inadequate sleep can have an impact on preexisting respiratory conditions by exacerbating symptoms of these disorders — for example, shortness of breath and wheezing — which can contribute to even poorer sleep quality.

>> **Weakened immunity:** Your body produces infection-fighting antibodies during sleep, so poor rest leaves you more susceptible to illness.

Addressing sleep deprivation early can help reduce these risks and protect your long-term health.

Consulting a Professional

If you've tried improving your sleep habits with tips from this chapter but continue to feel fatigued or struggle with disrupted rest, it's time to consult a professional. *Sleep studies* — which monitor brain activity, breathing, movement, heart rate, and blood oxygen and carbon dioxide levels — can provide valuable insights into what's happening during the night while you're sleeping (or trying to sleep). Treatment options range from behavioral therapies like cognitive behavioral therapy for insomnia (CBT-I) to medical interventions such as continuous positive airway pressure (CPAP) machines for sleep apnea.

TIP

Your primary care provider is a great place to start if you suspect a sleep disorder. They can refer you to a sleep specialist for further evaluation and treatment.

Getting help from a sleep specialist

When you see a sleep specialist, they not only discuss your sleep problems, medical history, and daily habits with you, but also conduct a physical examination. The physician focuses on evaluating your sleep issues to decide on whether you need a sleep study or other specialized tests such as

>> **Actigraphy:** A method to monitor human rest and activity cycles by using a device (actigraph) that usually resembles a wristwatch and records movement through an accelerometer. The actigraphy data can provide information regarding sleep patterns and sleep-wake cycles of activity over extended periods, which is most helpful for circadian rhythm issues.

>> **Home sleep tests (HSTs):** Tests that typically help diagnose obstructive sleep apnea, and directly or indirectly measure your airflow, breathing effort, blood oxygen levels, heart rate, and body position.

>> **Maintenance of Wakefulness Test (MWT):** A daytime test that measures your ability to stay awake when seated in a semi-darkened room. This test includes four 40-minute trials each spaced two hours apart. The goal is to demonstrate your ability to stay awake for the duration of the 40-minute trials, without environmental stimulation. This test has helped commercial drivers and pilots to return to duty after successful treatment.

>> **Multiple Sleep Latency Test (MSLT):** A daytime test consisting of a series of up to five scheduled naps designed to evaluate your propensity to fall asleep. If you need to take this test, it generally happens immediately following a night spent in a sleep lab to add upon the data produced during that overnight sleep test.

>> **Polysomnography (PSG):** A daytime or nighttime in-laboratory sleep study to measure the way your body functions during sleep. The data obtained is comprehensive and runs the gamut from measuring sleep efficiency (time spent asleep versus time in bed) to body positions, sleep stages, and abnormal breathing events.

Exploring treatment options

Sleep problems vary widely, so the treatment you receive depends on your specific issue. If you see your doctor or a sleep specialist, they may recommend one or more common approaches:

>> **Behavioral therapies:** Cognitive behavioral therapy for insomnia (CBT-I) is a gold-standard treatment for those struggling to fall or stay asleep or change their sleep schedule. This therapy helps you identify and eliminate unhelpful thought patterns and behaviors that disrupt sleep.

>> **Lifestyle adjustments:** Improving your sleep hygiene (habits) — such as sticking to a regular sleep schedule, creating a calming bedtime routine and environment, and limiting caffeine intake — can make a significant difference for many people.

>> **Medical interventions:** Conditions such as sleep apnea or narcolepsy often require medical treatment. Continuous positive airway pressure (CPAP) machines, for example, are highly effective for managing sleep apnea and medications (stimulants or suppressants) may help with other disorders such as narcolepsy or RLS.

REMEMBER

Don't hesitate to seek help for a sleep disorder. Whether your treatment involves therapy, medication, or a combination of approaches, you can find proven solutions to address even the most stubborn sleep challenges.

FINDING RESOURCES FOR SUPPORT

The process of improving your sleep might take time, but even small steps can lead to noticeable changes. Whether you incorporate relaxation techniques in your bedtime routine, adjust your sleep schedule, or seek professional help, every effort brings you closer to the rest you deserve. And navigating sleep challenges doesn't have to be a solo journey. Many resources are available to guide you toward better sleep:

● **Educational tools:** Books (like this one!) and reputable online resources, such as the American Academy of Sleep Medicine (AASM) at https://sleepeducation. org or the National Sleep Foundation at www.thensf.org, can empower you with knowledge and strategies to improve your sleep.

● **Sleep specialists and clinics:** Accredited sleep centers offer diagnostic tests, such as *polysomnography* (PSG, sleep studies), to pinpoint specific disorders. These tests

(continued)

(continued)

monitor brain activity, breathing, and muscle movements to provide a comprehensive picture of important changes in your body during sleep.

- **Support groups:** Connecting with others who face similar sleep challenges can provide emotional support and practical tips. Online forums, local meetups, and patient advocacy organizations are great places to start.

If you're unsure where to start, ask your primary care provider for a referral to a sleep specialist for further evaluation and treatment. They can help you navigate the options and determine the best path forward.

Chapter **9**

Smokes and Drinks: Time for a Rethink

magine taking up a truly enjoyable hobby. It's a little costly, but it feels good. Unfortunately, there's a downside: About half of the people who practice this hobby regularly end up dead due to its riskiness.

We're not talking about climbing Mt. Everest or jumping off cliffs. The hobby of smoking kills about half of long-term enthusiasts. That fact probably accounts for why most smokers want to quit smoking: They know what's in store for them down the road. Yet, giving up cliff-jumping is easier than giving up smoking. Wanting to quit is a start, but not enough by itself.

And what about drinking? Alcohol has been a part of human culture for millennia, dating back to biblical times, and is still part of many traditions and daily diets. In fact, some studies say moderate drinking is actually beneficial. However, drinking can lead to a range of adverse outcomes. In the short term, being drunk increases your risk of accidents, injuries, and impaired judgment. Longer-term, habitual drinking can lead to chronic health issues such as liver disease, heart problems, and mental health disorders.

In this chapter we explore the risks of both (and in the case of some types of alcohol, the potential benefits). If you want to be healthier, look and feel better, and live longer, and you currently smoke or drink, then it's time to rethink your habits and potentially reframe your behaviors to live your best life.

Facing the Big Risks of Smoking

Only one good thing can be said about cigarette smoking — it's good when you stop! In the United States, cigarette smoking is responsible for an enormous amount of unnecessary suffering and death every year:

>> Cigarette smoking is the leading cause of preventable death in the United States, claiming more than 430,000 lives per year.

>> Depending on the amount of cigarette smoking you do, it increases your risk of heart disease between 200 percent and 400 percent.

>> Smoking increases your risk of lung cancer by 15 to 30 times.

But guess what? None of this information is news to people who smoke cigarettes. As a friend of ours once said, "Everyone who doesn't exercise knows they should, and everyone who smokes cigarettes knows they shouldn't!"

WARNING

Cigarette smoke harms virtually every vital organ, but it's particularly dangerous to the heart and lungs. Incidentally, anyone who thinks they're safe using smoke-less tobacco, cigars, or pipes needs to think again.

Linking smoking and heart disease

We're astounded that so many people still don't appreciate just how serious the link is between cigarette smoking and heart disease.

Depending on how much they smoke, cigarette smokers increase their risk of developing heart disease two to four times more than nonsmokers. In fact, every cigarette that you light up increases your blood pressure, and the nicotine you take in causes coronary arteries to mildly constrict (close down). This problem is bad enough in a normal person, but for someone who suffers with angina, it can bring on significant symptoms. Smoking also increases inflammation and damage to artery walls, making it easier for artery-narrowing plaque to form.

In addition, cigarette smoking decreases the good cholesterol (HDL) in your bloodstream and increases the bad cholesterol (LDL). It also significantly increases your risk of developing peripheral vascular disease and aortic disease (which affects the main blood vessel leaving the heart).

Linking smoking with cancer and other diseases

Smoking accounts for many cancer deaths in the United States, including 90 percent of lung cancer deaths. Smoking also is associated with cancers of the mouth and throat, esophagus, pancreas, kidney, and bladder. Want more bad news? Cigarette smoking is associated with such annoying, chronic conditions as the common cold, stomach ulcers, chronic bronchitis, and many other lung diseases, and with catastrophic events, such as stroke.

Considering the dangers of secondhand smoke

People who live or work with active cigarette smokers are susceptible to *secondhand smoke* (also called *passive smoke, environmental tobacco smoke,* or *ETS*), which enters the air from lighted cigarettes or the exhalations of smokers. Every year, about 34,000 deaths from heart disease and over 7,000 deaths from lung cancer are attributed to secondhand smoke. Secondhand smoke also is responsible for between 150,000 and 300,000 respiratory tract infections annually.

Adding Up the Everyday Risks of Smoking

In addition to the biggest dangers of smoking, smoking affects day-to-day living as well. It sabotages actions you're trying to take to be healthier and live longer. It compromises your body's ability to absorb nutrients (and if you're making an effort to eat all the leafy greens, you want to get the benefits). And it makes you look older than your age (think "wrinkled leather" versus "fake ID").

Inhibiting exercise

Smoking makes it much harder to exercise. That's unfortunate because, as we talk about in Chapter 5, the benefits of exercise on overall physical health, well-being, and longevity are hard to deny.

Why is exercise more challenging for smokers? Because smoking

>> Narrows the arteries, reducing blood flow

>> Increases resting heart rate

>> Decreases lung capacity

>> Increases carbon monoxide in the bloodstream

>> Increases the body's production of phlegm

>> Decreases the body's ability to use oxygen

These effects of smoking obviously decrease your stamina and aerobic capacity. Smoking also damages muscles and their capacity for growth because of impaired circulation. That doesn't mean if you smoke you shouldn't exercise, but you need to proceed with care. Exercise seems to mitigate some, but not by any means all, of the risks from smoking. Quitting is best.

TIP

Some regular smokers who exercise claim that smoking doesn't impact their health. Sorry, dude; this is just denial and wishful thinking. Smoking may not have fully caught up with them or, more likely, they're experiencing some effects that will worsen with time.

TECHNICAL STUFF

But how about *smokeless* tobacco? Because of the stimulant effects of nicotine, many athletes have believed that chewing or snuffing tobacco could improve their performance. Indeed, smokeless tobacco does appear to have a few short-term, positive effects on athletic performance. It seems to improve concentration, decrease performance anxiety, and temporarily improve aerobic capacity. But what may help a bit in the short run can bite you in the long run. Smokeless tobacco has been associated with increased rates of mouth, tongue, gum, and cheek cancer. Caffeine has many of the positive effects and much less downside risk. Consider having a cup of coffee instead.

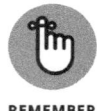

REMEMBER

If you smoke and plan to start an exercise routine, be sure to check with your primary-care provider first. Your health may already be compromised, and you may have to adhere to a graduated, careful regimen.

Eating and smoking

Some people start smoking because they want to lose weight. And, perhaps unfortunately, there's some truth that smoking and nicotine help control weight. Nicotine appears to have many impacts on the body, including increasing metabolism and suppressing appetite. In addition, smokers sometimes claim that they reach for a cigarette instead of a cookie or a donut (as if the cigarette is the lesser of two evils). Without nicotine, smokers who quit tend to gain moderate weight.

However, despite any perceived benefit to your waistline, smoking negatively affects nutrition. For example, tobacco smoke has the potential to decrease absorption of calcium and vitamins C, B, and E. Furthermore, smokers are less likely to eat a healthy diet full of fruits and vegetables. So if you're trying to adopt better eating habits so you can live a longer life with potentially fewer health issues, you're negating those benefits if you're a smoker.

WARNING

Concerns about weight gain are important. However, it's also important to remember that the negative health effects of smoking far outweigh the costs of gaining some weight.

Smelling and smoking

When it comes to the sense of smell, you get hit with two problems from smoking:

» **Smokers are six times more likely to have a diminished sense of smell than nonsmokers.** Heavy smokers lose even more of their sense of smell. Loss of smell can make food less appetizing, so meals may be less enjoyable. Or you may more frequently choose highly processed foods, which are created to be irresistible, but which are usually full of fat, salt, or sugars (or all three). Loss of smell even poses some danger: You may not be able to detect gas leaks or smoke and fire. You may not know your house has some horrible odor — not a good thing when having company over.

» **Smokers, well, um, they tend to smell to nonsmokers like cigarettes.** Cigarette smell is notorious for permeating curtains, furniture, bedding, cars, clothes, and even your hair. You may wonder why you don't smell it. Did we mention you lose your sense of smell?

Perhaps surprisingly, smokeless tobacco appears to reduce sense of smell and taste as well. No easy out here.

Aging yourself like a bad toupee

Smoking negatively affects the youthfulness and health of your skin. Several studies have been conducted in which identical twins (one a smoker and one not) were evaluated by researchers who didn't know their smoking history. Overall, the nonsmoking twins were judged as more attractive and had fewer signs of facial aging than their smoking counterparts.

So, if you want healthier, more vibrant skin, giving up smoking may be your next miracle beauty cream. And instead of having to pay over $100 an ounce for it, you actually get paid — by not having to buy cigarettes!

Smoking also affects appearance by causing

>> Yellowing of the fingers and fingernails

>> Thinning hair and hair loss

>> Acne breakouts

>> Stained teeth

>> Patches on the tongue

>> Belly fat

>> Increased risk of psoriasis

>> Sagging skin

TIP

Smokeless tobacco products don't cause as many of these problems, although they aren't entirely benign, as evidenced particularly by oral effects such as stained teeth and periodontal disease.

Recognizing the Risks of Vaping

Vaping has become a global phenomenon. In fact, although vaping devices (also called *e-cigarettes*) have been on the market since only about 2007, almost half of all U.S. high school students have already tried vaping and about a third report vaping regularly. And about 5 percent of adults currently vape. Those are astonishing figures given that vaping barely existed just 15 years ago.

The early vaping innovators were motivated to find safer alternatives to smoking tobacco. They claimed they wanted to decrease the risks of regular cigarettes, which represent the leading cause of preventable deaths in the United States. And many smokers do, indeed, look to vaping as a potential way to help them quit smoking.

REMEMBER

Compared to the risks of cigarettes, assessing the relative safety of vaping is complicated because of the variety of devices and substances that exist (there are literally hundreds of different types of devices that produce varying levels of heat and vapor), and because vaping is a relatively new phenomenon. There just hasn't been enough time for long-term studies yet.

VAPING: LEARNING FROM CIGARETTES' HISTORY

When people smoked cigarettes during the Roaring Twenties, they had little concern about the health consequences of their new habit. Serious warnings didn't start appearing until around 1950. In part, that's because many of the diseases associated with cigarette smoking take decades to develop. Vaping today is much like smoking cigarettes in the 1920s. Yes, there are far fewer known toxins in e-cigarettes, but we just don't have long-term data to know for sure what the risks are over time.

But what we know is this:

>> Like combustible cigarettes, e-cigarettes carry nicotine into the lungs and circulate through the cardiovascular system. The nicotine is carried by microscopic particles in the aerosol. These ultra-fine pollutants have been linked to high blood pressure, coronary artery disease, and heart attacks.

>> In a large survey of close to 100,000 participants, researchers found that e-cigarette users had significantly higher risks of heart attack and coronary artery disease than non-smokers or non-vapers. The risk suggested a 34 percent increased chance of having a heart attack for e-cigarette users.

This type of study demonstrates a possible association, but it can't truly establish a causal relationship between vaping and heart disease. And we acknowledge that regular smoking puts you at a much higher risk of cardiovascular disease than vaping does.

WARNING

However, despite a lack of long-term studies so far, vaping nicotine puts you at risk of becoming addicted to it, and quitting nicotine is much harder than avoiding it in the first place. And we know that the particles you inhale when vaping can damage your lungs, leading to a whole host of pulmonary issues, both chronic and sometimes fatal. So we do not consider vaping safe.

Tapping into Tools to Stop Smoking

Before you get too depressed about all the bad news associated with smoking, take a look at the bright side:

>> In the United States, about 50 million citizens are successful former smokers. After only one year of not smoking, the excess cardiac risk from smoking is cut

in half. Fifteen years after you stop smoking, your risk is similar to that of a person who never smoked.

>> Smokers who quit between age 35 and 44 gain an average of 9 years in life expectancy. Quitting between 45 and 54 gains a former smoker about 6 years in longevity. Even men who quit between the ages of 65 and 69 can increase their life expectancies, not to mention improve their health.

>> Quitting smoking is truly possible. With modern smoking cessation programs, 20 percent to 40 percent of participants successfully stop smoking. Stop-smoking aids now in the marketplace may help this success rate climb even higher (check out the next section for more).

TIP

A number of different options are available to help you stop smoking; see the following list as a start:

>> **Nicotine replacement therapy (NRT):** Using nicotine replacement products, such as nicotine patches, gum, lozenges, inhalers, and nasal spray, increases the likelihood of quitting successfully. In fact, NRT increases the rate of quitting by at least 50 percent. NRT helps people manage the withdrawal symptoms so they can concentrate on the emotional aspects of quitting. Those who are particularly dependent on nicotine (heavy smokers) are most likely to receive benefits from NRT.

>> **Social support:** Receiving encouragement and support from your physician and your family is important, but so is support from others who are also trying to quit smoking. Various smoking cessation groups (community-based and commercial) likely have meetings in your area. And you may even want to try an online support group like the one provided by SMART Recovery (www.smartrecovery.org).

>> **Quit lines:** Telephone *quit lines* let you speak with a counselor about your quitting plan and available resources to help you (800-QUIT-NOW is one example).

>> **Counseling:** Group and individual counseling also can help, including cognitive behavioral therapy (CBT). CBT teaches people new ways of coping and behaving, more effective problem solving, and how to change their thinking in more adaptive ways.

Other techniques that may help you quit smoking include acupuncture and hypnosis. In all instances, these aids should be used in conjunction with a comprehensive program prescribed by your physician and/or smoking cessation specialist. *Quitting Smoking & Vaping For Dummies* (John Wiley & Sons, Inc., 2020) provides additional options.

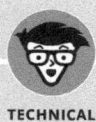

UNDERSTANDING NICOTINE ADDICTION: A CHAIN THAT BINDS

In the face of so many risks and repercussions of smoking, why doesn't every smoker just quit? Because nicotine is a powerfully addictive drug. Using nicotine causes changes in the brain that compel people to use it more and more. In addition, attempting to stop using nicotine causes unpleasant physical and emotional side effects. Good feelings when the drug is present combined with bad feelings when the drug is not present are the hallmarks of addiction. And many researchers judge nicotine to be as addictive as heroin and cocaine.

Nicotine replacements and heart disease

If you're diagnosed with any form of heart disease, never use any nicotine replacement product or e-cigarette without discussing it with your physician. In general, unsupervised nicotine-replacement therapy is not recommended for patients with heart or circulatory problems.

Weighing in on vapes as part of your quit plan

What about vapes (e-cigarettes)? Many users say that quitting smoking is why they tried vaping, and most e-cigarette brands advertise that purpose. However, the scientific jury is still out on whether e-cigarettes are actually helpful to many individuals in quitting smoking. In addition, the limited research to date on the safety of e-cigarettes is inconclusive. The many different types of e-cigarettes vary substantially in both the amounts of nicotine they deliver and also the additives and potential toxins they contain besides nicotine.

Health officials from various government agencies have warned against using e-cigarettes to stop smoking until more is known about the cause of serious pulmonary disease apparently following vaping. Talk to your healthcare provider if you feel you must consider e-cigarettes as part of your quit plan.

Developing a quit-smoking plan

A variety of sources offer excellent information to help smokers break the habit. Some particularly helpful resources were developed by the National Cancer Institute (NCI — your tax dollars at work in a good cause). You can review these resources online at www.smokefree.gov.

TIP

Here are our key recommendations adapted from the National Cancer Institute materials:

>> **Prepare yourself to quit.** After you decide to quit, list all the reasons why you want to quit, and get yourself ready. Set a target date for quitting, perhaps a special day such as a birthday, an anniversary, or the Great American Smokeout, which takes place annually on the third Thursday in November.

>> **Know what to expect.** Be realistic. You're going to experience some withdrawal symptoms, but they usually last only one to two weeks.

>> **Involve someone else.** Get the support of your family, friends, and physician. Maybe even ask another smoker to quit with you. You can't overestimate the importance of support.

>> **Before your quit day, change some of your habits.** Switch brands to one you find distasteful. Reduce your quantity of daily smokes. Make smoking inconvenient (only allow yourself to smoke outside, for example). And clean your clothes to get rid of the smell of cigarettes.

>> **On the day that you quit, adopt quit-day thinking.** Throw away all your cigarettes, matches, and lighters. Keep busy with plenty of activities. Remind your family and friends so they can be extra supportive. Think about something you'd like to buy, estimate its cost in terms of packs of cigarettes, and put aside that money for a future purchase. Celebrate at the end of your first smoke-free day.

>> **Immediately after you quit, adopt some new behaviors.** Develop a clean, nonsmoking environment. Buy fresh flowers now that you can really smell them! Drink large quantities of water. If needed, find something to keep your hands and fingers occupied. Start an exercise routine.

>> **Don't worry about gaining a little weight.** But do make sure that you have a well-balanced diet. As the appetite-depressing effect of nicotine disappears, avoid replacing cigarettes with calorie-dense candy, cookies, and snack foods. Try sugar-free gum or fresh fruits instead.

REMEMBER

If you slip and start to smoke again, don't be discouraged or give up. Remember, most smokers have to try several times before they finally succeed at quitting. Don't be too hard on yourself, and get back on the nonsmoking track as quickly as possible.

As you keep the faith — and fight the good fight — not smoking eventually becomes a part of you. You develop your own techniques and strategies for sustaining the positive feeling and pride that you get from having stopped smoking. Remaining vigilant about what triggers your smoking urge is important for a long time after you quit. When that old urge kicks in, make a mental note about what was going on when it happened. What were you doing? Where were you? Who were you with? What were you thinking? Check off the things that may trigger you to want to smoke and try counteracting them with specific strategies. Never give up — you can do it!

Navigating Booze and Your Body

Few people can successfully argue the positive effects of smoking or vaping. But what about drinking alcohol? Haven't there been studies that include the benefits of red wine to a healthy body and mind? Indeed. And not everyone who drinks alcohol — whether wine, beer, or spirits — develops a problem with it. This section seeks to give you the full picture so you can determine whether consuming alcohol is part of your healthy living plan.

The potential upside of drinking (red wine, that is)

The Blue Zones are regions in the world where people live significantly longer and healthier lives. One habit for many people in these areas is the tradition of "Wine at 5." Based on behaviors and longevity of Blue Zone residents, some scientists argue that the occasional glass of wine shared with friends or family can actually have some health benefits.

While the debate over the health benefits and risks of red wine continues, those who champion its virtues do so for one main reason: *Polyphenols* such as resveratrol. These are naturally occurring compounds in the skins of red grapes that have antioxidant properties. These antioxidants fight off oxidative stress and inflammation.

The evidence on alcohol's health impact is far from perfect (as is all research on diet and nutrition). But here's a good news story to balance out all the discussions of risky drinking (see later in this chapter for more):

>> A 2024 study using data from over 500,000 participants from the UK Biobank explored how different types of alcoholic drinks affect risks of death, heart disease, and kidney disease.

>> Participants shared details about their drinking habits, including what they drank (for example, champagne, white or red wine, beer, and spirits) and how often.

>> Over about 12 years of follow-up, 2,852 participants reported kidney disease, 79,958 reported heart disease, and 18,923 participants died.

The study found that total alcohol consumption showed a U-shaped curve for heart disease and death, meaning moderate drinkers had lower risks compared to heavy drinkers and non-drinkers (which included past drinkers).

"Safe" drinking limits were identified. These align pretty closely with the Australian guidelines, especially concerning weekly consumption limits:

>> Total alcohol: <11 grams/day for men, <10 grams/day for women

>> Red wine: <7 glasses/week for men, <6 glasses/week for women

>> Champagne plus white wine: <5 glasses/week

>> Fortified wine: <4 glasses/week

The results of the study tend to suggest you can get away with a few glasses *of wine* per week, but it's essential to drink responsibly.

The definite downside: Alcohol's effect on brain health

Risky drinking leads to changes in brain structure and network connectivity. Studies show that *heavy drinking* (three or more drinks a day for women and four or more for men) causes widespread brain changes, especially in areas such as the frontal cortex, hippocampus, and cerebellum.

People with alcohol use disorder (which you might know as *alcoholism*; see the upcoming section "Drinking Too Much or Too Often: Alcohol Use Disorder" for more information) show lower grey matter volume in key regions such as the prefrontal cortex, insula, and thalamus, with damage linked to the amount and duration of alcohol consumption. Alcohol also leads to white matter degeneration in structures such as the corpus callosum, affecting the brain's ability to process information. These brain changes can worsen with age, emphasizing the long-term impact of chronic alcohol use on brain health.

The good news is that some of the damage can be reversed if you stop drinking and get treatment early.

Other risks of excessive drinking

Excessive drinking harms virtually every system in your body. It can cause your pancreas and liver to become inflamed. It can cause anemia and increase your risk of infection. If your immune system is struggling to combat the illnesses that result from heavy drinking, it'll be less able to work on effectively fighting your cancer.

Realizing that even moderate drinking can be harmful

A 2022 study using data from 36,678 participants in the UK Biobank found that even light to moderate drinking is linked to negative changes in brain structure, including reduced brain volume and poorer white matter integrity. These effects are noticeable in people consuming just one to two units of alcohol daily (in the United States that's one beer, glass of wine, or shot of liquor *or less*), and the effects worsen with higher intake, highlighting the potential harm of moderate drinking on brain health.

Drinking Too Much or Too Often: Alcohol Use Disorder

REMEMBER

Alcohol use disorder, or *AUD*, is the term that's used nowadays to include what people commonly referred to as alcohol abuse, dependence, addiction, or alcoholism.

AUD is a chronic disease characterized by an inability to control your drinking despite negative consequences. It's recognized by the *Diagnostic and Statistical Manual of Mental Disorders* (the authoritative guide for diagnosing mental disorders, and published by the American Psychiatric Association) as a mental disorder, and it encompasses a range of physical, mental, and social symptoms.

Understanding the complexity of alcoholism involves recognizing its diverse manifestations, which can vary significantly from person to person. Physically, someone with AUD may experience the following:

>> Intense cravings for alcohol

>> Increased tolerance resulting in the need for more alcohol to achieve the same effects

>> Withdrawal symptoms when you try to reduce or stop drinking

Mentally, someone with AUD may experience the following:

>> Distorted thinking patterns

>> Reduced cognitive functions

>> Emotional instability

Socially, among other adverse outcomes, the disorder can cause

>> Alienation from family and friends

>> Job loss

>> Legal issues

Who's at risk for AUD?

Your risk for AUD increases with how much and how often you drink. Starting to drink at a young age, having a family history of alcohol problems, and experiencing mental health issues or trauma can all raise your chances of developing AUD. In short, AUD risk is influenced by a combination of biological, psychological, and social factors.

DISTINGUISHING BETWEEN HEAVY DRINKER AND ALCOHOLIC

Understanding the difference between a heavy drinker and someone with AUD is essential to identifying how severe someone's alcohol use is. A heavy drinker may participate in binge drinking or frequent drinking sessions but can retain control over their consumption. In contrast, someone with alcohol use disorder shows compulsive behavior and dependence, continuing to consume alcohol despite adverse consequences. Beyond the quantity of alcohol consumed, a heavy drinker may even be capable of setting limits, refraining from drinking when needed, and experiencing no severe withdrawal symptoms. However, this pattern of heavy drinking behavior can still lead to significant health risks, both physically and socially, and may serve as a precursor to more severe alcohol-related issues.

If you answer "yes" to questions such as these, you may have AUD:

>> Do you drink more or longer than you intended?

>> Have you tried to cut down but couldn't?

>> Does drinking interfere with your daily responsibilities?

>> Do you continue to drink despite problems with family or friends?

>> Do you experience withdrawal symptoms when not drinking?

The more symptoms you have, the more urgent it is to seek help.

Getting treatment for AUD

There are several ways to treat AUD, and what works for one person may not work for another. Options include:

>> **Medications:** Naltrexone, acamprosate, and disulfiram can help reduce cravings and prevent relapse.

>> **Behavioral treatments:** Therapy sessions that focus on changing drinking behaviors and developing coping skills can help overcome AUD.

>> **Support groups:** Peer support from groups such as Alcoholics Anonymous (www.aa.org) can be very helpful, especially when combined with other treatments.

REMEMBER

Recovery from AUD is possible, but it often requires ongoing effort and professional support. Early treatment can help a person develop skills to avoid triggers and manage stress, making it easier to maintain sobriety.

TIP

If you or someone you know is struggling with alcohol use, don't hesitate to seek help. A good online search term to find support is "alcohol addiction help near me" or "alcohol support services in [your location]".

Deciding Whether Alcohol Is for You

REMEMBER

What's a guy to think in the face of what feels like contradictory research about drinking? Is it a healthy activity when done in moderation, or should you be a teetotaler for the best chance at a longer, healthier life? Because your body, lifestyle habits, genetic history, and environment are unique to you, consult with a healthcare provider to determine whether moderate alcohol consumption can be part your best-life habits.

Chapter **10**

Monitoring Your Health

L iving your best and longest life starts with controlling risk factors. Even if you're the picture of perfect health — at least in the mirror — only regular checkups with your primary-care physician can tell you what's happening inside your body where many risk factors of deadly diseases silently get started.

Understanding the Role of a Primary-Care Physician

REMEMBER

Your primary-care physician (or PCP) is your main line of defense for good health. They may be an *internist* (a physician who specializes in medical illnesses of the internal organs), a *family practitioner* (a generalist who treats routine medical problems that are found both inside and outside your body), or a *specialist* (a doctor who specializes in treating certain areas of the body; for example, a *urologist,* who focuses on treating diseases of the bladder, kidneys, testis, and prostate).

Your PCP is your health hub — your main point of contact for your general health, and who looks at you as a whole being versus just a particular system or organ. Based on your history over time, PCPs can keep track of and identify changes in your health that may need investigating, potentially by other specialists. And if you need to see specialists, they coordinate your care with them when needed.

PCPs are also your first stop when you're sick enough to see a doctor, and they manage any chronic conditions you may be facing, such as high cholesterol and diabetes.

Selecting a primary-care doctor

Men depend on their primary-care doctor for most of their healthcare needs. So it's important to take care in choosing one.

First, look for a doctor who has superior knowledge about medicine, who listens, who asks pertinent questions, and who provides useful explanations and answers. Also look for a physician who displays genuine concern, cost-consciousness, and a determination to keep working on *any* medical problem that you have. Above all, your doctor needs to be someone who cares about you and inspires confidence, optimism, and hope in you.

TIP

You can ask friends, family, neighbors, and colleagues for referrals. Most hospitals, clinics, and private practices have websites with biographical information about their practitioners. You can also look at local websites where current or former patients review their providers, although remember that these reviews are subjective and may not provide a full picture.

Once you've selected two or three candidates, request a short get-to-know you meeting with each, either virtual or in person, to find out how the physician approaches the world and his or her patients. You'll get a feel for each candidate during this preinterview, and afterwards, you'll hopefully have enough information about each candidate to make a final choice.

TIP

Here are some questions you may want to ask during the preinterview:

>> What are your special areas of medical interest?

>> Can you tell me a little bit about how you approach medicine and patient care?

>> In managing health and disease risk factors, how important to you are lifestyle factors, such as nutrition, physical activity and weight management?

>> If you have an existing cardiac condition, ask these questions:

- What is your background in and knowledge of this particular condition?

- How do you typically manage heart disease risk factors? Do you focus on lifestyle measures first before using medications?

Be careful when asking these last questions, because even some of the very best physicians may be thrown off-guard by them, at least until they get to know you better.

After the conversation, when you're considering the answers you received and how the conversation went in general, don't forget that who you are as an individual plays a role of utmost importance in deciding which doctor is best for you. Some people like detailed and thorough explanations from their doctors. Others want a more regimented approach with less specific information. Don't be embarrassed to interview a few physicians to find the best fit for who you are. Remember, you're establishing a long-term partnership here, so you should not rush into it.

Hunting down a hospital

If you have any conditions that require testing or procedures at a hospital, choosing a hospital is a surprisingly important healthcare decision. If your primary-care physician refers you to a hospital for advanced testing or surgery, don't be shy about asking about the hospital's expertise and experience with these procedures. If we were facing open-heart surgery, for instance, we'd surely want to be in the care of a hospital team that specializes in that kind of surgery, performs it frequently (like every day!), and has an outstanding record of success and care.

TIP

Check out hospital ratings based on reports hospitals have to do for the government and for accreditation and certification. Medicare's Hospital Compare (www.medicare.gov/hospitalcompare/search.html) and ratings by Consumer Reports (www.consumerreports.org) are both reliable.

Knowing What to Expect at a Routine PCP Visit

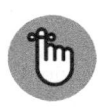

REMEMBER

No matter what type of doctor you see, plan annual visits so your doctor and you can stay on top of your health and lose no time in identifying anything of concern.

The next sections talk about how your visit will likely go, although your doctor may not follow this exact order, and some of the checks may be done by someone on their team.

Having a chat

Your doctor's checkup routine will start with a conversation about how you're doing and any changes since the last visit:

>> You'll talk about your overall health, lifestyle, and any changes since your last visit. During your first visit, this part will take more time as your doctor gets to know you. Your doctor will probably ask about your diet, exercise, sleep, and stress, as well as your use of alcohol, tobacco, and drugs. (Be honest when answering; holding back information just shortchanges the care your doctor can give you.)

>> You'll talk about your sexual health and any concerns you have. Don't be shy about asking questions if you have any; we've heard them all and are rarely surprised or shocked.

>> You'll discuss your family medical history (in detail the first visit, and then any updates in successive visits), and you'll talk about any new or lingering symptoms you're noticing.

TIP

Sometimes your doctor will collect some or much of this information as part of your pre-visit paperwork; if so, your conversation may focus on questions pertaining to any answers they want to hear more about.

Why does your doctor go into such detail about your medical and family history? Your body is a network of systems and organs working together. When one has a problem, others often feel the impact. Because your doctor understands these connections, knowing your past illnesses and those of your family can help your doc pinpoint the cause of any symptoms you're currently facing.

You might also be wondering how you're feeling right now is relevant — maybe you feel just fine! But a number of diseases or conditions don't have obvious symptoms — prostate cancer is an example, as is diabetes — and hearing how you're feeling may generate some clues for your doctor that warrant some additional conversation.

TIP

Even if you're experiencing a problem that seems pretty minor, report it to your doctor and let them decide if it's significant. For example, be sure to mention any problems you're having with urination, whether the problem is frequent urination, a slow stream, trouble with stopping and starting, pain with urination, or all of the above. Make sure that you report even minor urinary problems that continue, because they may be indicators of a developing serious medical problem. Your doctor can treat medical problems in the initial stages of development easier than they can treat them in the full-blown stages.

Checking your vitals and performing a physical exam

Your doctor will check your vital signs, including your blood pressure, your heart rate, your respiratory rate, and your temperature. They will also check your weight and BMI (*body mass index*, which estimates your total body fat based on your height and weight) for trends that may need discussing.

The physical exam continues as they assess your body, including:

>> Looking at your eyes, ears, nose, and throat

>> Checking your lymph nodes and thyroid

>> Listening to your heart and lungs

>> Pressing on your abdomen to check your organs

>> Testing your reflexes and basic neurological responses

>> Looking at your skin for unusual spots or moles

Your doctor may assess your testicular health, including asking you about regular self-checks you do at home (see Chapter 16 for instructions on performing this monthly self-exam).

Your doctor may also check your prostate health via a routine rectal exam (Chapter 16 gives details on what to expect during this exam). If you're 50 years old or older, you need to have this test yearly.

Ordering preventive screenings

Depending on your age and risk profile, your doctor may order some screenings to confirm whether your body is in tip-top shape or identify anything needing a closer look. The screenings your doc may order include these:

>> Blood work to check your cholesterol, blood sugar, and sometimes your liver and kidney function

>> Cancer screenings, including colonoscopy once you turn 45 (earlier depending on your family history) and prostate-specific antigen (PSA) blood test (annually once you turn 50)

>> Sexually transmitted infection testing if requested or indicated (see Chapter 13 for information on STIs)

>> Your doctor may also do a mental health check-in and ask about your mood, anxiety, and stress levels

Discussing a plan going forward

As your visit nears its end, you and your doctor will talk about any steps to take before your next annual visit, including

>> Any immunizations you're due for (see later in this chapter)

Any lifestyle changes you need to make (if you follow our recommendations throughout this book, you might get a high five instead of a to-do)

>> Any follow-up tests or specialist referrals you may need based on the visit

REMEMBER

If you're offered a chance to make next year's appointment, do it now — it's too easy to get caught up with life and in six months forget to call about making your next appointment.

VOLUNTEERING IMPORTANT INFO WHEN THE DOCTOR DOESN'T ASK

Be sure to volunteer important information even if, for some reason, your doctor doesn't ask you for it. Jot down some notes ahead of time, and refer to these notes when you see your doctor. Don't bring a scroll of complaints to discuss. Narrow your list down to three or four key issues or problems, if at all possible.

Here are some examples of information to volunteer during a physical examination:

- Symptoms pertaining to the urinary tract (pain, difficulty, frequency, or any other trouble with urination)

- Significant changes in your weight (such as a weight loss or gain of more than ten pounds when you haven't been trying to gain or lose weight)

- Changes in your overall sleep habits or energy levels (the problem may be that you're overworking, but it's also possible that a medical problem may be impairing your sleep or draining your strength)

- Instances of cancer in your family (especially your parents and siblings)

- Any pain you have, especially significant pain that's getting worse (for example, when prostate cancer spreads, it mostly goes to the bone; in rare cases, the first sign of prostate cancer can be bone pain)

Optimizing office visits

TIP

Office visits to the doctor are a pain, aren't they? Particularly if the doctor isn't located in your town and you need to travel to see them. So here are some tips for getting the most out of the visits.

» **Be efficient.** Respect your physician's time and expect that your physician will respect your time, too. Fill out any requested forms before the appointment (you may be emailed or texted a link to fill out forms online) or arrive a little early to fill it out in the office. Bring notes that track how you feel and any symptoms you're experiencing. For the first visit, bring a written list of the medications that you're taking, including the frequency and dosage (or bring a bag with the actual medicines in their containers). If you need to cancel your appointment, do so as early as possible — and the same goes for the physician.

» **Describe your symptoms.** Be prepared to tell your doctor about any symptoms that you have, when they occur, how severe they are, and how they affect you. If the visit is a regular checkup and you have no complaints, be prepared to tell your doctor what you're doing to maintain good health (the diet you're eating, your level of physical activity, any weight loss or weight maintenance program you're on, and so on).

» **Ask about your diagnosis, if that's the purpose of the visit.** It's important to ask specifically about your potential diagnosis and what tests the physician thinks are important to pin down this suspected diagnosis. Don't be afraid to ask that this information be provided in layman's terms.

» **Take notes.** Many times, patients leave the doctor's office and forget what they discussed. Visiting the doctor is often stressful, so don't be afraid to take notes during the discussion and, for that matter, bring someone with you. A second pair of ears helps. You can also record the conversation on your phone or other portable device you bring. Whenever possible, ask for instructions in writing.

» **Schedule a follow-up appointment.** If a follow-up appointment is necessary, ask the doctor specifically when to schedule it. Asking how to reach the physician in case of an emergency also is important.

Getting Vaccinated

WARNING

There's a lot of information — and misinformation — out there about vaccines. When large groups lose trust in the benefits of vaccination, many people, not just those who don't want to be vaccinated, can suffer. Diseases such as COVID-19 and measles can continue to spread. Those who have weakened immune systems that don't respond well to vaccines can be infected by others. It's important that we keep our eyes on the common enemy — infectious diseases.

Vaccines give your immune system a superpower. Through vaccines, your immune system learns how to stop bad guys it's never seen before. These bad guys cause infectious diseases. They're the *pathogens,* also called germs, which are so tiny that we can see them only with a microscope. These pathogens include bacteria, viruses, fungi, and parasites.

REMEMBER

Vaccines provide you with personal protection against these pathogens and the diseases they cause, but what works even better is if everyone is vaccinated. The superpower of a vaccine increases as more people jump on the bandwagon. With infectious diseases, we're all in this together. If everyone is vaccinated, a pathogen spreading person to person is stymied.

Vaccines may not provide 100 percent protection. Some people may not be able to take or benefit from a vaccine; they may be too young or have a weakened immune system. But if enough of us are vaccinated, odds are the pathogen just can't spread. It can't jump from person to person. It may infect one person and maybe another, but if most people are vaccinated, it won't keep finding new people to spread to and will fade away.

This is what *herd immunity* is all about — when enough people are vaccinated, we can push back the spread of some terrible and deadly diseases. Diseases can bounce back if fewer people are vaccinated.

Explaining how a vaccine works

Vaccines hold up a "Wanted" photo of the bad guy — the pathogen or germ. Each vaccine is a little different, but they all show our immune system something super recognizable about the pathogen. That way, if we're ever exposed to this pathogen, our immune systems will respond to it.

The "Wanted" photo can be some bit from the outside of the pathogen, like a specific protein or sugar. These bits act as a way to identify the pathogen, similar to the way a tattoo or birthmark helps you identify a person. The vaccine version may attach this "Wanted" photo to a warning, like a blinking red light, such as a protein that will create a stronger immune response.

Other vaccines may be the equivalent of a head-to-foot photo; some vaccines use the whole pathogen (in a killed vaccine) or in a live, but safe, similar version.

Distinguishing between antigens and antibodies

Antigens are what is memorable in the "Wanted" photo. An antigen is something very specific — like that birthmark or tattoo — that can't be missed. Your immune system uses that very specific marking to create an immune response and memory. This marking is usually a protein or sometimes a sugar on the outside of the pathogen.

Antibodies are what your body makes in response to antigens. After your body has been shown the antigen or "Wanted" photo, you keep a supply of memory immune cells that can make a whole lot more antibodies if the pathogen ever arrives. Specific antibodies go after just one specific antigen. Once that antigen is found again, your body floods it with copies of this antibody from those memory immune cells. The antibodies then attach themselves to their antigens, which are on the outside of the pathogen. The antibodies then stop this specific pathogen, like a virus particle or bacterium cell, from causing any more problems.

TECHNICAL STUFF

It typically takes a few weeks after exposure for the body to produce this response. Vaccination gives you a head start so you already have the ability to make all these antibodies if you need to. With a natural infection, you can get quite sick before you're able to scramble and create an effective immune response.

Breaking down other vaccine ingredients

Vaccines contain more than just the antigens — those "Wanted" photos that help your immune system identify pathogens (see the preceding section). Other ingredients are needed to make sure the vaccine works as it should:

>> Some of these "Wanted" photos don't create much of an immune response. The immune system needs to be alerted to the fact that this "Wanted" photo is important to remember. Vaccines may include an alert, which acts like a red blinking light, saying "pay attention here." This ingredient may even be directly attached to the "Wanted" photo. Such alerts when added to the vaccine mix are called *adjuvants*. A common adjuvant includes aluminum, also found in drinking water, antacids, and antiperspirants.

>> Vaccines also may contain stabilizers, much like some of our food does. These include sugars and gelatin that keep the vaccine ingredients well mixed, so they don't separate or deteriorate.

>> Vaccines can sometimes include preservatives to keep mold or bacteria from growing in the vaccine, much like we would have in a bottle of jam at home. Just as many foods are advertised as preservative-free, many vaccines are, too. Preservatives are particularly used in multi-use vaccine bottles, especially for the flu, as these are kept open longer to vaccinate multiple people. In some cases, this can include thimerosal, which contains mercury, but it's a

type of mercury that doesn't have the same worrisome risk as the mercury found in fish. Children's vaccines do not include mercury, except in rare cases with multi-use flu vaccine vials and some specific brands of tetanus shots for adolescents.

» Vaccines may also include trace amounts of chemicals used in their production. These substances are removed, but sometimes a very small amount remains. In order to include a whole virus or bacteria but make sure it's dead and won't make copies of itself, formaldehyde is used. The amount used in a vaccine is much, much less than we naturally have in our bodies.

» Sometimes antibiotics, usually not the sorts we're allergic to, are used to keep bacteria from growing during production. These antibiotics are removed at the end, so at most only a tiny amount remains. Eggs are used to grow some viruses used to make vaccines, and so egg proteins, in very tiny amounts, may be present in some specific vaccines.

Understanding the importance of vaccine schedules

Unfortunately, vaccines don't always fall into the "one and done" category. In many cases, a series of vaccines, given on a specific schedule, are necessary to provide you with protection against diseases. Although no one wants to get an injection more than once, skipping doses or spreading them beyond what's recommended can decrease the effectiveness of the vaccine and increase your chance of becoming ill.

Staying on schedule with vaccinations

Trying to keep track of vaccination schedules can be complicated. It can be easy to forget about vaccinations when you're busy working, moving a few times, and raising kids and worrying about *their* vaccination schedules. We make it easier by describing which vaccines are at which points in your adult life.

The need for vaccinations doesn't just disappear when you reach the magic age of 18. Your own health may take a back seat to things like job promotions, buying houses, and going to your kid's soccer games. But we know you want to keep yourself healthy and live long enough to enjoy retirement, maybe travel, and spend lots of free time with family and friends, and that means making a yearly pilgrimage to your healthcare provider's office for your scheduled vaccinations.

Vaccines for ages 19–26

REMEMBER

These are the years where you're most likely to be living in crowded conditions, whether it be a college dorm, military barracks, or an apartment with an ever-changing array of roommates and their friends. Because some diseases spread easily in crowded conditions like these, it's important to be up to date on vaccinations. Here's a schedule for you young guys:

>> **Your yearly flu shot.** The flu shot is the one vaccination that never ends. When you have the flu, you're sick. Like, really sick. You're also contagious. There are two versions of the influenza vaccine: the live attenuated vaccine, given as a nasal spray, and an inactive vaccine, given as an injection. The nasal spray vaccine is not always available, but when it is, most adults can get either form of the vaccine.

>> **The COVID-19 vaccine.** It's fair to say that none of us wants to go through another year like 2020, so as yearly vaccinations become available, you should get one.

>> **A Tdap or Td booster.** *Tdap* stands for tetanus, diphtheria, and pertussis, or whooping cough. *Td* is often given as a booster to adults but leaves out the pertussis portion. Tetanus remains a threat worldwide.

Vaccines for ages 27–49

REMEMBER

Although your life undoubtedly changes quite a bit over these two decades, your immunization schedule stays pretty much the same. You need the same three vaccines that you needed in your early to mid-twenties:

>> Influenza every year

>> COVID-19 every year, when offered

>> Td every ten years

Vaccines for ages 50–64

REMEMBER

Middle age continues the vaccine recommendations from earlier in adulthood:

>> Influenza every year

>> COVID-19 every year, when offered

>> Td every ten years

And, just for playing, you get this very important newcomer to your vaccine schedule once you hit age 50:

>> The shingles (recombinant zoster, brand name Shingrix) vaccine. This vaccine protects you against herpes zoster, better known as shingles.

>> This is the virus you got when you had chicken pox as a kid — the virus has been sleeping in your nerve roots ever since your mom hosted a chicken pox party back in the 1970s.

>> You'll need two doses of the Shingrix vaccine, spaced two to six months apart.

Vaccines for ages 65-plus

REMEMBER

The retirement age brings with it a new designation: elderly. You may not feel elderly, and you may not look it either, but at age 65, this is how you're classified. Here are the recommended vaccines for you silver foxes (even if all that's silver are your roots):

>> **Influenza.** If you've been blowing off getting an annual flu shot, now's the time to turn over a new leaf. The best time to get the vaccine is October or the second half of September to develop the needed antibodies.

You now face particular flu-related risks based on your age:

● Between 70 and 85 percent of deaths from flu and between 50 and 70 percent of hospitalizations from flu occur in people over 65.

● If you have the flu when you're over 65, you're at increased risk of developing pneumonia.

● You're three to five times more likely to have a heart attack in the two weeks after you catch the flu.

● Your risk of stroke increases by two to three times in the first two weeks after you have the flu.

● You're six times more likely to die in the weeks after you have the flu. Sign me up, doc!

>> **Tdap.** You're more at risk from tetanus, especially if you have diabetes. And being vaccinated for pertussis (the "p" in Tdap) avoids giving any baby grandchildren or other babies whooping cough, which can be deadly in wee little ones.

>> **Pneumococcal vaccines.** PCV13 (also known as Prevnar 13; usually given first) and PPSV23 (also known as Pneumovax 23; usually given a year later) protect against not only pneumococcus, a common cause of pneumonia, but also infections in the blood, heart, and around the brain.

Catching up if you weren't vaccinated as a child

It's never too late to catch up on vaccinations. If your parents or guardians didn't have you vaccinated or skipped some vaccines, it's not too late. If you decide to catch up on vaccines as an adult, it's not that difficult.

TIP

The CDC website at www.cdc.gov/vaccines/hcp/imz-schedules/downloads/adult/adult-combined-schedule.pdf lists which vaccines should be given if you're just getting started with your vaccinations as an adult.

3

What's Going on Down There: Mentioning the Male Member

Understand the anatomy and functions of the male reproductive system so you can keep your sexual self healthy.

Get a refresh on how babies are made and the options if tykes aren't on your to-do list right now.

Identify sexually transmitted infections and know how to avoid — or treat — them.

Get to the root cause of penis predicaments and figure out how to solve them.

Chapter **11**

Tuning the Male Organ

For a man, the penis is the star of the show in the bedroom (or in the living room, on the kitchen floor, or even in the aisles, so long as the theater is empty!). But as with any star, what you see on-screen is only the final performance. Lots of other factors go into preparing for each scene. In this chapter, you'll get the behind-the-scenes tour of the male anatomy and meet such important "extras" as the glands, tissues, and organs that allow the penis to stand tall and proud when the director yells, "Action!"

Knowing the Penis: Inside and Out

Conventionally, sexual intercourse occurs whenever a man puts his penis into a woman's vagina, although other variations exist. When the penis is in its normal, flaccid state, this feat is difficult (though not impossible) for a man to accomplish. (The technical term is called *stuffing*.) However, when the penis becomes erect and hard, most men learn quite quickly the technique of inserting the penis into the vagina — sometimes too quickly (for more about that, see Chapter 14).

How a man gets an erection is relatively straightforward. But to fully understand the process, you need to first examine a man's basic apparatus: his penis. This section is all about how and why a man gets an erection.

The three sponges (No cleaning involved)

Basically, a penis is composed of three structures (see Figure 11-1), which are made of a spongelike material that can fill with blood.

>> The two *corpus cavernosa* contain the central arteries and lie on the top half of the penis. They are cylindrical tubes and are larger than the other spongy structure.

>> The *corpus spongiosum*, which is under the two corpus cavernosa and surrounds the urethra, is the pipeline for both urine and sperm.

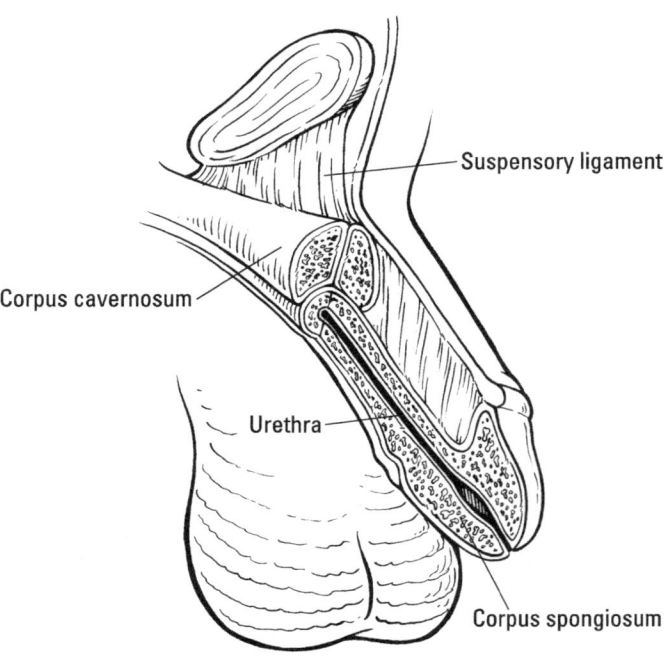

Suspensory ligament

Corpus cavernosum

Urethra

Corpus spongiosum

Illustration by Kathryn Born.

FIGURE 11-1:
The penis: not as simple as it looks!

When a man becomes excited — and we're not talking about watching his team score the winning touchdown here — the nerves surrounding his penis become active, causing the muscles around the arteries to relax and more blood to flow into the penis. The spongelike material then absorbs the additional blood, making the penis stiff and hard, or *erect*. This erection tightens the veins so the blood can't leave the penis, enabling the penis to remain erect. After a man ejaculates or if his arousal fades, *detumescence* occurs, in which the brain sends a signal to allow the blood to leave the erect penis, and it returns to its flaccid state.

At the base of the penis, the two corpus cavernosa split to form a Y, where the two ends connect to the pubic bone. This ligament controls the angle of the erect penis. We get many questions from men, each asking if something is wrong with him because the angle of his erect penis isn't straight out, parallel to the floor. We tell all of them not to go hanging any weights in an effort to change the angle, because they have nothing to worry about!

Penises become erect at all different angles — and the angle doesn't have any effect on the way the penis performs. As a man gets older, the ligament at the base of his penis stretches, and the angle changes. A man of 70, for example, may have an erection that points downward instead of upward, the way many a young man's erection does.

At the head of the class: The glans

The head of the penis, called the *glans*, is shaped like a cone (see Figure 11-2). The opening of the glans is called the *meatus* (pronounced "me-*ate*-us"), and at the base of the glans is a crownlike structure called the *corona*.

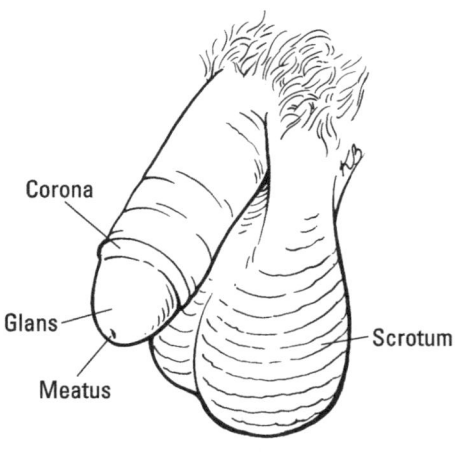

FIGURE 11-2: The glans brings it all to a head.

Illustration by Kathryn Born.

The glans serves several purposes:

>> The glans is a little thicker than the rest of the penis, particularly around the corona. This extra thickness serves as a seal to keep the ejaculated semen inside the vagina, near the cervix, after an orgasm. This is nature's way of making sure that the chances for fertilization are high. The glans also contains the greatest number of nerve endings.

>> The glans also creates extra friction, which, in this case, produces "good vibrations" that help promote orgasm and ejaculation.

>> Men aren't the only ones who benefit from the glans. With all the thrusting of the penis inside the vagina that goes on during intercourse, the woman's cervix may get damaged if it weren't for the glans, which acts as a shock absorber.

The foreskin: A real cover-up

At birth, the glans is covered by the *foreskin*, a sheath of skin that opens at the top. In an infant, this opening is very tight and usually can't be pulled back (or *retracted*, to use the medical term). Usually, the foreskin loosens up as the baby grows older. When a male has an erection, the foreskin pulls back entirely to fully reveal the glans. The skin of the glans is very sensitive, and the purpose of the foreskin is to protect it.

In Jewish and Muslim cultures, the foreskin is surgically removed in a procedure called *circumcision*. Circumcision has also become popular in many Western societies because the penis is easier to keep clean without the foreskin. Because of today's better hygiene, some parents and physicians believe that circumcision is no longer necessary, although the debate isn't entirely over. Figure 11-3 shows the difference in appearance between an uncircumcised and a circumcised penis.

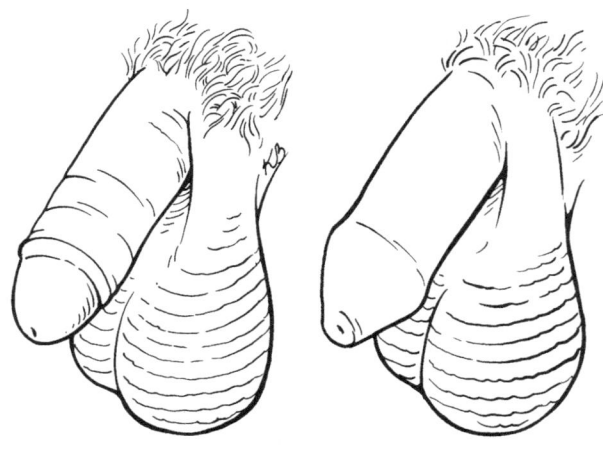

FIGURE 11-3: The penis on the right is uncircumcised, and the one shown on the left is circumcised.

Illustration by Kathryn Born.

TECHNICAL STUFF

Small glands underneath the foreskin secrete an oily, lubricating substance. If these secretions accumulate and mix with dead skin cells, a cottage cheese–like substance called *smegma* forms. In an uncircumcised man, this smegma can build up and lead to infections and, sometimes, even more serious diseases. An uncircumcised man should always take special precautions when bathing to pull back the foreskin and clean carefully around the glans.

TIP

If a man happens to be bathing with a friend, pulling back the foreskin may be a pleasurable task for him to assign to his partner. Some partners, who've seen the piles of dirty laundry stuffed into a corner of a bachelor's apartment, have general doubts about the personal hygiene of the average male. This can be one reason that they avoid performing oral sex. If oral sex is something that a man wants but his partner has avoided, having his partner make sure that his penis is absolutely clean may be one way of changing their mind. Even if it doesn't change their mind, at least he'll have a very clean penis.

Circumcision and sexual performance

Because the skin of the glans of a circumcised male grows tougher and less sensitive than that of an uncircumcised male, people often wonder whether circumcision affects sexual performance.

Some men who aren't circumcised erroneously believe that, because their skin is more sensitive, they are more likely to have premature ejaculation. We've even been asked by adult men if they should be circumcised to cure them of this problem. (Because premature ejaculation is a learned behavior that you can overcome — see Chapter 14 — we don't recommend having this surgery performed later in life.)

We're also asked by men who've been circumcised if a way exists to replace their foreskin. These men feel that, because the skin of the glans has been toughened, they're missing out on certain pleasures. We tell them that, as long as they're having orgasms, this isn't something that they should worry about. If they are not, this is probably caused by some other issue, not their foreskins.

Size and sexual performance

Of course, when considering the penis, what concerns a great many men the most is the size of their sexual organ; they focus on the length and width of the *shaft*, the main portion of the penis. They think that bigger is better.

Because men are more likely to get turned on by what they see, physical appearance is very important to them. That's why men are so concerned about penis size — just as some are concerned about the size of women's breasts. To men, the more there is of a body part that attracts them, the better. And, of course, seeing the male stars of porno videos doesn't help either, because these men aren't picked for their ability to act, but rather to inflate.

Now, if men asked their partners how they feel about penis size, they'd get another story. Some partners are actually frightened by very big penises, and many just don't attach very much importance to the issue. But these men who are all hung up about the size of their penises can't seem to get that straight — and, convincing them otherwise is a difficult job.

REMEMBER

Although you can't deny that men have different-sized penises, does the size of the penis make any difference? In most cases, the answer is a very big no. The size of the penis doesn't make any difference in the pleasure you can give your partner.

TIP

Men ask us all the time if some way exists to make their penises bigger. We know of only one way to do this, and we're passing it on only because it actually also promotes good health. Although most of the penis is visible, part of the penis is buried beneath the skin and is called the *crus*. If a man has a lot of fat in his pubic area, then more of the length of the penis is buried beneath the skin. With weight loss, a man can reverse this trend so a greater portion of the penis becomes exposed; thus, his penis can "grow." The approximation doctors use is one inch of penis length gained for every 30 pounds of excess weight lost. (Sorry, all you skinny guys, but losing extra weight won't help you.)

Some surgical techniques can enlarge a man's penis. One technique can make most of it, except for the head, fatter, which leaves the head looking disproportionate. The other technique makes the penis longer, but requires the doctors to cut certain ligaments so the penis doesn't point as high as before, which can cause the man to lose sensitivity. These side effects, as well as other risks, greatly reduce the value of these procedures, which is why very few surgeons perform them. In our estimation, the risks make such surgery not even worth considering. If you're intent on learning more of the gory details, however, make an appointment with a urologist.

MEASURING UP

You can measure a penis in several different ways, and a man usually chooses the method that makes his penis seem the biggest. Although the basic penis measurements are length and circumference, the mood of your penis at the moment you pull out that tape measure is a key factor.

Even if two flaccid penises look about the same size, they may be very different in size when they become erect. And a man may have different-sized erections depending on how aroused he is.

In the locker room, the man with the biggest flaccid penis feels the most cocky, but the real proving ground is in the bedroom.

One of the reasons that a man may think his penis is too small is the way he looks at it. (And no, we're not going to suggest that he put on rose-colored glasses.) Most of the time, he looks down at his penis, and when he does, his eyes play a trick on him called *foreshortening*, which makes his penis look smaller than it appears to someone else looking at it. To see his penis the way his partner does, all he has to do is stand in front of a full-length mirror and take in that view — we think he'll be surprised. If he takes a look both before and after he has an erection, we're sure his ego will get a nice boost.

Getting erection direction

The proportion of crus (penis under the skin) to exposed penis can cause variations in the direction that a penis points during an erection. Men with a shorter crus, and thus a longer penis, are more likely to have an erection that points downward, while an erect penis that has a longer crus will probably point outward, or even straight up.

Occasionally, a man tells us that he's concerned because his penis points in a certain direction when it's erect. As you can see from Frank's situation in the following case study, this phenomenon isn't unusual. Some men have a more pronounced curve than others, and sometimes the penis also bends to the left or to the right.

Frank

When Frank came to see us, we spent half an hour talking without broaching the real reason for his visit. He admitted that he didn't go out with women, but he blamed that on all sorts of things that didn't make sense to us. We could feel that more was bothering him than he was letting on, and we told him straight out that we thought he wasn't being truthful with us. That's when he told me that he was afraid of dating women because, if he got close enough to them to have sex, they would notice that his penis was misshapen.

We asked him to describe what his penis looked like. He said that, when he had an erection, instead of sticking straight out as did the erect penises he'd seen in porn videos, his penis had a very large curve in it. His description seemed to be within the bounds of normalcy, but we sent him to a urologist to make sure.

When we next saw Frank, he was a new man. The urologist had confirmed what we'd thought, and knowing that he wasn't going to be made fun of gave him the confidence to start dating. The next time we heard from Frank, about a year later, he shared that he was engaged.

TIP

If you feel that your penis has an abnormal shape, go to a urologist to make certain that this curvature doesn't indicate some problem.

In the vast majority of cases, the curve falls well within the norms of most men, and the concern is just a case of sexual ignorance. In other words, the man doesn't know that most penises are curved to some extent. Once in a while, a man does have a more pronounced curve than most. Even the majority of these men don't have a problem in bed, although a few may have to adjust the positions they use. In some cases, however, a man may have *Peyronie's disease*, a condition that can make sex impossible (although, rest assured, in most cases the disease goes away on its own after a short while, as we discuss in Chapter 14).

In any case, this problem is mostly in the minds of the men who come to us with concerns about the appearance of their erect penises. Because they believe that their penises look unusual, they're afraid to date. They worry that, when the time comes to undress, their partner will react negatively.

TIP

You have one simple way to avoid worrying about how a new partner will react to the shape of your penis, and this applies to the vast majority of other doubts that people have about their sexual abilities: Wait until you have established a strong relationship before you have sex with somebody. We're not saying you have to get married, but you'll find the experience of making love much better if you are in love and you integrate sex as an expression of your love rather than as a form of recreation.

So, whether your penis looks like a boomerang or is straight as an arrow, remember that the three little words "I love you" are far more important to your lover than the direction in which your penis points.

Grasping the Basics of Your Testicles

Although a man may not understand the inner workings of his penis, outwardly, he is at least on somewhat good terms with that part of his anatomy. But when it comes to testicles, too many men know almost nothing about them.

Be forewarned: By the time you've finished with this chapter, you will not only be seeing testicles differently, you'll also be feeling them in a whole new way.

Making the descent

As a baby boy develops inside his mother's womb, his testicles are still inside his body (in his abdomen). During the last few months before birth, the testicles poke their way outside, or descend, into the *scrotum*, a sac of skin located at the base of the penis. Occasionally, one or both of the testicles don't make the descent.

Some of these undescended testicles are of the hide-and-seek variety, meaning that during the first year or so, they kind of come and go. As long as they make an occasional appearance, everything will be just fine, and eventually they'll get up the courage to stay where they belong.

A testicle that remains inside the body (a condition called *cryptorchidism*) won't function properly because the temperature is too warm. A boy who has this problem may also be embarrassed by his appearance. For these reasons, medical intervention is usually called for, which may be a type of hormonal therapy but more likely will involve surgery. This condition also puts men at a higher risk of testicular cancer.

Manufacturing hormones

In addition to the testicles' vital role in the continuation of the species (which we discuss in the next section), men require functioning testicles for the hormones they produce, most importantly *testosterone*. Testosterone is called the "male hormone," and that name truly fits. If a boy is born without testosterone, his scrotum forms as the outer lips of a vagina and his penis as something akin to a clitoris.

Producing sperm

Despite the fact that a variety of contraceptive methods have allowed people to disconnect sexual intercourse from reproduction, the main purpose of having sex, from an evolutionary point of view, is to make babies. But, although the penis is required to penetrate the woman's vagina for the best chance at success, the man needs seeds to place within her to accomplish this important task. These seeds, called *spermatozoa* (or more often by their nickname, sperm), are manufactured in the testicles.

Sperm are rather amazing little creatures. They're the only parts of the body that do their work outside of it. You see, sperm don't survive well at high temperatures, particularly the temperature inside our bodies. This is why the testicles lie outside the body where they can be cooled by the soft summer breezes (at least for those of you who favor kilts or loincloths).

For the sperm to be successful at their task of making babies, they have to overcome many obstacles after making a long journey. You may well recognize their final shape — an oval head with a long tail that helps to propel them along — but sperm don't start out that way (see Figure 11-4).

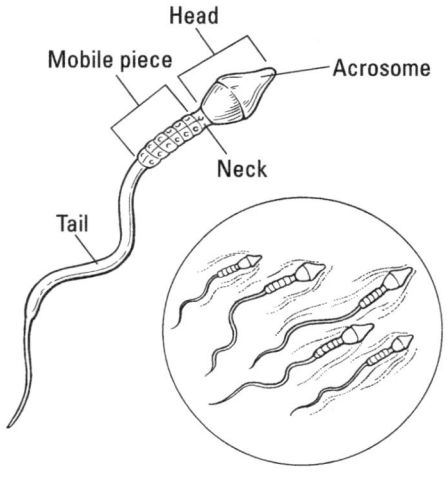

FIGURE 11-4:
The sperm: independent, a good swimmer, and a heckuva guy.

From humble beginnings

Early in their life cycles, sperm are called *germ cells*. (In this case, most people may have preferred a nice, long Latin name; but rest assured, these cells have nothing to do with what we commonly associate the word germ.)

Germ cells are produced in the *seminiferous tubules*, which are long, spaghetti-like tubes that are connected to each other, packed into a tight ball, and surrounded by a tough membrane. This package is called — drumroll, please — a *testicle*. (Between these tubes are cells that produce the male hormone testosterone.) As the germ cells travel along the tubes, slowly but surely they turn into sperm.

Their metamorphosis complete, the sperm leave the testicle and head for the *epididymis* (more on that in the next section) on their way to the *vas deferens*. Take a look at Figure 11-5; it's amazing that sperm can find their way without any help from GPS.

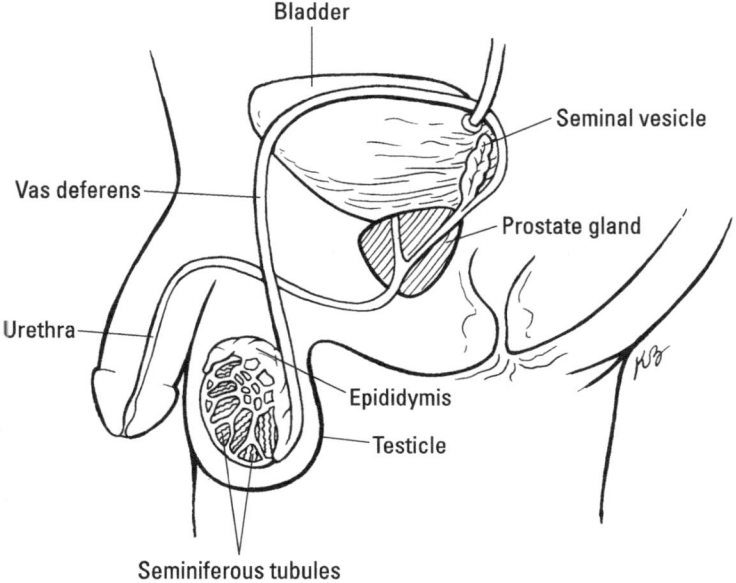

Illustration by Kathryn Born.

FIGURE 11-5:
The sperm leave the testicle and head for the epididymis and vas deferens.

Meiosis: Small division

Now that you've had a chance to look at Figure 11-5 and can picture in your mind's eye the journey that the spermatozoa take, we have to tell you about one more important transformation that they make.

TECHNICAL STUFF

All of our cells have the complete code of genetic material, called *DNA* (the long term is *deoxyribonucleic acid*, but DNA is much easier to say), unique to each individual. But although the germ cells start out with all of this DNA, along the way they undergo a process called *meiosis* (pronounced "my-*oh*-sis"). Here are some of the important effects of meiosis:

>> When a germ cell undergoes meiosis, it forms two new cells, each of them having only half of the DNA code: 23 bits of genetic material (called *chromosomes*) instead of the normal 46.

- >> When a sperm teams up with a female egg, which also only has 23 chromosomes, their genetic materials intertwine, and the resulting baby ends up with a package containing a total of 46 chromosomes that's a mixture of both the mother's and the father's genetic material.

- >> When the male germ cells divide, the sex chromosomes divide also. The male has one X and one Y chromosome; the female has two X chromosomes.

- >> Whether the sperm that reaches the egg first has an X (female) or Y (male) chromosome determines whether the baby will be a girl or a boy.

TECHNICAL STUFF

You may appreciate knowing one more thing about sperm: Not only can sperm move around on their own outside the body, but they're also fully armed, like little guided missiles. Over the head of the sperm lies the *acrosome*, which is full of enzymes that help the sperm penetrate an egg if it should be so lucky as to meet one on its journey.

When they're ready, the sperm leave the *testes* (another name for testicles) and enter the *epididymis*, which is a series of tiny tubes that lie on top of the testes. (Check out Figure 11-5 if you missed it.) Fun fact: If unfurled, these tubes would reach 60 feet in length. During their journey through the epididymis, sperm learn to swim. They enter the epididymis with useless tails and leave it as little speed demons. (See, the advice that practice makes perfect lies at the very heart of human life.)

Vas deferens

If you go back to Figure 11-5, you see that the sperm's next stop on their voyage is the *vas deferens*, a tube that ejects the sperm into the *urethra*, through which semen and urine pass. In the urethra, the sperm are mixed with fluids from the *seminal vesicles* and the *prostate* (which we discuss in more detail later in the section called "Previewing the Prostate Gland"); then they make their way out into the world through ejaculation.

The combination of these fluids and the sperm is called *semen*. The amount of semen ejaculated during orgasm is generally around a teaspoonful, though it varies depending on when the man last ejaculated. The semen is whitish in color, has a distinctive smell, and is thick when it first comes out. Sperm only comprise about 5 to 10 percent of the volume, but they're the only part of the semen that can cause pregnancy.

Too few sperm (male infertility)

Just because your testicles look normal doesn't mean that they are fully functioning. If a couple tries to conceive but can't seem to do it, one of the first things that doctors look for is a problem with the sperm. The most common problems are a *low sperm count* (which means the man isn't producing enough sperm) or the sperm he is producing lack sufficient motility (that is, the ability to swim to the egg). The basis for the problems may be abnormal sperm production, which can be difficult to treat or can be as simple as changing from tighty whities to boxers because heat is known to decrease sperm count. Another cause can be a blockage somewhere along the line, which may be corrected through surgery.

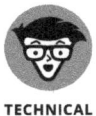

TECHNICAL
STUFF

Interestingly enough, most semen analysis is done by *gynecologists*, specialists in the female reproductive system. A gynecologist is usually the first person a woman consults when she has problems getting pregnant. Commonly, the gynecologist asks that the man's sperm be analyzed. If the tests reveal a problem with the sperm, the man is sent to a urologist for further evaluation.

Examining yourself to identify cancer

WARNING

Testicular cancer isn't the most common cancer that men in general face, but it's the most common cancer diagnosed in men ages 15–35. It can be a deadly disease if not found early enough, but it's easily curable if found in time. Flip to Chapter 16 for more information on testicular cancer and how to perform regular self-checks.

Previewing the Prostate Gland

The *prostate gland*, located below the man's bladder, produces some of the fluids that are contained in the semen, giving semen its whitish color. The prostate continues to grow throughout a man's life. A 20-year old's prostate is about the size of a walnut, whereas a 50-year-old's is about twice that size, or more. The *urethra*, which carries semen and urine out of the body, runs through the prostate.

WARNING

In addition to their testicles, another area that men should have checked — and all too often don't — is the prostate. The prostate has a nasty habit of becoming cancerous, which can be quite dangerous, though it is easily treated if discovered in time. Chapter 16 goes into detail about the prostate, prostate cancer, and the all-important exam to identify any serious concerns.

Chapter **12**

The Birds, the Bees, and (Dodging) Babies

S ex. Once you're under its power, you're a captive for life. It starts when you're young. When you're a teenager and your hormones are surging, almost everything you do is connected to sex in one way or another. And although your sexual voltage goes down a notch or two as you get older, many of your daily activities are still influenced by sex:

» You take a shower in the morning and style your hair to increase your sexual attractiveness.

» You choose clothes that will draw the attention of other people.

» You send sexual messages with your body language, from the way you walk to the angle you hold your head.

And it doesn't matter whether you're single or married, young or old, all of us are interested in how others react to the image we project. We want to be noticed. We want to know that we can still attract someone, even if we've been monogamously involved in a relationship for 50 years.

In this chapter, we give you a brief course in Reproduction 101 so the basics are clear. We also cover various birth control options so you can have some frisky fun and save pregnancy for when you're ready to start or add to your family. And we discuss several birth control myths and the actual facts for each.

Thinking About Sex and Why We Have It

Is sex just the means by which we reproduce? Is it a yearning that makes us go a bit crazy until we can satisfy those urges? Or could it be the key to exchanging extreme pleasure? Maybe it's a way of cementing a relationship. What makes sex so amazing is that it's all of those, and more.

We have special organs that are made to have sex; they fit together and have many nerve endings so as to make sex feel good. So ultimately, we have sex in order to participate in a very pleasurable activity and sometimes to keep the human race going, too.

Throughout most of humankind's history, sexual intercourse and making babies were almost always linked, but today they needn't be. Being able to have an orgasm without worrying about creating a baby has changed the nature of sex, and that's what this chapter is about.

Moving From Fun to Fertilization: Reproduction Basics

Although some couples must go through a great deal of trouble to have a family, possibly turning to medical science or adoption for help, the process of making a baby is relatively easy in most male–female relationships. The man needs only to place his erect penis into the woman's vagina and ejaculate. A baby may not result the first time — though it can — but eventually one of the man's sperm will unite with the woman's egg, and, voilà, a baby is conceived.

Because baby-making can be so easy, your partner may become pregnant without either of you intending that outcome. So we can't underscore the following enough:

TIP

If you absolutely, positively don't want to make a baby, then don't have sexual intercourse — remain abstinent.

Yes, we know there are ways of preventing pregnancy from occurring — that's a key purpose of this chapter! — but none of these methods is foolproof. (Believe it or not, in at least one recorded case, the man had a vasectomy, the woman had her tubes tied, and she still became pregnant.) So remember, *the only method that works 100 percent of the time is abstinence.*

Sperm meets egg: A reproductive love story

The process of making a baby hasn't changed over the millenia: A sperm from the penis must meet an egg inside of the vagina (test-tube babies notwithstanding). When the sperm and the egg unite, the egg becomes *fertilized*.

Timing plays an important role in this sperm + egg meetup. Female humans differ from nearly all the rest of their sex in the animal kingdom because, rather than wanting sexual intercourse only when they can conceive (that is, when they're in *heat*), women can want sexual intercourse at any time. But unlike other female mammals, they're able to make a baby, or *conceive*, only at certain times — in most women's cases, they're fertile from one to three days a month.

WARNING

Just because a woman is fertile only a few days a month doesn't mean those are the only days that unprotected sexual intercourse can make her pregnant. A woman's reproductive organs are much more complicated than that.

TECHNICAL STUFF

Unlike a man, who continually makes sperm (more than 26 trillion a year!), a woman has all her eggs already inside her at birth. These eggs — about 200,000 of them — reside in a woman's two *ovaries* (see Figure 12-1). About every 28 days, a fluid-filled sac in the ovary, called a *follicle*, releases one of the eggs.

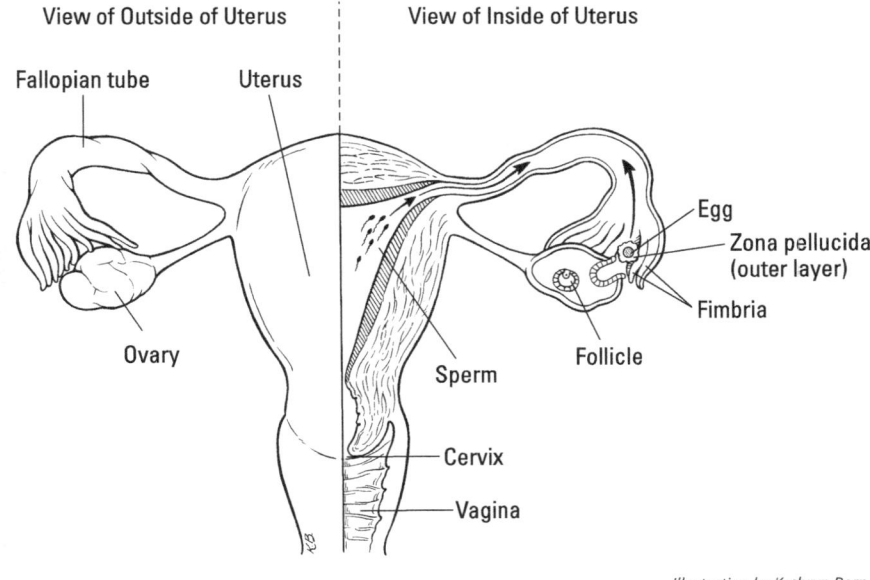

View of Outside of Uterus   View of Inside of Uterus

Fallopian tube   Uterus

Egg
Zona pellucida
(outer layer)

Fimbria

Ovary   Follicle

Sperm

Cervix

Vagina

FIGURE 12-1:
The egg begins an incredible journey in search of a sperm to produce a child. No wonder sex has been called "making whoopee"!

Illustration by Kathryn Born.

The sperm's journey

Everyone's talking about what happened last night at Club Fallopian. Mr. Sperm bumped into Ms. Egg, and now they're really stuck on each other! Ba dum DUM.

Just as people have to meet each other before they can form a relationship, the process of fertilization can't begin until a sperm gets up into the *fallopian tubes* and meets the egg. This introduction takes place as a result of *sexual intercourse*, which is defined as a man placing his penis in a woman's vagina. When the man has an orgasm, he releases millions of sperm into the back of the woman's vagina. These sperm bind to the cervical mucus and swim right up through the entrance to the uterus (called the *cervix*), through the uterus itself, and then into the fallopian tubes — each sperm hunting for an egg. And if an egg happens to be floating along, the fastest sperm takes the prize.

WARNING

Keep in mind two very important points about sperm:

>> Sperm can live from two to seven days inside a woman. So although the egg may have only a short time during which it can be fertilized, sperm that a man deposited in the woman up to a week before can still fertilize the egg and cause pregnancy.

>> Even before a man ejaculates, his penis releases some liquid (the proper name is *Cowper's fluid*, because the Cowper's gland produces it, but it's popularly referred to as "precum"), which serves as a lubricant to help the sperm go up the shaft of the penis. Any sperm that may not have been ejaculated during the man's previous orgasms may be picked up by the Cowper's fluid. Although that number is less than the millions of sperm in the ejaculate, how many sperm does an egg require for fertilization? One fast one.

Because of Cowper's fluid, a man may deposit sperm inside a woman's vagina before he has an orgasm. That's why the pullout, or withdrawal, method is not an effective means of preventing pregnancy. (See "Myth: Pulling out is adequate protection" later in this chapter for more on this.)

The egg does some traveling, too

Little finger-like appendages on the end of the fallopian tube called *fimbria* lead the egg into the tube, through which it makes its way into the *uterus*. If, during this trip, the egg encounters some sperm swimming along, then the first sperm to reach the egg and penetrate the hard outer shell (the *zona pellucida)* will enter the egg and begin the life-creating process called fertilization.

A fertilized egg continues down the fallopian tube on a journey that takes about three days. During the first 30 hours, the chromosomes of the egg and the sperm merge, and the cells begin to divide. This new entity is called an *embryo*. When the embryo finishes its journey and enters the uterus (see Figure 12-2), it gets nourishment from uterine secretions, and the cells inside it continue to divide, causing the embryo to grow. Approximately six days after fertilization, the egg "hatches," emerging from its hard shell and then burrowing its way into the uterine wall, or *endometrium*.

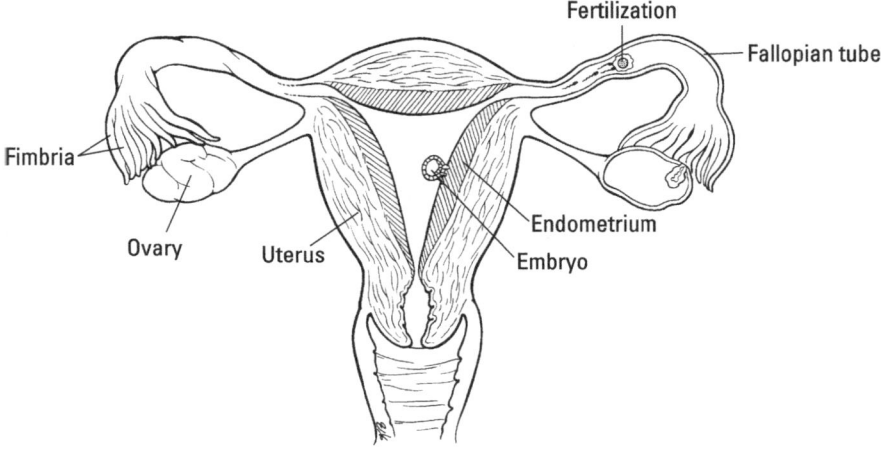

Fertilization

Fallopian tube

Fimbria

Ovary

Uterus

Endometrium

Embryo

FIGURE 12-2:
The embryo nests in the wall of the uterus after fertilization. Happy landing!

TECHNICAL STUFF

The embryo releases a hormone called hCG. When the hCG reaches the mother's bloodstream, it signals that she is pregnant and causes the ovaries to continue producing the hormones estrogen and progesterone, which are necessary to maintain the pregnancy.

If the egg is not fertilized, it passes through the uterus. About two weeks later, the uterus sheds its lining (the *endometrium*) in a process called *menstruation*. A new lining then begins to grow, ready to receive a fertilized egg the next month.

MAKING BABIES MAKES GOOD SEX, TOO

One more thing about sexual intercourse and its pleasures: As great a feeling as you get when having an orgasm during sexual intercourse, we think that most couples will tell you that they got even more pleasure from the intercourse they had while trying to make a baby. You get an extra kick from knowing that the possible result of this union between two people who love each other is another little human being.

Becoming a baby

After an embryo burrows its way into the endometrium, it grows until it has a human shape and all its organs — a process that takes about 12 weeks. At this point, the embryo is renamed a *fetus*. (Also, by this stage of the pregnancy, many couples give the fetus funny names — none of which, hopefully, will land on the final birth certificate.)

The fetus grows inside the uterus until approximately nine months after the egg was first fertilized. Then, in a process called *giving birth*, a fully formed baby comes out of the uterus and through the vagina into the world (unless doctors have to remove the baby surgically, which is called a *cesarean section*, or c-section).

TIP

If you want to know more about the specifics of pregnancy, pick up *Pregnancy For Dummies*, 4th Edition (John Wiley & Sons, Inc., 2014). And for a dad's-eye view, check out *Dad's Guide to Pregnancy For Dummies* (John Wiley & Sons, Inc., 2022).

So an important possible consequence of sexual intercourse is the making of a baby that will be born nine months later. Of course, giving birth to a baby is only the beginning of providing the care a child requires. Having a child is a very big responsibility — not one to be taken lightly, and certainly not one to be ignored when having sexual intercourse.

HOW CAN YOU TELL THAT YOUR PARTNER IS PREGNANT?

During early pregnancy the only sure way is to take a test, which you can buy at your local drug store. But a woman will undergo many physical changes that will at least give an indication of a possible pregnancy, and these often occur before the most obvious sign, a missed period. (Not that all missed periods indicate a pregnancy, but if you had unprotected sex, the odds of a missed period being an indicator of pregnancy grow much stronger.) One of the first possible signs is a tenderness in the woman's breasts. Another is morning sickness, as many women during the first trimester suffer bouts of nausea, particularly in the morning. Fatigue and more frequent urination are other signs that it's time to buy a pregnancy test or visit your gynecologist.

Considering the Benefits of Contraception

Having intercourse has two potential outcomes: causing pleasure and making babies. You will have moments in your life when you'll want to combine those two, but most of the time you're going to want one without the other. That's where contraception comes in. And the less worried you are about causing an unintended pregnancy, the more you'll enjoy sex — sort of a two-for-the-price-of-one deal. This also works the other way, so if you opt to have sex without using contraception, and you don't want to get pregnant, you'll enjoy sex a lot less.

WARNING

In addition to not wanting to cause an unintended pregnancy, you'll also want to avoid catching a *sexually transmitted infection* (STI; also called a *sexually transmitted disease*, or STD). We have an entire chapter on this subject (Chapter 13), but because preventing pregnancies and diseases can be related, we want to mention some facts here.

Some of the contraceptive methods we cover in this chapter do a great job of preventing pregnancy, such as the birth control pill, but don't offer any protection against STIs. The condom is really the only method of birth control that also offers protection against disease, but it's not the most effective method of birth control. So you may have to use two types of contraceptive to maximize both effects.

We recognize that all of this can be a bit cumbersome, which is why so many people just don't bother to use any form of protection, at least from time to time. That's one of the reasons why there are so many unintended pregnancies and why STIs are so rampant. So if you're going to engage in sexual intercourse, please make the effort to learn how to prevent pregnancies and STIs, and we guarantee you that you'll enjoy sex a lot more.

Reducing Your Chances of Becoming a Dad

Whether you're not ready to start a family now, you're taking a break between Thing 1 and Thing 2, your family's complete, or you've decided kids aren't on your bucket list, at some point you'll likely want to enjoy sex without making a baby. To prevent pregnancy, you've got four basic types of contraceptives to choose from:

>> Sterilization

>> Hormonal methods

>> Barrier methods

>> Natural family planning

Each of these types has varying degrees of success at preventing pregnancy. Some require more diligence than others to make them as successful as they can be. You can buy some over the counter without a prescription, and others need a doctor's visit and possibly a procedure.

WARNING

Only one of these methods of birth control, the condom, significantly reduces your risk of catching a sexually transmitted disease. The condom is not the most effective method of birth control (although it's certainly better than nothing), but it's a vital piece of equipment in the war against HIV and other STIs (see Chapter 13). So regardless of the birth control that you like to use, if you're not with one steady partner, or if your one partner has more partners than just you, you should always have some condoms on hand — and use them!

Sterilization

Sterilization methods come in two basic types: one for men (*vasectomy*) and one for women (*tubal ligation*).

Both the male and female methods of sterilization have certain advantages over other kinds of birth control:

>> They're one-time operations.

>> They're very effective.

>> They don't have side effects.

>> They don't affect sexual functioning.

>> They eliminate worries about pregnancy.

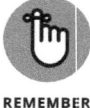

REMEMBER

The main disadvantage of sterilization is that it's permanent. If you later change your mind and want to make a baby, it's difficult — and in many cases impossible — to do so.

The snip: Vasectomy

The male version of sterilization, the *vasectomy*, is a surgical procedure that's performed on an outpatient basis. In a vasectomy, the tubes that carry the sperm (the *vas deferens*) are cut and tied (see Figure 12-3). Only very rarely do the tubes grow back together, so that only 1 out of 1,000 men who are sterilized causes a pregnancy in the first year after the operation.

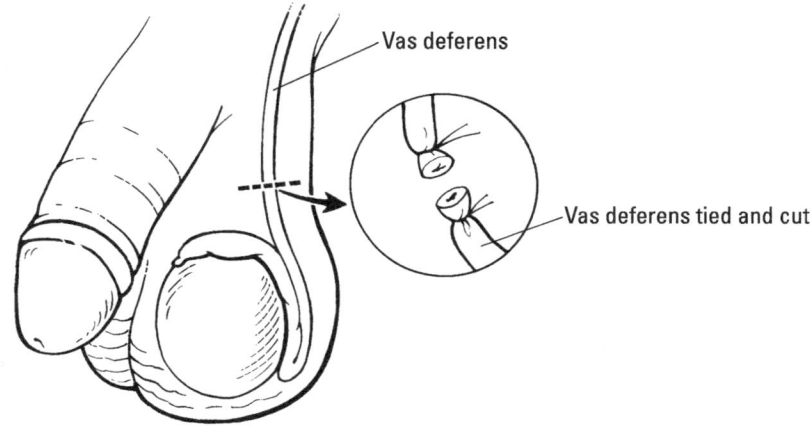

Vas deferens

Vas deferens tied and cut

FIGURE 12-3:
A vasectomy gives "tying the knot" a whole new meaning.

Illustration by Kathryn Born.

WARNING

One difference between the male and female sterilization is that some sperm remain in the man's system after the operation, so you must use another method of contraception for at least the first 20 to 30 ejaculations. You can be certain that all the sperm have passed from his system by getting a simple lab test done on the semen. Ask your doctor for more details.

Some men worry that undergoing a vasectomy will in some way reduce their sexual prowess, but this fear is ungrounded. A man feels no difference in sexual performance after a vasectomy because he can still have erections and ejaculate.

The only change after a vasectomy is that, after the system has been cleaned out, the semen no longer contains any sperm. Because sperm make up only 5 to 10 percent of the volume of the ejaculate, a man who undergoes this procedure won't be able to tell any difference, nor will his hormones be affected in any way. The testes continue to manufacture sperm, but instead of being ejaculated, the body absorbs the sperm.

Vasectomies are much less expensive than tubal sterilizations. Trying to reverse the procedure, however, costs much more than having the procedure done in the first place, and is not necessarily covered by insurance. Reversing the procedure requires microsurgery, and the rate of success depends on several factors including how long ago the vasectomy was performed and the age of the man.

Tying the tubes: Tubal ligation

A common name for the female method of sterilization is *tubal ligation*, although tubal sterilization can actually be performed in a variety of ways, not all of which call for tying the tubes.

The tubes in this case are the fallopian tubes, in which the egg is fertilized by the first sperm that finds it (see earlier in this chapter). If these two tubes are cut and tied, the eggs and sperm should never be able to come together (see Figure 12-4). In rare instances, the tubes grow back, and a woman can become pregnant, but this only happens in about 12 out of 1,000 cases.

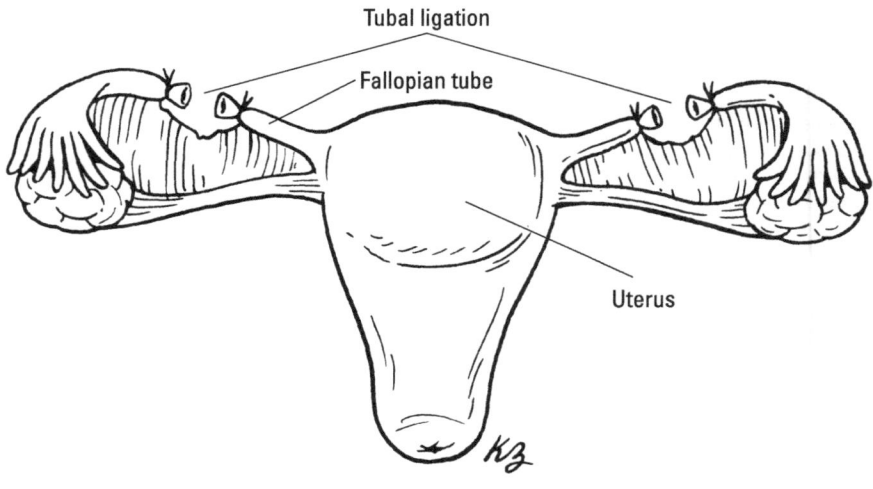

Tubal ligation

Fallopian tube

Uterus

Illustration by Kathryn Born.

FIGURE 12-4:
Tubal ligation is the female equivalent of a vasectomy.

Women have several kinds of tubal sterilization from which to choose:

>> One of the two most common types of tubal ligation is called an operative *laparoscopy*, where a surgeon inserts a rodlike instrument, called a *laparoscope*, through a small incision and cuts and ties the tubes. Complications are rare.

>> A *mini-laparotomy* is the other popular method. It is similar to the laparoscopy and is done within 48 hours of giving birth, when the abdomen is still enlarged and viewing is easier for the surgeon.

>> Other options exist and require major surgery and longer recovery periods, and are usually performed because of additional medical factors.

With any of the tubal methods of sterilization, the woman's organs function normally, so she still ovulates, has her full set of female hormones, and has her monthly period. The eggs, which continue to be released monthly, simply dissolve the way any unused cells do. (Remember, the egg is microscopic in size, so it really can't do any damage floating inside of you for a while.)

After sterilization, sexual functioning also remains the same, or is sometimes improved because the woman no longer has to concern herself about becoming pregnant.

As with vasectomy, tubal ligation requires a surgical procedure, but most women can undergo it on an outpatient basis (either in a hospital or clinic), under local anesthesia, and in under 30 minutes. The costs can vary from $1,000 to $6,000, but this is a one-time charge as opposed to other methods that involve a cost for every use, such as the condom or birth control pill. Insurance may cover some or all of the cost, depending on the individual policy.

The Pill and other hormonal methods

The ancient Greeks had this weird idea that our temperaments and bodily functions were controlled by what they called *the four humors*: blood, mucus, yellow bile, and black bile. Turns out they were right, although they got the details slightly wrong.

The human body secretes close to 50 different hormones in the endocrine system. These *hormones* are chemical substances that go directly into the bloodstream to our various organs and control how they work. The hormones that affect the sex and reproductive systems are absolutely vital to their functioning, and, conversely, by controlling these hormones, we can now affect the functioning of our reproduction with great accuracy. The contraceptive pill works exactly like that, inhibiting pregnancy through the use of hormones.

REMEMBER

The birth control options we cover in this section are all designed for women (see "On the horizon" later in this section for a quick intro to male hormonal birth control in development). So if you and your partner use one of these highly effective methods, you need to trust that she's following all medically advised practices so the birth control works as it's intended to. If you don't have a trusting relationship with your partner, then use a condom to help protect yourself and minimize any unintended surprises down the road.

WARNING

We must repeat the warning concerning STIs. The hormonal methods like the Pill offer absolutely no protection against HIV or any other sexually transmitted infection. A man must use a condom in conjunction with his partner's homonal birth control of choice if any risk exists that either may catch a disease from the other.

The Pill

The Pill is a very effective method of birth control — almost as effective as sterilization, in fact — assuming full compliance (that is, the woman takes the Pill regularly and without fail). Because the Pill made having sex almost risk free, it's credited with starting the sexual revolution in the 1960s, when the use of oral contraceptives became widespread.

These days, the Pill comes in two types:

>> *Combination pills,* which contain both estrogen and progestin, keep the ovaries from releasing eggs.

>> The so-called *mini-pills* contain only progestin.

The Pill can prevent ovulation, but the primary way it prevents conception is by thickening the cervical mucus so the sperm can't penetrate it. The Pill also makes the uterine lining less receptive to the implantation of sperm.

TIP

A woman taking the Pill must remember to take it every day, and preferably at the same time of the day — say, every morning — for the hormones to work best. (When using the combination pill, the woman goes off the hormones for seven days a month to allow for withdrawal bleeding, which simulates normal menstrual flow. In most cases, however, she continues to take placebo pills during this time to enforce the habit.)

WARNING

The failure rate of the Pill relates closely to compliance, so it's important to follow a doctor's instructions exactly as prescribed.

TECHNICAL
STUFF

Some women fear that the Pill may cause cancer of the breast or uterus because the hormones used have been linked to these cancers in animal studies. Whether or not such a risk once existed, no scientific evidence indicates that this is the case at the doses presently prescribed. In fact, the Pill has been shown to reduce the risk of cancer of the ovary or endometrium.

Most women of child-bearing age can take the Pill, except women

>> Who are smokers over the age of 35. These women should refrain from taking the Pill because it can cause some risks to the cardiovascular system.

>> Who have some other physical conditions, such as diabetes or a history of blood clots, that make the Pill unsuitable for them.

Because of these risks, a physician must prescribe the Pill. The initial doctor's visit usually costs between $35 and $175, and the pills themselves cost between $0 and $50 per month. The costs for both may be lower at a clinic or through Planned Parenthood, and depending on the insurance coverage a woman has.

WARNING

If a woman uses other drugs — including antibiotics — while on the Pill, she should check with her doctor to make sure that these medications won't interfere with the Pill's effectiveness. In many cases, her doctor will advise to use an additional form of protection at this time.

Birth control shot (Depo-Provera)

An alternative to the Pill is *Depo-Provera*, which was reformulated so it now contains less hormones. The higher dose of hormones was thought to cause a loss in bone density. Depo-Provera is nicknamed "the shot" or Depo, and is something a woman gets every 12 weeks, which is given under the skin instead of into the muscle.

Although its side effects are the same as the Pill's, unlike the Pill, if a woman doesn't like the side effects or wants to have a baby, she can't simply stop taking Depo-Provera. Instead, she must wait until the full 12 weeks have passed for the effects of the shot to go away.

The costs of the injection range from around $0 to $150, depending on location and insurance coverage. But, again, a clinic may charge less.

Birth control implants (Nexplanon)

Nexplanon is a thin plastic rod, about the length of a toothpick, that's implanted in a woman's arm and releases progestin to prevent pregnancy. It's effective for up to three years.

In tests, Nexplanon was proved to be very effective, partly because a woman can't forget to take it. But at the end of the three years, she has to remember to have the device removed and a new one implanted.

Getting the implant costs anywhere from $0-$2,300, depending on insurance and if a woman gets it implanted at a clinic.

Vaginal ring (NuvaRing)

The *NuvaRing* is a small flexible ring that a woman inserts into her vagina and leaves in place for three weeks. She removes it the fourth week. It releases synthetic hormones, like the Pill does, and is very effective, more so than the Pill because a woman doesn't have to remember to take it every day. The ring is designed to stay in place, but if it slips out and isn't put back in within three hours, then an unintended pregnancy could take place.

The cost of using the ring is about the same as using the Pill, and any side effects are also similar because both methods involve regulating a woman's hormones. Only the method of application differs.

The patch (Xulane and Twirla)

Another way of delivering the same hormones is through the birth control patch. The patch is applied to the buttocks, stomach, upper arm, or torso once a week for three out of four weeks. Some women develop an irritation under the patch making it unsuitable for them to use.

Because the patch delivers more hormones than the Pill and the hormones are delivered through the skin instead of orally, the FDA ordered the patch's manufacturer to add a warning to the box about possible risks, though no data indicates that the patch is any more risky than the Pill. We suggest a woman consult with her doctor before deciding to use the patch, just to be sure.

The costs and effectiveness for the patch are pretty much the same as for the Pill or ring.

The intrauterine device (IUD)

The IUD is a small plastic device containing either a hormone or copper that is inserted into a woman's uterus. IUDs work either by preventing the fertilization of the egg or by preventing implantation of a fertilized egg in the uterine wall, and they are highly effective at preventing pregnancy. The IUD does not change either the hormone levels or the copper levels in a woman's body.

Inserted into the uterus through the cervix during menstruation, the copper IUD can be left in place for up to 12 years. The hormonal IUD must be replaced after 3-8 years, depending on the brand.

The cost of an exam and insertion ranges from $0 to $1,300 depending on where you get it and your insurance coverage.

On the horizon

Several versions of a male contraceptive pill are currently under study. Like the Pill for women, one of these male contraceptives involves adding hormones. In this case, the male contraceptive pill adds a synthetic version of the male hormone testosterone, which causes sperm production to shut down for about a week. But, because taking this hormone orally can cause liver damage, the male contraceptive pill may never be an actual pill but rather an injection. There is also a male gel that is being tested, which suppresses sperm production and is applied daily to each shoulder blade.

The condom, diaphragm, and other barrier methods

The aim of the barrier methods is to block the sperm from getting at the egg. Applying military tactics to this job, the logical place to begin is at the narrowest opening: the cervix. Casanova first tried a barrier method using hollowed-out halves of lemons at the cervix, but these days latex has pretty much taken over from the citrus family.

The condom

When the Pill first came out, people suddenly relegated the lowly condom to the back of the shelf. But the condom's ability to protect its user from transmitting diseases pushed it again to the forefront.

The condom is a sheath that fits over the penis, blocking the sperm from being released into the vagina. Most condoms are made of latex, although some are made out of animal tissue (usually lambskin) or polyurethane. The latter two were created mostly for those who are allergic to latex. Although the polyurethane condoms are more expensive, they're thinner and stronger than latex condoms, nonporous and nonpermeable to all viruses (including HIV), hypoallergenic, safe to use with oil-based products, and heat conductive, which is supposed to make them transmit sensations between partners better.

WARNING

Lambskin condoms have microscopic holes that, while small enough to stop the sperm in mid-backstroke, are big enough to allow viruses safe passage into the vagina. These condoms, therefore, do not offer adequate protection against HIV.

Condoms are widely available at drugstores, at many supermarkets and convenience stores, and in dispensers in many public restrooms. And you can also order them online. When you purchase a condom, it comes rolled up in a package. You place the condom on the erect penis and roll it down along the shaft, leaving a small pocket at the top to collect the semen (see Figure 12-5). Be sure to smooth out any air bubbles.

You can buy condoms in various colors, different sizes, and with unique packaging. You can also purchase dry or lubricated condoms (even flavored ones!). Some lubricated condoms include a spermicide for added protection (except if the spermicide causes irritation; it then actually increases the risk of disease transmission).

Speaking of sizes, condoms had long been sold like socks in that they were pretty much a one-size-fits-all piece of equipment. But that's certainly changing and some websites sell condoms in as many as 70 different sizes, and you can measure your penis so you get the perfect fit. Of course, most men settle for the store-bought brands, but even these provide size options. Men with smaller penises may have a problem with some condoms slipping off during intercourse. They should purchase condoms with a "snugger fit." Among the brands that make this type are Lifestyles and Atlas TrueFit. Men who are more amply endowed risk splitting a regular condom, but a brand from Trojan called Magnum aims at this market. If you have problems finding these variously sized condoms in your area, shop online for a wider variety.

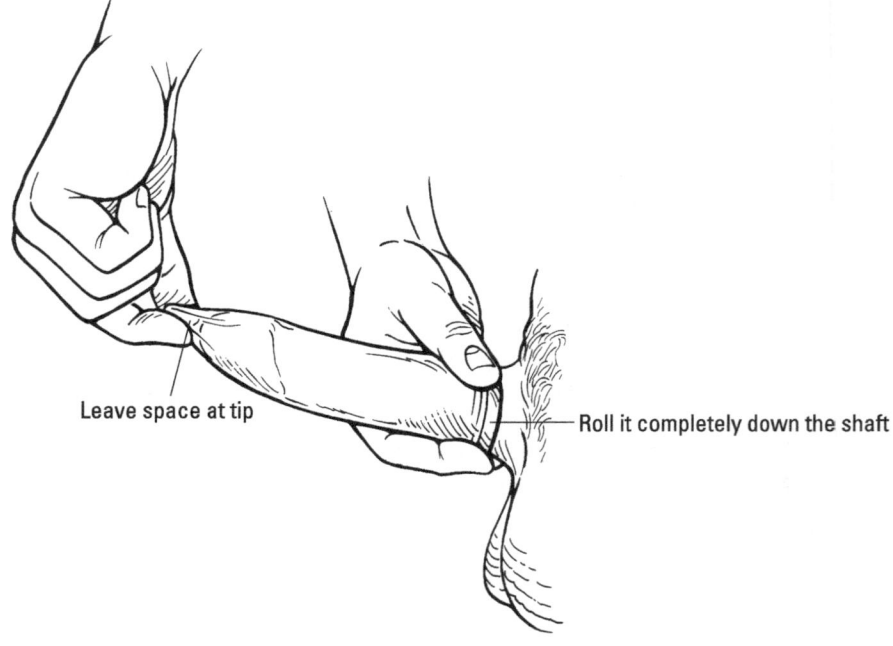

FIGURE 12-5: Although how to use a condom may seem obvious, many people wind up paying a high price for not knowing as much as they thought they did.

Leave space at tip

Roll it completely down the shaft

Illustration by Kathryn Born.

WARNING

If you use a dry condom and decide to add a lubricant on the condom itself, to the penis, or to the inside of the vagina, make sure that the lubricant is a water-based one, like KY Jelly. Oil-based lubricants, like Vaseline, or other products made from mineral or vegetable oils, including Reddi Whip and coconut oil, can break down the latex and make the condom porous. This breakdown can happen very quickly, so don't use any of these products with a condom.

REMOVAL IS TRICKY

The trickiest part of using a condom can be removing it. Always be very careful to make sure that the condom doesn't leak because, if the sperm escape from their little rubber prison, they can make their way up into the vagina and pull off the escapade that you're trying to prevent.

>> Either partner should hold onto the base of the condom to keep it on the shaft of the penis while the man pulls his penis out.

>> To minimize the risk of leakage, you should remove the condom before the man loses his erection entirely.

THE SUCCESS RATE OF CONDOMS

Although the condom is relatively risk free to the man (unless he happens to be allergic to latex), it offers less protection from pregnancy compared to other options. Of 100 women whose partners use condoms, approximately 12 will become pregnant during a year of typical use because condoms can break during use or semen can spill from them during the removal process. Obviously, the more careful you are using a condom, the more protection it offers. The biggest reason for condom failure, however, is failure to use it in the first place. In other words, a couple may say that their method of birth control is always the condom, but they only use condoms occasionally.

WARNING

If you rely on condoms to protect against pregnancy or STIs, you must use them all the time.

CONDOMS DON'T LAST FOREVER

Condoms have expiration dates on them, which vary based on the materials the condom is made from and if it's preloaded with spermacide. After that date, the condom is less effective at preventing pregnancy (or STIs), so treat an expired condom as you would expired milk, and throw it out.

WARNING

Irrespective of the expiration date, exposure to heat, humidity and moisture, and sunlight or fluorescent light can accelerate a condom's demise and make it less effective.

Some men carry condoms in their wallets on the off chance that they'll get lucky, and we appreciate the effort to be prepared. Unfortunately, a wallet can be a warm and cozy place for a condom waiting its turn to shine. We don't want to put a time limit on how long a condom can stay in a wallet before you need to declare it damaged goods. That decision depends on a lot of factors, including how hot it is outside and how big a tush you have. Better storage options include a jacket pocket, a small toiletries bag, or a compartment in your backpack — anywhere cooler than 100 degrees F (37 degrees C).

By the way, this storage advice doesn't apply only to wallets. Men have a number of places where they may keep a "safety," including the glove compartment or trunk of their car, the bathroom medicine cabinet, a tool kit, or even in a kilt. Whatever that place is, if it's subject to extremes of cold or heat, humidity, or exposure to light, assume that, after a while, the condom will no longer be reliably "safe."But if you store them properly, in a cool dry place, you can rely on the expiration date.

The internal condom (also known as the female condom)

An internal condom, also called the *female condom,* allows women to protect themselves against sexually transmitted infections. The female condom is a loose-fitting pouch with a closed end that a woman inserts deep inside her vagina. Like a diaphragm, a woman can insert the female condom ahead of time or right before intercourse. The closed end must be lubricated first. The open end is left outside the vagina, and the male inserts his penis into it when entering the vagina for intercourse. The rate of effectiveness is slightly less than that of a condom men wear.

By the way, for those of you who may want to double your level of protection by using both a male and female condom at the same time, don't — they could stick together and tear.

Although condoms for men can cost as little as 50 cents, the female condom costs $2-$3. This may seem unfair, but the reason turns out to be one of those Catch 22s. Female condoms aren't very popular, and their lack of popularity keeps their price up. They're more cumbersome to put in, which also reduces their use.

The diaphragm, cervical cap, and sponge

The *diaphragm* is a shallow, dome-shaped cup with a flexible rim to allow for insertion because it needs to be folded to be placed into the vagina. The *cervical cap* works the same way as the diaphragm, the difference being one of shape. The *contraceptive sponge* is another similar barrier method where a sponge replaced the rubber diaphragm or cup. All three of these methods of birth control have fallen out of use, in part because a number of other methods are more effective.

Foams, creams, and gels

Many contraceptive foams, creams, and gels are available over the counter. They don't require a prescription, and apart from possible temporary allergic reactions to the chemicals they're made of — which may affect the woman, the man, or both — they have relatively few side effects.

They're also relatively ineffective when used by themselves. Of 100 women who use a contraceptive foam, cream, jelly, or suppository, 21 will become pregnant during the first year of typical use, although if perfectly used, that number drops to 3.

The spermicides in these products do offer some protection against HIV and other STIs, but we don't recommend that you rely solely on these products to remain disease-free. And if you use them several times a day, they can cause irritation that can actually make catching HIV easier.

Most of these products come with applicators to place them inside the vagina. The exact application varies per product, but in general a woman should have the product in place at least ten minutes before intercourse (though this process can be integrated into foreplay). A couple must reapply the product each time they intend to repeat sexual intercourse. Another drawback, which is why they're rather unpopular, is that they're messy.

The vaginal contraceptive film

Another way of applying a spermicide is the vaginal contraceptive film (VCF), a 2-×-2-inch paper-thin sheet that contains *nonoxynol-9* (a chemical that kills sperm). You place it on or near the cervix, where it dissolves in seconds, releasing the spermicide. Like other spermicides, when used perfectly only 6 percent of women using VCF become pregnant. Under normal use, however, the number jumps to 25 percent.

TIP

These products are easy to buy and easy to use, but they're much more effective when used in conjunction with a condom.

Getting into a rhythm: Natural family planning

Certainly the best way to avoid becoming pregnant is *abstinence*, or never having sexual intercourse.

Another way is to be abstinent during the time of month when the woman is fertile and can become pregnant (see earlier in this chapter for a discussion of these times). This reliance on the fertile time of month is called *natural family planning* (or the *calendar* or *rhythm method*, or *periodic abstinence*, or *fertility awareness method*).

Natural family planning is based on the regular patterns of fertility that most women have. And that's the number-one drawback these methods share. Many women are not all that regular, and even those who are regular sometimes have irregular months. When that happens, an unintended pregnancy can result.

To use any of these methods, you and your partner must first try to predict when she'll next ovulate. Unless a woman already knows that she's "regular," meaning that her period always comes at the same time in her cycle, her first step is to determine what pattern she follows. If her pattern tends to be very irregular, natural family planning carries more risk of pregnancy for the two of you.

Calendar method

Your partner's fertile period is not just the day that she ovulates. The egg lives for one to three days, but sperm can live inside the vagina from two to seven days. This means that, if you've had sexual intercourse before the time that your partner ovulates, any of those sperm may still be hanging around the fallopian tubes when the egg comes along, ready to ambush the egg and impregnate the woman.

To be safe from pregnancy, both of you should think of a nine-day period as being risky — five days before your partner ovulates, the day of ovulation, and three days after that. During that fertile period, you should either abstain from sexual intercourse or use a barrier method.

The other 19 days that comprise the cycle are considered to be "safe," and — theoretically — you can have sexual intercourse during those days without using any other method of birth control and not become pregnant. But nothing is ever certain when those sneaky eggs and sperm are involved, so be aware of the risks.

WARNING

By now this should be a reflex, but we'll give you this warning once again. Even if you and your partner are presumably safe from becoming pregnant, that doesn't mean that you're safe from getting a sexually transmitted infection. Unless you're certain that your partner is 100 percent disease free, you should make sure that a condom is in place before attempting intercourse.

Basal body temperature

You and your partner can use other fertility indicators in conjunction with the calendar method. One is *the basal body temperature method.*

A woman's temperature rises slightly (between 0.4 and 0.8 degrees) when she ovulates. If she takes her temperature every morning before she gets out of bed using a special high-resolution thermometer, and if she discovers a rise one day (and she's sure she doesn't have an infection of some sort to account for the rise), then you both can presume that she's ovulated and should refrain from unprotected sex.

Of course, any sperm deposited ahead of time can still impregnate your partner. Therefore, this method only serves as a proof that the calendar method is working.

If the two of you want to get pregnant, and especially if you've been having difficulties, the basal body temperature is a good predictor of when you should be having intercourse to make a baby.

Cervical mucus

Another way a woman can check whether she's ovulating is to examine her cervical mucus, which thins out when she's ovulating to allow the sperm to pass through. By continually checking the cervical mucus, your partner can notice when it begins to thin out, indicating that she's ovulated. Interpreting cervical mucus is difficult without training, so we recommend that you and your partner take a class — offered by some hospitals — on how to identify the changes in cervical mucus if you plan to try this technique.

As with the basal body temperature method, the cervical mucus method is a reliable way of telling when a woman has ovulated, which is useful information if you're trying to become pregnant. By itself, however, examining the cervical mucus does not let a woman know when she's about to ovulate. Therefore, any sperm already deposited in her vagina can impregnate her.

The sympto-thermal method

When you combine the three previously discussed methods — the calendar method, the basal body temperature method, and the cervical mucus method — the conglomerate is called the *sympto-thermal method.* This method can serve as a relatively accurate guide for deciding when to abstain from sex or use a barrier method.

How effective is periodic abstinence?

Under normal usage, of 100 women using the periodic abstinence method — meaning they refrain from having intercourse during what they believe is their fertile period — 20 will become pregnant. However, if perfect use can be obtained, the number drops to 3.

WARNING

Because outside factors can play havoc with natural family planning, perfect use is rare.

>> A lack of sleep can cause a woman's temperature to vary.

>> The consistency of a woman's cervical mucus can change if she has a vaginal infection, of which she may not be aware.

>> Either one of a woman's ovaries may decide to evict an egg for nonpayment of rent at any old time.

Emergency contraception

What should you do if you wake up one morning knowing that you had unprotected intercourse or a contraceptive failure, such as a broken condom? A couple methods are available that can prevent a potential pregnancy after you've had sex.

Emergency contraception pills (ECPs), which have been nicknamed *morning-after pills*, can be taken up to 120 hours after sexual intercourse, with all of them being most successful in the 24 hours following unprotected sex. The most common brands include Plan B One Step (available without a prescription) and ella (prescription only). They work mainly by preventing or delaying ovulation — if there's no ovulation, there's no egg for a sperm to join up with. ECPs aren't as successful at preventing pregnancy as other methods, so don't use them as your regular method of birth control.

Another emergency contraception option is a ParaGuard IUD, which can be inserted up to five days after having unprotected sex. It is considered even more effective than the pills. See "The intrauterine device (IUD)" earlier in this chapter for more info on IUDs.

Facing Facts about Birth Control Myths

WARNING

Okay, so your head is filled with all the facts about birth control. What worries us now is that you may still have some other "facts" floating around up there, which are really myths that can get you into big trouble. Following are some of those myths, debunked.

Myth: Pulling out is adequate protection

The most dangerous of myths is this one, which has caused more pregnancies than any other: the epic tale of the withdrawal method.

Through the ages, men have sworn to probably millions of women that they have great control over their ejaculations and that, as soon as they feel their orgasm coming, they will remove their penis from the vagina so she won't get pregnant.

This theory has a lot of holes in it:

>> In the first place, a lot of men who think they have matters under control don't. They wind up ejaculating before they can pull out.

>> Some men, in the heat of excitement, forget their promise and don't pull out.

>> Some men lie and have no intention of pulling out.

>> Even if the man does pull out before he ejaculates, it's already too late. The pre-ejaculatory fluid produced by the Cowper's gland may pick up sperm left inside the urethra from previous ejaculations, and those sperm are already making their way up into the uterus long before their brethren are being expelled onto milady's stomach or thighs.

WARNING

So, although *coitus interruptus* — the fancy Latin name for this not-so-fancy method of birth control — may be better than nothing, it's not much better. And, of course, it offers no protection against the spread of sexually transmitted infections.

Myth: You can't get pregnant the first time

A myth that has gotten a lot of couples in trouble is that a woman can't get pregnant from her first attempt at sexual intercourse.

In reality, a virgin's egg is no more difficult for a sperm to penetrate than any other egg. And sperm on their first journey through a vagina and into a cervix are as mobile as any others. So first-timers, whether male or female, have to take the same precautions as everyone else.

Myth: You can't get pregnant if the woman doesn't orgasm

Some people believe that if the woman doesn't have an orgasm then she can't become pregnant.

It's true that the vaginal contractions of orgasm cause the cervix to dip into the pool of sperm-laden semen at the bottom of her vagina and can help foster pregnancy. Nevertheless, some of the sperm are going to make their way up the cervix whether the woman has multiple orgasms or none at all.

Myth: Standing up stops sperm

Some people think that sperm can't defy gravity, so if the couple has sex standing up, the woman won't get pregnant.

Wrong again, folks. Those sperm are strong swimmers and can go upstream as well as down.

Myth: Periods prevent pregnancy

Some people trust that if a woman is menstruating, then she can't become pregnant.

Although menstruation does limit the odds of becoming pregnant, it's not a 100 percent, surefire way to prevent pregnancy. Some women have irregular bleeding, which isn't true menstruation. Misinterpreting this bleeding can throw off your strategy for preventing pregnancy.

Chapter **13**

It's All Fun and Games Until Something Itches

I n a perfect sexual world, terrific partners would be easy to find, everyone would have great orgasms easily, and no one could get sick from having sex. Of course, we don't live in a perfect world, sexually or any other way, and so one out of four Americans between the ages of 15 and 55 will catch at least one sexually transmitted infection (STI — formerly known as STDs, *sexually transmitted diseases*).

"Did they say *at least* one?" Yes. Because more than 30 sexually transmitted diseases exist, oftentimes the people who engage in the behaviors that lead to getting one disease wind up getting more than one. Unlike the sexual revolution of the 1960s and 1970s, with so many diseases around these days, you can say that society is now in the middle of a sexual invasion, with the result that having multiple partners can lead to mucho trouble.

WARNING

If you've had sex many times with many partners, don't assume that you're disease free just because you don't have any symptoms:

» Many people with STIs (especially women) don't show any symptoms at all.

» Other people with STIs have only a slight fever, which they don't connect with an STI, and no more symptoms for years. Although having an open sore certainly means that you're highly contagious, the fact that you have no symptoms at all doesn't mean that you can't give someone else the disease.

>> Just because your partner has no outward signs of having a sexually transmitted disease doesn't mean that your partner is disease free; because your partner may never have had any symptoms, they can pass something on to you in all innocence.

If you want to remain healthy, you must act as if there's an invading army camped out all around your bedside (or couch, or kitchen table . . . we don't judge).

Exploring the Facts and Figures

Before we dive in to the STIs that men most commonly face, we want to provide some context for you.

Because the sexual invasion encompasses so many different STIs, it's a complicated battle to fight. Furthermore, since the arrival of HIV (described later in this chapter), the consequences of failure could be deadly.

REMEMBER

STIs aren't young men's issues or older men's issues, they're all men's issues. However, some male populations are more at risk than others. According to 2023 data from the Centers for Disease Control and Prevention:

>> Men ages 15–24 are more likely to be diagnosed with chlamydia, gonorrhea, and syphilis than older men.

>> Gay, bisexual, and other men who have sex with men are disproportionately impacted by STIs compared to men who have sex only with women.

Our advice, therefore, is to find yourself one partner, have yourselves tested for all the major STIs to make sure that you're both healthy, use condoms if you have any doubts about your respective health, and practice safer sex.

Identifying STIs: Battle Scars No One Wants after a Night of Sex

Despite our advice, we know many of you will have more than one sexual partner throughout your life, so when you're sexually active you could encounter some sexually transmitted infections. In this section, we cover the main infections you might encounter, starting with those that are most commonly reported for men. And we also cover some infections that are more common in women but which you're at risk of getting if you have sex with women.

Although the figures used in this book apply to the United States, which keeps careful statistics, they generally hold true throughout the developed world. Developing countries vary widely in the incidence and prevalence of STIs. As they say, to be forewarned is to be forearmed; read this list carefully so you can become as familiar as possible with the enemy.

And two quick points before we get into the details of STIs:

>> **If you have a sexually transmitted disease or even *think* that you may, see a doctor.** This advice may sound obvious, but too many people don't seek medical help, probably because of embarrassment. They may be embarrassed because they don't want to reveal their sex life or because they don't want to submit to an exam of their most private parts, or both.

>> **Don't self-prescribe medication or use your friend's.** If a doctor has prescribed a medication for one person, a friend of that person with similar symptoms might ask to use that medicine too. Sharing prescriptions is a bad idea. Even doctors sometimes have difficulties diagnosing which STI is which. By taking the wrong medication, you may make your situation worse.

Genital warts and HPV

Approximately 14 million people are infected in the United States every year with genital warts, which are caused by the *human papillomavirus (HPV)*. HPV has become so common that it is estimated that 80 percent of sexually active people contract it at some point. Among people between the ages of 15 and 49, only one in four Americans has *not* had a genital HPV infection, though in most cases the virus is harmless and exhibits no symptoms. Genital warts are spread through vaginal, anal, and oral intercourse. They can also be passed on to infants during childbirth.

>> Not always visible, the warts are soft and flat; they grow on the genitals, in the *urethra* (the tube that carries urine and semen out of the body), in the inner vagina, in the anus, or in the throat.

>> The warts often itch and, if allowed to grow, can block openings of the vagina, anus, or throat, causing discomfort.

>> Because genital warts can be microscopic and therefore unseen by the naked eye, they can easily be passed to sexual partners.

High-risk strains of HPV do exist and in women can cause cervical lesions, which, over a period of time, can develop into cervical cancer if untreated. Doctors can detect HPV lesions with annual Pap smears. The use of Pap smears has drastically reduced the incidence of cervical cancer.

Even better than early detection is prevention. A vaccine exists against some of the types of HPV that cause 70 percent of cervical cancer and 90 percent of genital warts. Developed by Merck, the vaccine is called Gardasil, and health officials recommend that boys aged 11 to 12 as well as all girls and women between the ages of 9 and 26 be vaccinated.

Doctors can treat genital warts in several ways, including topical medical creams, some of which require a prescription and some of which don't.

Over-the-counter medications for other types of warts should not be used on the genitals.

In cases of either large or persistent warts, other treatments may include surgical removal, freezing using liquid nitrogen, or cauterization by electric needles. Because doctors have no cure for HPV, genital warts can reoccur, and the virus can remain in the person's cells indefinitely, though often in a *latent* (or not active) state. Most people who have reoccurring genital warts have only one more episode. Even in rare cases of people with multiple reoccurrences, the body's immune system usually develops immunity within two years. On the other hand, removing a person's genital warts does not mean that they can't transmit the disease.

Although condoms offer some protection against the spread of HPV, they provide no guarantee against its transmission because they don't cover the entire genital area.

Chlamydia

Chlamydia affected 1.6 million Americans in 2023, with young people ages 15–24 being most reported. And in 2020, the World Health Organization (www.who.int) estimated 128.5 million new infections, to give you a sense of the prevalence globally. It can be transmitted through vaginal, anal, or oral sex. It is even carried in the man's Cowper's fluid ("precum").

>> The first symptoms of chlamydia in men are usually painful urination and pus coming from the urethra. Chlamydia often has no overt symptoms in women.

>> Symptoms may start within a few days after sexual exposure.

>> In men, the organism is thought to be responsible for half the cases of *epididymitis*, an infection of the epididymis (a series of tiny tubes that lie on top of the testicle), which can cause painful swelling of the testicle.

>> In women, the disease can cause scarring of the fallopian tubes, sterility, infertility, ectopic pregnancy, or chronic pelvic pain.

Although doctors can successfully treat chlamydia with doxycycline or other antibiotics (a single-dose version is available), they often have difficulty diagnosing the disease because of the lack of visible symptoms. People who have chlamydia and don't take all the medicine for the full time that it's prescribed often get the disease again (because they aren't fully cured the first time). Because gonorrhea often accompanies chlamydia, doctors usually treat the two together.

Although most people who have chlamydia have no symptoms and thus don't even know they have the disease, they can still suffer the long-range consequences. Because chlamydia is so common, people who have sex with multiple partners, especially if they don't use a condom or dental dam, should be tested whenever they change partners or after any unprotected sex with a new partner.

Gonorrhea

In the United States, the number of reported cases of gonorrhea declined slightly from 2022 to 2023, but over 600,000 cases of gonorrhea still were reported in 2023. Fifty percent of women and 10 percent of men with the disease show no symptoms, so they don't know they have it. When symptoms do occur, men may have pain during urination or a puslike discharge from the urethra. Women may have a green or yellow-green discharge from the vagina; frequent, often burning urination; pelvic pain; swelling or tenderness of the vulva; and possibly arthritic-like pain in the shoulder.

>> Gonorrhea can be spread through vaginal, anal, or oral sex.

>> Gonorrhea can cause sterility, arthritis, heart problems, and disorders of the central nervous system.

>> In women, gonorrhea can cause pelvic inflammatory disease, which can lead to ectopic pregnancies, sterility, or even the formation of abscesses.

Penicillin was the treatment of choice for gonorrhea, but because more recent strains of the disease have become penicillin-resistant, doctors now use a drug called ceftriaxone. Gonorrhea is often accompanied by chlamydia, and so doctors often treat them together.

Syphilis

Syphilis was first noticed in Europe in the 15th century, coinciding with the return of Christopher Columbus from the New World. No one knows for sure whether the disease came from America or West Africa, but it caused a tremendous epidemic with a high fatality rate.

Although syphilis isn't as prevalent as it once was, in 2021, men reported higher rates of syphilis than women across all age groups, with the highest rate reported by men aged 25-29.

Syphilis is caused by a spiral-shaped, snail-like microscopic organism called *Treponema pallidum*. Because syphilis resembles so many other diseases, it is known as "the great imitator." The disease progresses over a long period of years with different stages along the way.

>> The primary syphilitic lesion is the *chancre*: a circular, painless, and firm sore that appears at the site of the invasion either on the lips, mouth, tongue, nipples, rectum, or genitals anywhere from 9 to 90 days after infection.

Six to ten weeks later, the chancre heals by itself, followed by a symptomless time (latent period) of anywhere from six weeks to six months before symptoms of secondary syphilis appear.

>> Secondary syphilis is marked by rashes of various types that don't itch and that heal without scars. These rashes indicate that the microbes have traveled through the bloodstream and lymphatic system to every organ and tissue in the body.

Secondary syphilis is followed by another symptomless period, which can last a lifetime, or the disease can reappear after a number of years.

>> Tertiary syphilis attacks the nervous system and can destroy skin, bone, and joints as well as interrupt the blood supply to the brain. Syphilis can be deadly in this last phase.

Syphilis is passed from one person to another during vaginal intercourse, anal intercourse, kissing, and oral/genital contact. The disease is especially contagious while the sores are present in the primary stage.

WARNING

Treatment with long-acting forms of penicillin is effective for primary, secondary, and latent syphilis; however, the damage caused by tertiary syphilis can't be reversed by penicillin therapy.

Human immunodeficiency virus (HIV) and AIDS

If you've heard of only one sexually transmitted disease, that one is likely the *acquired immunodeficiency syndrome* (AIDS), which is linked to infections by the *human immunodeficiency virus* (HIV). Why is so much more attention given to this disease than to any other STI? The answer is quite simple: AIDS has the potential to be deadly, and it has no cure and no vaccine.

HIV now infects a little more than 1 million people in the United States (although 1 in 7 don't know it) but close to 40 million people worldwide. Of the nearly 1.3 million new cases acquired in 2023, about 39,000 occurred in the United States. In 2023, 630,000 people around the world died of AIDS, about half the total of 2010.

HIV is most commonly passed on through sexual activity or by shared needles. HIV can also be passed through transfusions of contaminated blood products (though since 1985 all blood is screened for HIV in the United States), from a woman to her fetus during pregnancy, and through breastfeeding.

Although HIV has been detected in small quantities in body fluids such as saliva, feces, urine, and tears, to date no evidence exists that HIV can spread through these body fluids, despite extensive testing. You can't contract HIV or AIDS by touching someone who has the disease, by being coughed or sneezed on by that person, by sharing a glass with that person, or through any other routine contact that may take place.

WARNING

HIV/AIDS poses serious risks, so you should take it seriously. Consider the following:

>> HIV infections weaken the body's ability to fight disease, causing acquired immunodeficiency syndrome (AIDS) and other health problems.

>> A person can be infected by HIV and not show any symptoms for up to ten years.

>> If AIDS develops, a variety of different ailments may attack the body, leading to death.

Two known human immunodeficiency viruses exist, HIV-1 and HIV-2. They both cause disease by infecting and destroying blood cells called *lymphocytes* that protect the body against infection. HIV-1 is most common in Western countries; HIV-2 occurs most frequently in Africa.

Diagnosis, symptoms, and treatment

Doctors diagnose HIV infection with tests to detect HIV antibodies in the blood. These antibodies usually appear in the bloodstream three to eight weeks after infection, though it may take as long as three months for these antibodies to show up. Because of this window of time, a person can have a negative HIV test and still be able to pass the disease to others. In addition, the first 60 days after being infected with the virus is a period of high contagion. For that reason, you should always use a condom; it's impossible to really know whether or not a partner can infect you.

Initial symptoms of HIV infection may resemble those of a common nonsexual disease, mononucleosis: high fevers, swollen glands, and night sweats. After that you may go through a period, which commonly lasts for years, during which you have no symptoms. Eventually, as the body's immune system weakens from fighting HIV, some *opportunistic microbe* — an organism that the body's immune system would normally dispose of — causes an infection, such as pneumonia, that just won't go away. At this point, a doctor usually discovers that the person is infected with HIV and diagnoses a case of AIDS. Whether or not someone infected with HIV will develop AIDS depends greatly on whether or not they get treated, and sadly, that may depend on their financial situation. Life expectancy has been greatly extended when HIV is treated, but the cost of this treatment is significant (outlined later in the chapter). Life expectancy is shorter for those people infected by transfusions of blood or blood products and for people who don't get good medical care.

Medical science has, as yet, produced no vaccine against HIV/AIDS, nor has it found a cure. The medical field has developed many different drugs that can now help prolong the life of a person with HIV and manage the various symptoms. Three basic categories of drugs exist. First are the *antiretroviral drugs* (ART) that inhibit the growth and multiplication of HIV at various steps in its life cycle. Doctors prescribe these drugs in groups known as *cocktails.* Other drugs fight the opportunistic infections that may occur because HIV lowers the immune system's ability to fight them.

REMEMBER

While a person infected with HIV and taking ART cannot be said to be cured, their *viral load* (the amount of HIV viruses in their system) is much lower, to the point where it is believed the virus cannot be transferred to another person. In addition, someone having sex with an HIV-positive person could take a Pre-Exposure Prophylaxis (PrEP) that would further reduce any risk of infection.

Studies have shown that male circumcision can reduce a man's chances of being infected by HIV by 60 percent. It is believed that the warm, moist environment under the foreskin can be a breeding ground for HIV. While this is not a guaranteed preventative measure, it is a factor to be considered among high-risk male populations.

Good news and bad news

That doctors today can offer treatments that both prolong the life of someone infected with HIV and prevent virus transmission is wonderful news. But HIV diagnoses among some gay and bisexual men (particularly those aged 25-44) increased from 2018 to 2022, suggesting a return to risky behavior that had been declining. By not practicing safer sex, these men, while less at risk of dying of AIDS, are at risk for catching many other STIs.

And although big steps have been taken in the fight against AIDS, one mustn't forget the cost of treatment. The actual cost will depend on the amount of contagion, but $10,000 a year is on the lower end. Since many young people, who are most likely to get infected, don't have health insurance, this can be quite a burden. And even those with insurance may face significant co-pay costs, depending on their health plan.

Hepatitis B

Hepatitis B is one of two sexually transmitted diseases for which a preventive vaccine exists. (A vaccine is available for human papillomavirus [HPV]. See the "Genital warts and HPV" section in this chapter for more details.) Hepatitis B is very contagious, 100 times more so than HIV. Hepatitis B can be transmitted through intimate contact as well as sexual contact, so sharing the same toothbrush, exchanging bodily fluids during sex, or sharing needles can transmit the disease. Healthcare workers are particularly susceptible and almost always get vaccinated.

>> Hepatitis B can cause severe liver disease or death, but the virus often has no symptoms during its most contagious phases.

>> Reported cases have fallen from about 240,000 a year to only 20,000, though it's estimated that more than a million carriers of the disease remain.

Normally your immune system can get rid of hepatitis B, but if you're diagnosed with chronic active Hep B, several drugs can help you get rid of the infection, including Entecavir and Tenofovir.

Herpes

Herpes, which is caused by the *herpes simplex virus* (HSV), is another incurable STI. Herpes actually has two forms: herpes simplex–type 1 (HSV-1) and herpes simplex–type 2 (HSV-2). HSV-1 is most often associated with cold sores and fever blisters "above the waist." The World Health Organization (www.who.int)

estimates that 64 percent of people globally have HSV-1, or oral herpes, and that 20 percent of adults worldwide have HSV-2, or genital herpes, though most are not aware of it, and their symptoms are too mild to notice, but they can still pass the disease on.

The most common symptoms of genital herpes arise from a rash with clusters of white, blistery sores appearing on the penis, mouth, anus, vagina, cervix, or other parts of the body. This rash can cause pain, itching, burning sensations, swollen glands, fever, headache, and a run-down feeling. The first symptoms may be more severe than the symptoms of later outbreaks because the immune system is not as well prepared to fight off the disease the first time around. However, a person may have no symptoms whatsoever, and their first outbreak may occur months or even years after exposure. HSV-2 symptoms can occur on the thighs, buttocks, anus, or pubis. People who suffer only mild symptoms may mistake them for some other condition, such as insect bites, jock itch, yeast infections, hemorrhoids, or ingrown hair follicles. Some lesions may be so small that they remain invisible to the human eye. And if a small lesion appears inside a woman's vagina, she will never see it.

These symptoms may return at regular intervals, sometimes caused by stress, menstrual periods, or other factors that aren't well understood. Although these symptoms can lead to discomfort, they aren't dangerous, and herpes doesn't affect the immune system or lead to other health problems.

Because of oral sex, doctors are finding that some cases of genital herpes are actually caused by HSV-1, the virus that causes oral herpes, and that some cases of herpes located on the mouth have been caused by HSV-2, genital herpes. For those who believe oral sex is safe sex, this should serve as proof that it's not.

WARNING

Most people think that herpes is contagious only when the sores are present, but studies have shown that some people may spread the disease during the few days just before an outbreak called *prodrome*, when they have no sores, and possibly even at other times even in people who have never had an outbreak. An infected person may figure out how to recognize the warning signs that occur during prodrome, which may include itching, tingling, or a painful feeling where the lesions will develop.

>> During pregnancy, herpes may cause miscarriage or stillbirth, and the disease can be passed on to newborns, especially if the mother contracts the disease during her third trimester. A mother who has herpes before this usually passes on her antibodies to the baby.

>> If the sores are active during childbirth, they pose serious health consequences for the babies. To avoid these consequences, doctors usually

perform cesarean sections when active sores are visible during the time of childbirth.

>> If you have herpes, you should always use a condom when having sex, unless your partner already has the disease.

WARNING

Although you should always use a condom, condoms can't entirely protect you from herpes. If a man has the disease and the only sores are on his penis, then a condom offers some protection to his partner. However, secretions may leak over the pelvic area not protected by the condom. And if the herpes virus is being shed from another part of the body, such as the hips or buttocks, a condom offers no protection at all.

Herpes can spread beyond genital contact to other parts of the already-infected person's body. If you touch a herpes sore, always wash your hands thoroughly before touching anyone else or any other part of your body.

WARNING

Be aware that oral herpes can be transmitted by kissing, sharing towels, or drinking from the same glass or cup.

Developments in the treatment of herpes include new, more accurate tests, and although doctors still have no cure for herpes, new medications are effective at keeping the virus in check. Zovirax (acyclovir) has been available since the 1970s and can now be obtained in generic form. Valtrex (valacyclovir) and Famvir (famciclovir) have a more active ingredient and are better absorbed and need to be taken less frequently. See a doctor if you suspect that you have the disease, both to make sure that herpes really is the cause of the symptoms and to learn how to live with herpes and not spread it to others. If you are infected, the doctor can give you a set of rules to follow to help keep you from spreading the virus to other people or other parts of your body. Studies also have shown that if someone whose partner has herpes takes Valtrex, their chances of becoming infected are much less.

REMEMBER

Researchers now believe that herpes lesions act as an entryway for HIV, so that people infected by herpes are much more likely to become infected with HIV if they come in contact with the virus. So although herpes itself may not be deadly, having herpes can have deadly consequences.

The U.S. Centers for Disease Control and Prevention (CDC, www.cdc.gov) does not recommend testing for HSV because the tests are expensive, often lead to false positives, and seemingly don't change people's behavior. The CDC does recommend that you ask your doctor whether you should be tested, and because part of that decision will rely on telling your doctor your complete sexual history (such as whether you've had multiple partners), it's important that you be honest when having this discussion. And if you're diagnosed and have any feelings of guilt, shame, or depressions related to the diagnosis — all of which are not uncommon — talk with your doctor so you can get mental health support as well as physical.

Pubic lice

Pubic lice, also called *crabs,* is spread primarily through sexual contact, and less likely by coming in contact with infected bedding and clothing. Their bites cause intense itching. Because they are visible to the naked eye, you can check yourself if you have any symptoms. The lice are the size of a pinhead, oval, and grayish, unless they are filled with your blood, in which case they are more orange.

You can treat pubic lice yourself with over-the-counter medications including Kwell, A-200, and RID. In addition, you should thoroughly wash in hot water or dry-clean all bedding and clothing that has come into contact with the lice.

Molluscum contagiosum

The *Molluscum contagiosum* virus can cause a small, pinkish-white, waxy-looking, polyplike growth in the genital area or on the thighs. It is spread by sexual inter-course but can also be spread through other intimate contact. While Molluscum contagiosum growths will usually disappear on their own, it can take up to five years. Doctors can usually treat it by removing the growths either with chemicals, electric current, or freezing.

Trichomoniasis

Usually called "trich," trichomoniasis is one of the most common vaginal infec-tions, causing about one-fourth of all cases of *vaginitis* (inflammation of the vagina). Men rarely have symptoms, and many women have no symptoms. Symptoms that men may experience include pain when urinating or ejaculating, an increased urge to urinate, discharge from the penis, and irritation around the head of the penis or foreskin.

Doctors can treat trichomoniasis with antibiotics, and any sexual partners should be treated as well to prevent reinfection. The biggest danger from being infected is the higher risk of HIV if it is present in a partner.

Candidiasis

Often called a yeast infection, candidiasis is actually caused by a fungus, *candida*, that normally lives in people's mouths and intestines, as well as in the vaginas of many healthy women. When the body's normal acidity doesn't control the growth of this fungus, an overgrowth can occur. Candidiasis is the result. Its symptoms can include itching or irritation of the penis, testicles or vulva; a yeasty odor; a thick, white, cottage cheese-like vaginal discharge; and, sometimes, a bloated feeling and change in bowel habits.

>> Candida can also appear in the mouth, throat, or tongue; when it does, the disease is called *thrush*.

>> Candida is not usually spread as an STI, but it can be — more likely through oral sex than intercourse. Unfortunately, some couples transmit it back and forth in what can seem to be a never-ending cycle.

Among the factors that can lead to abnormal growth of candida are birth control pills, antibiotics, pregnancy, diabetes, HIV infection (or any other immune system dysfunction), douching, a woman's monthly period, and damp underwear.

Prescriptions for antifungal creams, ointments, or suppositories are the normal cures. Single-dose oral antifungals have also recently become available and are highly effective. Over-the-counter products may work, but should only be used by women for vaginal yeast infections.

WARNING

Some of the medicines used to treat a yeast infection may weaken latex condoms. If you use condoms as a form of birth control and disease prevention, consult with your pharmacist or doctor.

Being Safer about Sex

Doctors have no vaccine against HIV/AIDS. They have no cure for herpes. You can get STIs that have no symptoms but can later leave you sterile. Are you scared of catching an STI? If you're not, you should be — scared enough to practice safer sex.

We deliberately use the term *safer sex*. Truly *safe* sex means celibacy. Safe sex *can* also mean monogamous sex with an uninfected partner, but, sorry to say, one mistake by one of you (perhaps even before you met because some of these diseases don't make themselves known for years) can lead to both of you becoming infected, so we're really back to *safer* sex.

Certainly the fewer partners you have, the less risk you have, but catching a disease can happen in only one instance with an infected partner.

WARNING

Remember, when you sleep with someone, you're also sleeping with the germs of every partner that this person ever had.

Remembering that condoms give good, not great, protection

And what about condoms? Condoms offer protection — that is absolutely true. But condoms do not offer absolute protection against AIDS or the other STIs. Why?

>> Condoms sometimes break.

>> Condoms can break down in the presence of oil-based products.

>> Condoms sometimes leak when you take them off.

>> People sometimes forget to use condoms.

>> Even people who do use condoms for intercourse often don't use them for oral sex, which — while less risky — is not safe.

Some STIs are spread through contact with other parts of the genitals, including any leakage of vaginal fluids.

So the best preventive measure is a combination of responsible sexual behavior and condom use.

Having a relationship before you have sex

We know that finding one person to fall in love with when you're both young and sticking with that person for the rest of your life is difficult. That situation is ideal for preventing STIs, but it's unrealistic to assume that everybody can do that. You may not be ready for a long-term relationship when you're young, or at some point you may get divorced, or your partner may pass away. Most people have multiple partners throughout their lives, and so most people are at risk.

No matter what age you are, having a relationship with someone before you have sex with them allows you to first build emotional intimacy. This, in turn, makes it easier to talk about STI risks, and if you or your partner has AIDs or an STI, the closeness you've developed in your relationship makes it easier to navigate the steps you can take together to minimize risk of sharing that STI.

Avoiding being a silent partner

In our society, more people are willing to engage in sexual activity together than to talk about it, and a good deal of the blame for sexually transmitted infections comes from this failure to communicate.

You all know the Golden Rule about doing unto others as you would have them do unto you. If you planned to have sex with someone and they had a sexually transmitted infection, wouldn't you want them to tell you in advance? The same applies to you: If you have a sexually transmitted infection, you have to tell any potential partners. Notice that we said *potential* because we won't hide the fact that, if you tell somebody that you have an STI, that person may suddenly run in the opposite direction. On the other hand, with an infection like herpes or HIV, if you warn the other party and they take the proper medical precautions, the odds of that partner contracting your infection are greatly reduced. That doesn't mean some potential partners won't reject you because of your honesty, but you have to accept that. You cannot go around infecting other people.

Some of you may want to be honest but are saying to yourselves right now, "How do I talk to a potential partner about STIs?"

The answer is very simple: You just do it. If you have the gumption to have sex with somebody, then don't tell us that you can't work up the courage to open this subject. We're not saying doing so is easy. We *are* saying it's not impossible, and that you have to do it.

Timing your AIDS and STI talk

Despite our recommendation to do so, we know that not everybody waits to form a strong relationship before having sex, so the issue of STIs can come up before the two people involved are really a couple. They may have to ask some very intimate and personal questions of each other before they really know each other all that well.

Now you may believe that if a couple is ready to *have* sex, then they should be ready to at least talk about it. But these days sex can precede real intimacy, so a discussion about STIs must also be inserted at an earlier stage. If both parties clearly want to have sex and deliberately look for a simple assurance of probable good health, then this conversation may be no more than a speed bump on the way to the bedroom. But if one person is not confident of the other person's desire to have sex, how should the discussion of AIDS and other STIs be handled?

Let us give you some possible scenarios.

Paul and Juliette

Paul and Juliette have had five dates, and they haven't had sex yet. Their last date was with another couple. They'd gone out dancing, and during the last few slow dances, Paul had held Juliette very close. He'd had an erection, and rather than pull away from him, Juliette had pushed her pelvis into his. To Paul, it was a clear sign that Juliette was ready to have sex with him, but because their friends were driving, Paul had to content himself with a goodnight kiss when they dropped Juliette off at her place.

During the week, he called Juliette and asked her to dinner. He picked a place that was about six blocks from where she lived. When he arrived, he parked his car and suggested they walk. After a little bit of banter, he sucked in his breath and asked her: "Do you think it's too early in our relationship to be talking about AIDS testing?" She answered, "No, Paul, I don't," and the discussion that needed to take place did.

By posing the question this way, Paul didn't presume that they were going to have sex. He left it to Juliette to decide. If she'd wanted to wait longer, she could easily have told him so. But, because she was ready to have sex with him, the discussion was able to proceed smoothly. They were both interested in the same goal.

Fran and Tony

Fran met Tony the day after he moved into her apartment complex. She saw him again later at the grocery store, where he was stocking up on supplies. She ended up cooking him dinner that night. He was very busy those first few weeks setting up his apartment and starting a new job, but they did get together for a drink a few times and once for a quick dinner at a local Mexican place.

Tony finally had a weekend off. This time he offered to take her to a French restaurant that Fran really loved. They had a great meal and shared a bottle of champagne that went to Fran's head a little bit. When they got back to the apartment complex, instead of heading their separate ways, as they'd done previously, Tony invited Fran inside and she accepted. They had some bourbon while sitting on his new sofa, and soon Fran found herself wrapped in his arms. Her clothes started coming off, and not too much later he was leading her to the bedroom, their clothes scattered over the living room floor.

As they lay down on the bed, Fran asked Tony: "You don't have any . . . uh . . . diseases, do you?"

"No way," he said, "I'm not one of those guys who'll sleep with just anybody." A little voice inside of Fran started to whisper something, but at that point she was somewhat tipsy, very aroused, and totally naked, and so she didn't bother listening.

What that little voice inside of Fran was trying to tell her was that, although Tony was saying that he wasn't that kind of guy, here he was ready to hook up with someone he barely knew. Was that really the first time he'd done that?

REMEMBER

Most people in Fran's position would have done exactly what she did — give in to the moment. That's why you must have the STI and AIDS discussion long before that moment arrives. Don't wait until you're in a situation where it could be embarrassing to suddenly pull back, but also difficult to resist going ahead when desires are high. Especially exhibit caution when drugs or alcohol are involved. You have to be realistic about sex and know that your ability to resist temptation is not infinite. You have to protect yourself in many ways, not just with a piece of rubber.

Speaking of rubber, what if Tony had added, "And anyway, I'm using a condom"? Would that have made it okay?

Not necessarily, because condoms can break or fall off or leak. Even if a condom stays on in one piece, a condom still may not be enough to protect you from STIs — several STIs can be passed simply from contact with an infected person's pubic area (as explained earlier in the chapter).

REHEARSING THE TALK

TIP

If you think that you might have difficulties having such a talk, why not ask a friend to role-play with you so you can practice what you'll say. By rehearsing this talk, you'll find it much easier to actually have it. And don't get down on yourself because you feel awkward — STIs are an awkward subject, without a doubt, and talking about them doesn't come easily to anybody. Knowing that your potential partner will also be feeling strange won't necessarily make it easier to bring up, but maybe it'll give you more courage.

SETTING YOURSELF SOME BOUNDARIES

Whether or not you listen to our advice about forming a relationship before jumping into bed, you can make it easier to avoid the type of situation that Fran faced (see earlier in this section). How do you avoid that?

TIP

Make yourself a resolution that you'll never get undressed until you're sure that doing so is safe. If she grabs hold of your zipper or he starts to unbutton your shirt, tell your partner to stop and explain why you're stopping them. Tell them that your reluctance isn't because you don't want to become intimate — assuming that you do — but because you need to talk about safer sex first.

BODILY CONTACT IS NOT THE ONLY RISK

You may have heard that you can't contract an STI from a toilet seat, and that's true — but what about a sex toy? If your toys, such as a vibrator, are only used by you, then they're safe. But if you share toys, either sterilize them in between partners or cover them with a condom.

And this goes for drug paraphernalia, particularly needles, as well. Since you can't cover them with a condom, never share a needle with anyone. And remember that shared joints or hookah pipes/bongs can also harbor viruses.

After having this conversation, you may both decide to renew your activities, possibly stopping at a prearranged point or maybe going all the way, depending on what you said. Whatever the final outcome, at least you'll know that the decision was calculated and not left to chance.

Discovering a potential partner's character

Although it's difficult to have the STI talk, besides protecting yourself from disease, you gain another benefit from having this talk, and that's what you'll learn about a potential partner's character. We're pretty sure you want a sexual partner to be honest, aboveboard, and caring. We want to tell you that when you bring up the subject of being tested for STIs, you're going to learn a lot about how honest, aboveboard, and caring this person really is. By the time the conversation is over, you'll know whether you want to get extremely intimate with this person.

One of the authors of *Men's Health For Dummies* wrote a book about herpes, and spoke to many people who have herpes and who've had to have this talk many times. These interviewees all reported the same thing — yes, they were nervous to begin STI conversations, but they all said that what they discovered about these potential partners was invaluable. And although some of these people were rejected because they acknowledged having herpes, they also ended up rejecting potential partners because of the way that person handled the STI discussion.

Minimizing your risks

After reading the descriptions of sexually transmitted diseases in this chapter, it's possible you'll decide that maybe sex isn't worth the risk, and therefore planning for various scenarios isn't needed. That reaction may fail you when you most need it.

What do we mean by that? At some point, you'll be with somebody you're very attracted to sexually and who's attracted to you. Maybe you'll be in your apartment, or maybe in the other person's. And you'll be kissing, hugging, and stroking each other. Temperatures will start going up. Clothes will start coming off. An erection will be on the loose. A comfortable bed will be nearby. You'll both be absolutely ready to have sex, and you won't have a condom handy.

In that scenario, will you remember this chapter and all these unpleasant and potentially deadly sexually transmitted infections? Will you be willing to say no, or to put your clothes back on and go find a 24-hour drugstore? Or will you say to heck with the risks and jump into bed?

TIP

Although some of you may have the fortitude to place caution ahead of passion, many of you won't. For that reason, you have to be prepared ahead of time. Carry a condom in your wallet or pocket, and keep one in your glove compartment or bedside table. (And remember that heat can degrade condoms, so regularly swap out unused ones for new if some of your storage spots are consistently warmer than room temperature. See Chapter 12 for more condom cautions.)

REMEMBER

We want to make sure that you have the best sex possible. And an integral part of great sex is healthy sex, protected sex. Although, in the heat of passion, you may well be willing to take any risk, afterwards, if you catch one of these infections — especially AIDS — you'll regret that orgasm for the rest of your life. So have great sex, and be careful. In fact, have terrific sex and be very careful.

IN THIS CHAPTER

» **Curing premature ejaculation**

» **Combating erectile dysfunction**

» **Identifying delayed ejaculation**

» **Treating the permanent erection**

» **Getting bent out of shape over Peyronie's disease**

» **Restoring desire**

Chapter **14**

When Your Equipment's Not Cooperating

The word macho and sexual dysfunction aren't good teammates, which is why many men refuse to acknowledge any difficulties they may have in the sexual arena. The problem with insisting on maintaining a tough guy image is that instead of getting the help they may need, many men suffer needlessly, and that usually means their partner suffers as well.

But, as reluctant to admit it as you or any man may be, many men do suffer from a sexual problem of one sort or another, at least at certain times in their lives. Sometimes sexual problems can result from disease, such as testicular or prostate cancer. (We discuss these in Chapter 16.) But, lucky for you, the most common male sexual problem isn't a physical problem at all, but a learning disability.

This chapter covers those problems you may be embarrassed to talk about — premature ejaculation, impotency, curved penises, delayed ejaculation, and lack of desire — as well as the one problem you may secretly be glad to have on some level — permanent erections. As our knowledge of the human body has advanced, better treatments have been developed for many of these conditions, and we talk about those too.

TIP

We hope that if you have any of the problems mentioned in this chapter, or if you ever develop them, you won't turn your back on them but instead will take some positive action. Many men act as though their genitals are separate from the rest of their bodies and not totally under their control. But, of course, that is ridiculous. So if something is bothering you, take charge and get the problem fixed.

Understanding Premature Ejaculation

The subject that people ask us about most often is premature ejaculation. Men who suffer from the problem seek our help, as do their partners, who also suffer as a result of the problem.

People have all sorts of ideas about why a man can't keep his erection as long as he wants to and what he can do to make himself last longer, but we don't think most of these so-called treatments are effective. We give you a surefire solution for premature ejaculation in the section, "The real cure: Recognizing the premonitory sensation."

Defining the dilemma

What is *premature ejaculation* (PE)? The definition that we use is that a man is a premature ejaculator when he can't keep himself from ejaculating before he wants to. Notice that we said before *he* wants to, not his partner. That distinction is important. And the cause is not physical, but mental. In other words, it's not the man's penis that is "malfunctioning," but his brain.

Just how long is the period of time a man needs to last? The time frame depends on the man. If your partner reaches their orgasm after 20 minutes of intercourse, you want to aim to last for that amount of time. If they don't climax through intercourse at all, then maybe you only want to last for 10 minutes. What's important is that you learn how to gain control of when you have your orgasm, so you can decide when to ejaculate instead of ejaculating because of circumstances beyond your control.

As with many sexual dysfunctions, different degrees of premature ejaculation exist. Some men are so severely afflicted that they can't last long enough to have penetrative intercourse. Some men even climax in their pants at the very thought that they may have sex. But even a man who can penetrate his partner and last 15 minutes may fall under the umbrella of premature ejaculator if he wants to last 5 extra minutes and can't do so.

Does circumcision make a difference?

The penis of a man who hasn't been circumcised is often more sensitive than a circumcised man's (see Chapter 11). The reason for this is that the *glans,* or head, of a circumcised penis gets toughened by coming into contact with the man's underwear all day without the protection of the foreskin. (We say underwear, but if you prefer to go commando, it doesn't matter what you call the cloth your penis rubs against — the effect is the same.)

We don't know of any scientific study on the effects of circumcision with regard to premature ejaculation, but for most men who ejaculate prematurely, the problem is in their heads on top of their necks — not the heads of their penises. So we don't believe that circumcision makes a significant difference. Most certainly a man who isn't circumcised can learn how to prolong his climax just as effectively as a man who is.

The age factor

A young man's *libido* (sexual drive) is stronger than an older man's, so premature ejaculation is a problem that sometimes disappears, or at least decreases, with age. Mind you, we said *sometimes.* We've heard from men in their 80s who've suffered from premature ejaculation all their lives. And when we say that the problem lessens, we've also heard from men who were able to last 3 minutes instead of 2, so how much better is that? Our advice is not to wait for age to take care of this problem, but rather to act as soon as possible.

TECHNICAL STUFF

By the way, there are two types of PE — primary (meaning you've always had this condition) and secondary (meaning that you develop this condition later in life). Sometimes secondary can be psychological in nature, but sometimes there's a medical cause, such as the inflammation of the prostate, in which case medical treatment needs to be sought.

Home remedies

Talking to your doctor about penis problems can be uncomfortable for even the most confident guy, so many men decide to handle their PE situation by tinkering with their technique, rather than by seeking professional help. As you may expect, the results are mixed, so we don't recommend any of these ideas as certain solutions. But, if you're a DIY kinda dude, read on.

The "slide" technique

Probably the most common method that men use to control their orgasmic response is to think of something that isn't sexy. Woody Allen immortalized this technique in a film where, in the middle of making love, he yelled out, "Slide!" He was thinking about Jackie Robinson running the bases, instead of the woman he was with, in an attempt to delay his orgasm. (By the way, the film is *Everything You Wanted to Know About Sex But Were Afraid to Ask.*)

This technique can work to some degree, but it's not a good way of making love. This method makes a chore out of the sex act, rather than something pleasurable; your partner may sense that wall you put between you and the act and think you want to distance yourself from them.

Rubber love

Condoms do cut down on the sensations that a man has, and some men can control their premature ejaculation by using condoms. If one condom doesn't work, they put on two or more.

We certainly recommend that people use condoms — sometimes we sound like a broken record about it — but our goal is to prevent the spread of sexually transmitted infections (STIs — see Chapter 13 for more information). Using these same condoms as a crutch, lessening your pleasure, is a shame when a better PE solution exists. And using two condoms could actually make the condom less effective at protecting against disease and pregnancy (the condoms might tear when rubbing against each other).

Snake oil

You can find products on the market that supposedly lessen the sensations in the penis so the man can last longer. In the first place, we don't know whether these over-the-counter products really work, although you can buy prescription medications that deaden whatever body part you apply them to. But, even if all these products do the trick, just as with condoms that lessen sensation, why decrease your pleasure when you can have a permanent cure that doesn't need any numbing?

By the way, any cream that successfully numbs your penis would also reduce sensations from anything you place it in, so be sure to wipe it off before beginning intercourse, or else put on a condom.

Masturbation: Taking matters into your own hands

A method adopted by some young men is to masturbate before going on a date that may lead to sex (who can forget that scene in the movie *There's Something about Mary* when Mary unintentionally gets creative with "styling cream?"). The goal of this pregaming is to decrease the intensity of their desire for sex in the hopes of gaining some control.

Although this method sometimes works, it has several drawbacks:

>> Masturbation may not always be possible. What if the two of you are living together or married? Or what if your date pays a surprise visit ahead of time?

>> Another drawback is that of timing. What if you masturbate in anticipation of having sex after the date, but your partner wants to have sex before you go out, and you can't get an erection?

>> And then there's your enjoyment. The second orgasm may not be as pleasurable as the first, and, with all the worrying about when to masturbate, the sensory experience of sexual intercourse ends up being diminished.

TIP

When it comes to curing premature ejaculation, our advice is to keep your hands to yourself and practice some of the techniques found later in this chapter.

Different positions

Some men say that they have more control over their orgasms in one sexual position or another. The *missionary position* (when the man is on top) is probably the one in which men have the most problems when having sex with a woman, but not always. We even had one man write to us saying that he could control his climaxes if he was lying on his right side but not his left.

TECHNICAL STUFF

Some researchers have found that greater muscular tension can increase the tendency toward premature ejaculation, which means the missionary position (in which the man holds himself up with his arms) may accentuate premature ejaculation. But, because we really believe that this condition is a psychological one rather than a physical one, some psychological factors — different for each individual — may also come into play regarding positions.

If you find you have more control using some positions than others, then sticking to those positions is a possible solution — but not the most satisfactory one in the long run. If you limit yourself to that one position, sex may become boring. There's a solution that lets you try all the positions in the Kama Sutra if you want to! Which leads us to the next section with our recommended PE approach.

The real cure: Recognizing the premonitory sensation

The real cure for premature ejaculation is for you to be able to recognize the *premonitory sensation.* What is that, you ask? The premonitory sensation is that feeling that a man gets just before he reaches the point of no return, also called the *moment of inevitability.*

Each man has a certain threshold of pleasure; after he crosses it, he can't stop his orgasm. A fire engine may go through the bedroom, and he would still have an orgasm and ejaculate. But, right before he reaches that point, if he so desires, he can cool the fires and not ejaculate. And if he wants to abandon his status as premature ejaculator, he must learn to identify this sensation.

How do you learn to recognize this premonitory sensation? By treating your orgasm with kid gloves and approaching it very carefully. You're not the Road Runner, with his uncanny ability to stop dead in his tracks just before a cliff. Most men are more like Wile E. Coyote, trying to screech to a halt but ultimately plummeting into the canyon.

The idea, then, is to learn how to slow down the process before you get too close to the edge. Exactly how you do this depends on several factors, the biggest being whether you have a cooperative partner, with the emphasis on *cooperative.* Someone you've had sex with only a few times, and not very satisfactory sex at that, may not be willing to be as supportive as you need. But if you have someone who loves you, and who wants to make your sex life together better, then you're probably well on your way to curing the problem.

TIP

Although curing premature ejaculation as a couple may be easier, making progress alone isn't impossible. In other words, you can practice recognizing the premonitory sensation through masturbation and begin to develop some control. (Not every man can learn this control via masturbation, because sometimes a partner's presence is the cause of the overexcitement in the first place.) Practicing this technique alone probably takes more effort and more self-control, but it's certainly worth your time to see if it works for you.

The start-stop technique

One simple technique for treating premature ejaculation is called the *start-stop technique* — it involves learning how to recognize the premonitory sensation and stopping before you get to the point of inevitability. You do this by slowly increasing your level of arousal, stopping, allowing yourself to calm down, and then heading back upward again. Some people advise assigning numbers to the levels, from 1 to 10, with 10 being the point of no return. If that numbering system helps you, fine. If it distracts you, then just concentrate on the sensations.

When a couple comes to us looking to solve a case of premature ejaculation, we usually forbid them from having intercourse for a set time, as a way of removing the pressure from the situation. We don't want them to remain sexually frustrated, so we allow them to give each other orgasms after their lessons, but not through intercourse.

During a couple's first lessons, the partner uses their hand to arouse the man and stops the motion when he signals them to. Slowly, he begins to exercise more and more control. Depending on the man, this whole process can take a few weeks or a few months, but the process is almost always successful.

The squeeze technique

A variation of the start-stop technique is called the *squeeze technique.* With this method, rather than merely stopping stimulation to the penis, the man's partner gently squeezes the *frenum* of the penis (the strip of skin connecting the glans to the shaft on the underside of the penis) until the man loses his urge to ejaculate. Because the start-stop technique is usually effective, the squeeze technique isn't as commonly used.

TIP

Another useful aid in controlling premature ejaculation can be the *pubococcygeus (PC) muscle,* which, when squeezed, has a similar effect to the man's partner squeezing the base of the penis. The first thing you have to do is find this muscle. Put a finger behind your testicles. Pretend that you're going to urinate and then stop yourself. You'll feel a muscle tighten, and that's your PC muscle. If you exercise this muscle regularly by squeezing it in sets of ten, it will get stronger, and you can then use it to help control your ejaculations.

IS IT REALLY THAT SIMPLE?

When we describe the start-stop and squeeze techniques to some men, they look at us and say, "Is it really that simple?" The answer to their question is yes and no. The techniques are very simple, but involve some discipline, and that discipline is not always so simple.

Learning to exercise control isn't always easy. Look at all the people who can't stop themselves from overeating or smoking cigarettes. If premature ejaculation is a habit that has become highly ingrained, you can't assume that you can make it go away without some effort on your part. But, if you do put in the necessary time and effort, you can gain control over when you ejaculate.

Going for help

The start-stop and the squeeze techniques are often successful ways a man can end his premature ejaculation with the help of his partner or sometimes on his own via masturbation. But these self-help methods don't work for everyone — some men need the extra guidance provided by a sex therapist. In that case, our advice to you is to go and find one.

TIP

Another treatment option is selective serotonin reuptake inhibitors (SSRIs), otherwise known as antidepressants, which can help men overcome premature ejaculation (delayed orgasm is a side effect of some SSRIs). One of these has been created especially to treat PE, called Dapoxetine. Because it's short acting, it can help with PE without acting as a true antidepressant. Although this drug is sold specifically as a treatment for PE in other countries, it hasn't yet gotten the Food and Drug Administration's (FDA) approval for that function in the United States. In the meantime, your doctor could prescribe another antidepressant for "off label" use to help with PE.

Tackling Erectile Dysfunction

Erectile dysfunction (ED), also called *impotence,* is the term used when a man is unable to have an erection, and it's the second most common male sexual problem. The causes of ED can be either psychological or physical, and the degree of ED can vary from a simple loss of rigidity to a total inability to have an erection. Although ED can strike at any age, it becomes much more common as men grow older. Among men in their late 70s and beyond, some symptoms of ED are almost universal.

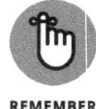

REMEMBER

Given the importance most men place on erections, we're quick to note that ED doesn't necessarily mean the end of a man's sex life. Depending on the cause of the problem, several possible solutions are usually available.

The precursor: Loss of instant erection

The most important point we can make about erectile dysfunction has to do not with ED itself, but with its precursor. The reason its precursor is so important is that it affects every man, at least every man who reaches a certain age in life, so pay careful attention to this section.

It sneaks up on you

Young men get erections all the time, often when they least expect to and at embarrassing moments. A variety of stimuli can cause these erections — something visual, such as the sight of an attractive person in short shorts; a fantasy about that person in the short shorts; or even just a whiff of scent that reminds the young man of that person in the short shorts. This type of erection is called a *psychogenic erection,* meaning it is stimulated by something that triggers the brain to release hormones that cause an erection.

At a certain age — and that age differs with every man, but ranges from his late 40s to early 60s — a man loses his ability to have a psychogenic erection. That ability usually doesn't disappear all at once; he begins to get fewer psychogenic erections and may not even notice at first. But eventually the decrease becomes apparent to him, and at some point, his psychogenic erections cease altogether.

This change can be a precursor to ED, but it's not ED because the men experiencing this change can still have erections. The only difference to a man's sexual functioning at this stage in life is that he needs direct physical stimulation to his penis to get an erection. He or his partner have to use their hands or mouth to make his penis erect.

Spreading the word

The loss of psychogenic erections wouldn't prove much of a problem if men expected the change, the way that women expect the hot flashes that accompany the start of menopause. Surprising, at least to us, is that so many people still have no idea that this change is part of the natural progression of growing older. This lack of knowledge causes the real problem.

WARNING

Many men think that they must be impotent when they can no longer get erections the way they used to. Rather than seeking help, they begin avoiding sex. When this happens, partners think that their husbands either are no longer attracted to them or that they are having an affair. Some couples fight over this problem; others withdraw from each other.

This breakdown of a relationship is so sad to us because it's not necessary. All that these couples have to do is include foreplay for the man. If they do this, then they have no problem.

TIP

We think that one of the reasons the loss of psychogenic erections isn't so widely known is that the condition doesn't really have a name. People may call it a symptom of so-called *male menopause,* but men don't like that phrase (and we really don't blame them) because it's really not appropriate. We need to coin a catchy phrase for this syndrome; then the media will pick up on it, and a lot of unhappiness can be prevented. We think a good name would be The Male Cooling Off Period.

Dealing with ED in older men

As a man gets older, his erections begin to get weaker and weaker, and he may need more and more stimulation to get an erection. Some older men can get an erection but can't keep it long enough to have intercourse. Sometimes they can get an erection, but the erection isn't stiff enough to allow for penetration.

These are all real, physical problems, but they don't necessarily spell the end of a man's sex life. If men understand that age causes these problems, and they take appropriate action, many men can continue to have sexual relations through their 90s.

The morning cure

For many men, the best solution to their problem with impotence is just to change their sex habits to suit their age. The easiest suggestion we can offer older men is to have sex in the morning instead of at night. Because you're probably retired and have no children at home, you have no reason to always try to have sex at night, except the force of habit. However, here are good reasons that illustrate how changing your routine can help you to become better lovers:

>> Older gentlemen are often tired after a long day. Getting the blood to flow into the penis is what an erection really is, so the more tired you are, the more difficult it is for this process to work correctly. In the morning, you have more energy, and so you can get erections more easily.

>> The male sex hormone, testosterone, is at its peak level in the morning and at its weakest at night. Because this hormone is instrumental in effecting erections, trying to get an erection in the morning makes a lot of sense.

Now, we don't recommend trying to have sex first thing in the morning, because the older you are the longer it takes you to get your body warmed up for "action" such as sex. Because you probably don't have to be on a rigid schedule, we suggest waking up, having a light breakfast, getting your blood flowing, and then taking your partner back to bed for a sexual interlude.

Some older men resist this suggestion at first. For some reason, doing all that planning doesn't suit them. But if they listen to us, many men find that the fires that had died down start burning once again.

The stuff technique

If some men think having sex after breakfast is strange, imagine how hard-headed some men are about the idea of trying to have sex without first having an erection. But sometimes this technique works the best.

TIP

The *stuff technique* is just what it sounds like. The man, with the help of his female partner, stuffs his nonerect penis into her vagina. Sometimes, after a man begins to thrust, the blood flows into his penis and that elusive erection finally rises to the occasion. The best position for doing this will depend on the physical condition of both partners. And because this technique doesn't always work — or may never work for some men — try it for a few minutes, and if it doesn't seem like an erection will occur, then drop it.

Managing short-term impotence

Unlike ED, short-term impotence is almost always psychological in nature. Many, many men, at one time or another, suffer from impotence — meaning that they can't have an erection when they want one. In fact, sometimes because they want an erection so badly these men fail, as Jimmy discovers in the following example.

Susan and Jimmy

Susan was a transfer student, and Jimmy spotted her the very first day he returned to college in his senior year. She had the type of looks he'd always dreamed of, and, to his amazement, when he struck up a conversation with her, she responded.

Jimmy had slept with a few other girls during his college years, but the thought of actually sleeping with Susan drove him wild. He managed to play it casual for a while, and, after a week went by, he asked her out on a date. She accepted, and they had a great time. They had a few more dates, each one advancing further than the last, so that, on his fifth date with her, Jimmy was pretty sure that they were going to have sex.

The anticipation was almost torture to Jimmy, and he had an erection for much of the day. They went to a dance and, with their bodies clinging to each other during all the slow dances, Jimmy felt that he was as ready for sex as he ever had been.

Jimmy had never had problems getting an erection, but as they were walking back toward his dorm, he started having doubts about his ability to please Susan. He was sure that someone as good-looking as Susan had had sex with all kinds of guys, and he began to question whether or not he could stand up to the test. By the time they got back to his room and took off their clothes, Jimmy was in a state of pure panic, and his penis reacted accordingly by staying limp. Jimmy was more embarrassed than he ever thought possible.

Anticipatory anxiety has caused many a Jimmy to experience similar problems. *Anticipatory anxiety* means the fear or expectation of a possible failure causes an actual failure. If a man starts worrying about his erection, usually doing so is enough to prevent him from having one. And the more he worries, the more likely that he will fail the next time he tries. Many men, because of one failed erection, have suffered through years of misery.

Visiting a urologist

In younger men, having erectile difficulties is usually psychological rather than physiological, so curing the problem is usually easy with the help of a sex therapist.

If a young man comes to us with a problem such as this, the first thing we do is send him to visit a *urologist,* which is a medical doctor who specializes in the care of the *genitourinary tract,* the urinary tract in men and women and the male genital tract.

>> One reason we send men who experience impotency to a urologist is to make sure that their problem isn't physical.

>> The other reason we send them off to have their physical plants checked out is that just getting that clean bill of health is often enough to clear up the problem.

   You see, many of these men worry so much about something being wrong with them that just hearing from a doctor that they're A-OK is enough to give their penises the psychological lift they need.

Even if the doctor's visit itself doesn't address a man's ED, it's a very good first step.

Building confidence

After sending an impotent client to a urologist, our next job is to build up his confidence in his penis back to what it was before he ran into trouble. Sometimes just getting him to masturbate does the trick. Sometimes we have him do certain confidence-building exercises with his partner. These exercises usually involve prohibiting intercourse for a while, but allowing the couple to engage in other sexual activity. The man can usually get an erection when he doesn't have the pressure of needing an erection to penetrate his partner. After he gets his erection back, transferring that confidence to having erections when he plans to have intercourse is usually easy. In the majority of cases, if he's willing to work at it, we can help him get back to his old self.

Studying sleep habits

If the man is physically sound but doesn't respond to treatment, the next step is to find out whether he has erections while he's asleep.

TECHNICAL STUFF

During the course of the night, a healthy man gets several erections during REM or "dream" sleep. He's not necessarily having an erotic dream or any dream at all, but having erections is definitely part of the male sleep pattern. This phenomenon even has its own name, *nocturnal penile tumescence,* and initials, NPT. Having initials means it's really official.

Because a man usually doesn't have performance anxiety while he's asleep, a man who suffers from impotence while he's awake but doesn't have a physical problem usually has erections while he sleeps.

TIP

The simple, at-home test to find out whether you're having erections during your sleep is to wrap a coil of postage stamps around the base of your flaccid penis. (A few turns around the penis should be enough to keep it in place.) If you find the circle of stamps broken when you wake up, you probably had an erection. (Once in a while the tooth fairy goes astray, but usually she's too busy putting coins under children's pillows.)

If the coil of stamps doesn't work, and we still suspect nighttime erections, a sleep lab is the next step. At a sleep lab, physicians substitute the stamps with plastic strips and Velcro connectors, which are more reliable indicators than postage stamps. And doctors have even more precise devices, if needed.

If all this testing doesn't turn up any sign of erections, then we have to send the client back to the medical community. But for many men, these tests do uncover some erectile functioning, which probably indicates that the problem is psychological in nature. This is not true 100 percent of the time, but it certainly deserves following up. The basic aim is to build back the man's confidence to the point where he can have erections while he is awake — and even with a sexual partner around.

Monitoring your erections as a clue to your health

As you probably know, smoking and obesity increase the risk for heart disease. But studies have proved that long before troublesome symptoms present themselves, a man is likely to notice differences in his ability to have an erection, and these challenges can be caused by either being out of shape or from smoking. So this leads to a few conclusions:

>> If a man notices any changes to his erections, he should immediately consult with his physician to be checked for any signs of heart or circulatory disease.

>> If a man would like to keep ED at bay and he smokes, he should stop.

>> And although exercise is good for many reasons, a man who strengthens his heart through cardio workouts also maintains his ability to have erections. A recent study showed that men who expended energy equivalent to running 1.5 hours a week reduced the chances of encountering problems with ED by 30 percent as compared to men who didn't exercise.

>> That same study found that men who didn't exercise and were also overweight were 2½ times likelier to develop ED than men who led active lifestyles and were of normal weight. So by keeping your weight down, you can help to keep you-know-who up.

Giving Mother Nature a boost

If none of the techniques discussed in the previous sections help you to deal with your impotence, then you may have to help Mother Nature with medical or mechanical assistance. In fact, a majority of erectile dysfunction problems occur as a result of serious medical conditions including diabetes, hypertension, or prostate cancer surgery. These conditions are much more common in older men, though they can happen in men of any age.

Oral medications

The FDA's approval of the drug Viagra in 1998 significantly enhanced the medical world's arsenal of weapons for treating ED. Developed by the drug company Pfizer, this little blue pill is effective in 75 to 80 percent of men who suffer from ED. The biggest exception is men with heart conditions who take nitrates such as nitroglycerin because the combination of the two drugs can be deadly. But there are many medical causes of ED, especially as a side effect to medications for other conditions. So it's absolutely necessary to check with a physician to make certain that by taking a drug for ED caused by another drug you're taking, you're not negating the healing effect from that initial, ED-causing drug.

Viagra (the brand name of the generic drug *sildenafil*) must be taken one to four hours before sexual activity and requires sexual stimulation to take effect. Patients who take Viagra may have some mild side effects, such as headaches or seeing halos around objects, but they don't seem to bother most men who take the drug.

Viagra has become very popular, and, disturbingly, not just with men who suffer from ED, but also with men who don't have ED but believe it will increase their sexual pleasure. The following are some of the reasons taking Viagra may be dangerous for men who can have erections:

>> Viagra is a prescription medicine. Men who don't have ED and take it do so without a prescription.

>> Viagra has side effects. Men with ED may be willing to endure those side effects as a trade-off for having erections. But because the FDA hasn't given Pfizer approval to use Viagra on men without ED, it's not yet known what those side effects can do to them over the long term.

>> Some men get *priapism,* a permanent erection (see "Priapism — The Case of the Permanent Erection" later in this chapter), from taking Viagra. Although no concrete studies have been done, men who can get erections normally but choose to take Viagra may be more prone to priapism than men who can't have erections naturally.

Sildenafil has now been around long enough that it can be purchased in generic form; as a result, the price has dropped to just dollars per pill. However, Viagra is the most counterfeited drug in the world, and the counterfeits don't contain sildenafil but instead contain all sorts of other ingredients, such as blue printer ink, which are neither effective or good for you. So while we don't want you to overpay, we also want you to get the real drug and not a fake.

Other pharmaceutical companies have developed drugs that have the same function, including Levitra (vardenafil) from Bayer & GlaxoSmithKline, Cialis (tadalafil) from Lilly ICOS, and Stendra (avanafil) from Metuchen Pharmaceuticals. Cialis can be effective for up to 36 hours, which is why some call it the "weekend drug." Stendra is fast-acting (as little as fifteen minutes) and can be taken without the food and alcohol prohibitions of some of the other drugs.

We're not going to suggest which of these pills may be right for you. And please don't try to order any of these online without first checking with your doctor. They all have side effects, and you don't want to do any serious harm to yourself. Plus, you want to make sure you're purchasing the actual drug and not an online counterfeit. Finally, men who take one of these drugs without having ED may end up becoming dependent on them, ultimately developing ED much sooner than they otherwise would have. These drugs are not recreational drugs but serious medicine, and that's why it's best to decide with your doctor the right solution for you.

Unfortunately, these pills aren't right for up to 30 percent of all men who suffer from ED, so read on for information on other options.

Penile implants

Penile implants are either hydraulic or non-hydraulic. The *non-hydraulic prostheses* are basically semi-rigid rods that doctors surgically implant within the erectile chambers. Although they are reliable, they have one major drawback — after the surgery, the penis is always in a rigid state. You can push your penis down when you're not having sex, but the erection may still be visible, which can be embarrassing.

REMEMBER

The surgery required for this type of penile implant does leave soreness in the area, and you can't have sex for several weeks. But most men report very good results and are quite happy. The only men who seem to complain are those whose hopes were too high, and who expected to have erections as strong as the ones they had in their youth. This won't — and can't — happen because the erection is permanent, and it needs to be at least somewhat concealable.

On the other hand, the *hydraulic prosthesis* has a fluid reservoir and a mechanical pump that a man uses to fill the prosthesis and create an erection whenever he wants one. Men report liking the system, and recent improvements have made the devices very reliable. Like the non-hydraulic implant, it requires a surgical procedure. Unlike the non-hydraulic implant, you only have an erection when you want one, which is more like the natural erection.

Injection therapy

Another method that was developed in the 1980s is self-injection therapy. Both Caverject and Edex use the drug *alprostadil*, which is similar to the oral medication used to treat ED. A man injects his penis with this medication and the muscles relax, thus allowing blood to flow into the penis and cause an erection. Although the thought of injecting yourself in that particular spot may not sound appealing, the penis is relatively insensitive to pain, so you can barely feel the injections. Most men who use this system have reported good results. Possible side effects include scarring and, rarely, *priapistic erections* — sustained erections that won't go away without medical treatment. (You can flip ahead in this chapter for more on priapism.) Because the drug is injected right into the penis and doesn't affect other organs as much as oral medications do, this method may be appropriate for men who can't take a pill. Check with your doctor.

It takes between five and twenty minutes for one of these injections to become effective and lasts for about an hour. Men should not use them more than three times a week, and always wait 24 hours before using it again.

Vacuum constriction

Another method of relief for impotence is the use of *vacuum-constriction devices.* Basically, a man places a vacuum pump over the penis, and as the air is pumped out, blood flows in, creating an erection. He then places a ring at the base of his penis to hold the blood in place.

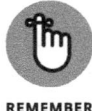

REMEMBER

We've received letters from couples saying that vacuum pumps work wonders (and at least these devices don't require surgery). But certain side effects have kept vacuum-constriction devices from becoming popular:

>> The erections these devices produce aren't as rigid as those produced with a prosthesis.

>> Sometimes mild bruising occurs as a result of using these devices.

>> Some men have difficulty ejaculating after using these devices.

But vacuum-constriction devices are a possible alternative for someone who doesn't want to, or can't, undergo surgery or use a drug, and who doesn't care to stick a needle into his penis every time he wants to have sex. Also, giving your penis an erection is actually good for it because an erection brings fresh blood into the arteries of the penis. So for men who no longer have nighttime erections, the use of a vacuum device can be looked at as a means of exercising their penis.

THE DOWNSIDE OF "UP" THERAPIES

Whether a man takes a pill, injects himself, or uses a vacuum pump to get his erection, the fact that he can have an erection doesn't necessarily mean his partner will be ready to have sex. If a man without ED approaches his partner for sex and they turn him down, he may be frustrated but he also knows that he'll have plenty of additional erections, perhaps even during the course of that same day. But a man who pops a pill or injects himself may be a lot more demanding because he's gone to some "lengths" to obtain his erection. If he doesn't first consult with his better half, that partner may not enjoy any resulting sexual interplay. So, a couple should decide together which method will work best for them and when to use one of these ED therapies, instead of the man making the decision on his own.

Couples who've historically had a good sex life and look at ED as a major problem in their relationship don't mind using one of the options we describe. But partners who haven't enjoyed sex very much, or who've lost interest in their later years, may consider the inability to have sex a godsend. Their attitude may seem wrong, but no one can know what their life has been like, so one can't jump to conclusions.

For these reasons, we believe no man should use one of the methods for overcoming ED without first having a long talk with his partner.

Dealing With Delayed Ejaculation

Premature ejaculation and erectile dysfunction are the two main male sexual problems, but some men encounter other, rarer problems, such as delayed ejaculation. Unlike premature ejaculation, where a man can't stop himself from ejaculating, *delayed ejaculation* means he can't make himself ejaculate without significant stimulation and time, or sometimes he can't ejaculate at all.

Although being able to last a long time is something our society puts great value on, delayed ejaculation is definitely a case of too much of a good thing, at least for the man . . . even if he brags about his lasting powers to cover up the problem. Obviously, a man who can't ejaculate winds up feeling frustrated and angry and may actually begin to turn off to sex.

Sometimes a medical problem causes delayed ejaculation, in which case only a urologist can help. Sometimes the cause is medication, such as those used to treat depression and anxiety. Sometimes the cause is psychological, and a sex therapist can treat the problem. A relationship problem can be one of the psychological causes, which may lead to a man unconsciously holding back his ejaculation. In that case, fixing the relationship is key to curing the problem. Determining the reason for the man's delayed ejaculation is important in determining the best solution to address it.

Exploring Priapism — The Case of the Permanent Erection

Like delayed ejaculation, priapism is another one of those too-much-of-a-good-thing conditions. In *priapism,* a man develops a permanent erection. This erection can result from the man taking or injecting himself with medication because he suffers from impotency, or can result from some disease that thickens the blood, making it impossible for blood to leave the penis after it has entered. Sickle cell anemia is one such disease.

Although priapism was named after the Greek god of fertility, that fact certainly doesn't make the man afflicted with this problem feel good about his masculinity for very long. Priapism is not only painful, but the man usually ends up in the emergency room. (An erection that lasts more than four hours definitely calls for a trip to the hospital.) Doctors can now treat priapism without surgery, but the condition still requires medical care.

Treating Peyronie's Disease — The Bent Penis

Peyronie's disease inflicts some men with their worst possible nightmare — they go to sleep with a functioning penis and wake up the next morning with a penis that bends so severely when it becomes erect that intercourse becomes impossible (see Figure 14-1).

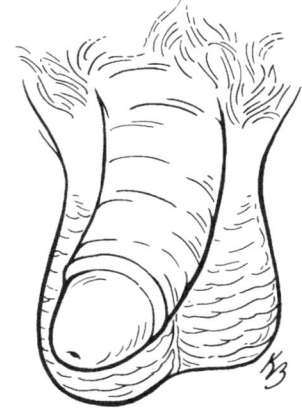

FIGURE 14-1: Peyronie's disease throws a curve in men's sex lives.

Illustration by Kathyrn Born.

The cause of Peyronie's disease is unknown; in many instances, it arises as a result of an injury. In early stages of the disease, men usually experience pain associated with having an erection. Sometimes that pain begins before the actual curvature starts and serves as an early indicator of the problem.

How bad can Peyronie's disease get? Bad enough for doctors to describe severe cases in which the erect penis looks like a corkscrew. On the other end of the spectrum, the bend may be very slight, not affect the man's ability to have intercourse, and not cause any concern. In mild cases of the disease, if the man has any pain, it usually goes away on its own; all the doctor has to do is reassure the man that in two to three months all will be well.

Sometimes the curve disappears on its own. Because the disease is basically a scarring process, some men have reported positive results from taking vitamin E, although no scientific proof exists that this technique works. Surgery can sometimes remove the scarred tissue, but surgery can also result in a loss of the man's ability to have an erection, so he would then need to have a prosthetic device implanted.

TIP

The best advice we can pass on to any readers who have Peyronie's disease is to visit a urologist who can help you. Some men are so embarrassed by their condition that they refuse to get help, but urologists have helped many men with this problem, so you have no reason to be shy.

Lacking Desire

Another problem we'd like to tackle is lack of sexual desire. One of the most common causes of this problem is stress. You come home late every night from work, or you've lost your job, or whatever, and sex is the last thing on your mind. If your partner is amorous and then starts to complain about being rejected, you become even tenser and want to have sex even less. A vicious cycle builds up, and your sex life can deteriorate down to nothing.

Men who take antidepressants and antianxiety medication may also face a lack of desire, as these medications can have that as a side effect.

Can you fix a problem such as this by yourself? Maybe, but it's not easy. One of the components of this problem is usually a lack of communication. And breaking down the barriers that have been set up can be very hard to do. Our recommendation is to visit a sex therapist or marriage counselor.

Some of the causes of loss of sexual desire aren't emotional but are physical. A good sex therapist always asks that the man see a medical doctor first to rule out any medical problems.

4

Less Risk, More Life: Outsmarting Leading Causes of Death

Get to know heart disease and its causes so you can determine your risk and modify your lifestyle.

Become familiar with the types of cancer that are most dangerous to men and identify if you're at risk for any.

Understand why unintentional injuries are so often fatal to men and what you can do to avoid accidents.

Recognize types of strokes and figure out how to reduce your chances of having one.

Understand how chronic obstructive pulmonary disease (COPD) and asthma are particularly risky to men's long-term health so you can focus on prevention.

Spot any predisposition you may have for diabetes and Alzheimer's disease and turn those yellow lights to green.

Chapter **15**

Clogged Pipes or a Broken Pump: Heart Disease

As you read this book, your heart is beating away in your chest, sustaining your life. Although it's about the size of a clenched adult fist and weighs less than a pound, your heart beats 40 million times a year and generates enough force to lift you 100 miles into the atmosphere. What an amazing — and absolutely essential — machine!

So consider these facts:

» An estimated 250 million people worldwide have coronary heart disease.

» One American dies of heart disease every 40 seconds — amounting to almost 600,000 deaths every year. Heart and circulatory diseases cause nearly 1 in 3 deaths globally.

>> Heart disease is an equal-opportunity killer. It's the leading cause of death worldwide, and until the coronavirus pandemic, heart disease had been the leading cause of deaths globally for at least 30 years.

REMEMBER

But here's the good news: Extensive research proves that you can preserve and maximize the health of your heart with some simple lifestyle changes. If you want to live a longer, fuller life, check out these facts:

>> People who are regularly physically active cut their risk of heart disease in half.

>> People who stop smoking cigarettes can return their risk of heart disease and stroke to almost normal levels within five years after stopping.

>> Overweight people who lose as little as 5 to 10 percent of their body weight can substantially lower their risk of heart disease.

>> Simple changes in what you eat can lower total blood cholesterol and LDL-cholesterol, both of which contribute to heart disease.

Heart disease describes multiple conditions that affect the heart. The most common type in the United States is *coronary heart disease,* abbreviated *CHD* (also known as *coronary artery disease,* or *CAD*). We focus on CHD the most because it's the most common; we also touch on other types of heart disease, including arrhythmia, heart failure, and heart valve diseases.

Regardless of your age, ethnicity, and current heart health, you can reduce your risk for heart disease, which just may extend your life and certainly makes the life you live better.

Getting to Know Your Heart and How It Works

You need to know how your heart and cardiovascular system are supposed to work to understand what's up when they don't — when heart disease and its many manifestations enter the chat. The heart's one of the most important organs of the body, and naturally its job is a little complex. Get familiar with your heart and its inner workings in the following sections.

Pumping for life: The heart's anatomy and function

TECHNICAL STUFF

The heart is located in the center of your chest cavity, just to the left of the midline of your body. Figure 15-1 illustrates the exterior of a healthy heart and Figure 15-2 illustrates the interior. You need to understand the following important parts:

» **The heart muscle:** Called the *myocardium* (pronounced my-o-*car*-dee-um), this muscle contracts and relaxes to pump blood throughout the cardiovascular system.

» **The coronary arteries:** Three large coronary arteries and their many branches deliver a continuous supply of oxygenated blood to the heart. Narrowing of these arteries causes chest pain; blockage causes heart attack.

» **The pumping chambers:** The heart's job is to pump blood to the lungs to get oxygen and to pump the oxygenated blood to the rest of the body. To fulfill these tasks, the heart has a left and a right side (shown in Figure 15-2), each with one main pumping chamber called a *ventricle* located in the lower part of it. Sitting above the left and right ventricles are two small booster pumps called *atria* (or *atrium*, when you're talking about just one).

The right ventricle pumps deoxygenated blood from the body to the lungs to receive a new supply of oxygen and back to the heart, through the left atrium to the left ventricle. The left ventricle pumps oxygenated blood through the arterial system to the rest of the body where it feeds every single living cell. Various disease conditions can damage each of these structures.

» **The valves:** Four valves regulate the flow of blood in and out of the heart and from chamber to chamber. They act a bit like cardiac traffic cops by directing the way blood flows, how much of it flows, and when to stop it from flowing. Disease and injury can cause heart valves to leak, narrow, or otherwise malfunction, disrupting the heart's ability to pump blood efficiently.

» **The electrical system:** This electrical system is controlled by a group of specialized cells that spontaneously discharge, sending electrical currents down specialized nerves and tissues, causing the heart to contract. When any of these electrical structures becomes diseased or disordered, *arrhythmias*, or heart rhythm disturbances, occur.

» **The pericardium:** The entire heart is positioned in a thin sac called the *pericardium*. Fluid within the sac lubricates the constantly moving surfaces. Inflammation of the pericardium from an infection or other cause causes *pericarditis*. Build-up of excess fluid inside the pericardium can cause problems with how the heart functions, a condition called *cardiac tamponade*.

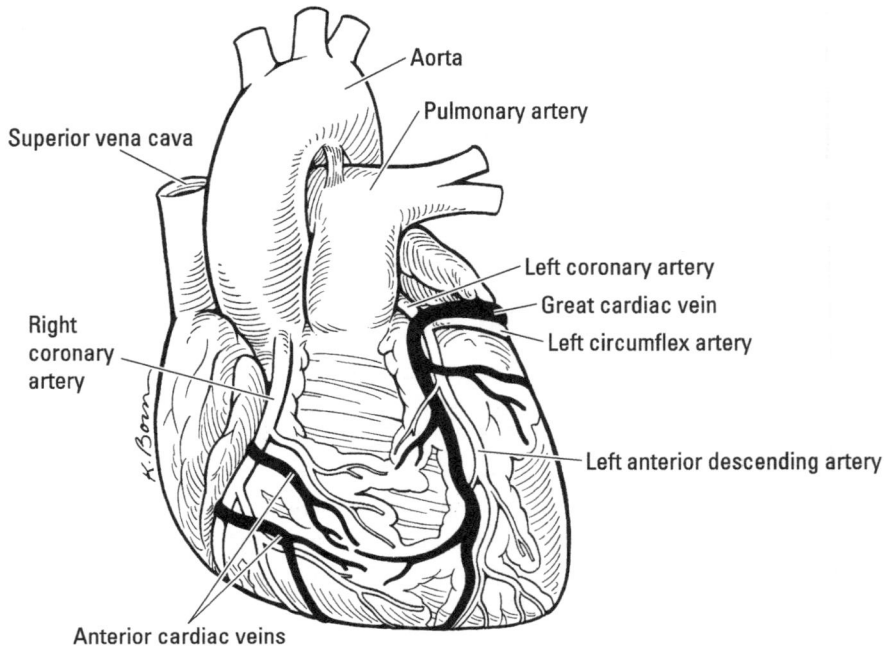

FIGURE 15-1:
A typical
healthy heart.

Aorta

Pulmonary artery

Superior vena cava

Left coronary artery
Great cardiac vein
Left circumflex artery

Right
coronary
artery

Left anterior descending artery

Anterior cardiac veins

Illustration by Kathryn Born.

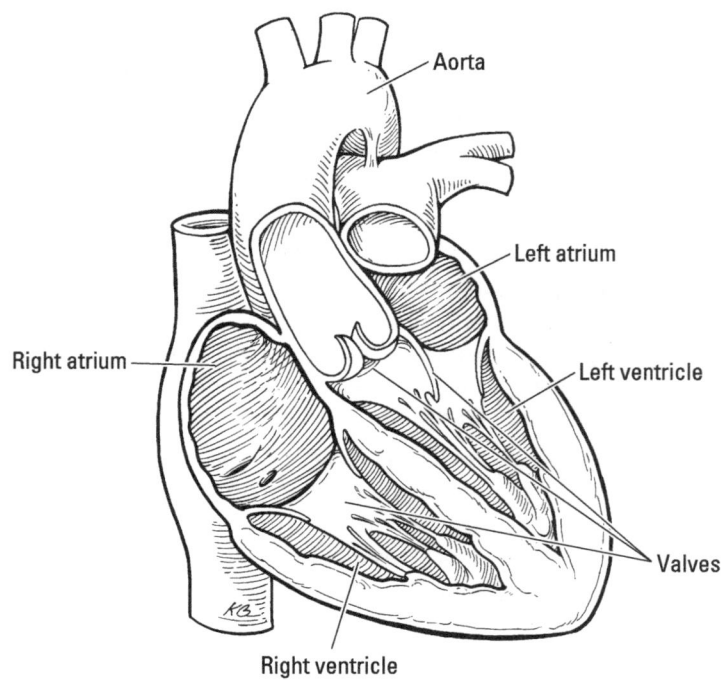

FIGURE 15-2:
The interior of a
normal heart.

Aorta

Left atrium

Right atrium

Left ventricle

Valves

Right ventricle

Illustration by Kathryn Born.

Connecting every cell in your body: The cardiovascular system

A pump is useless without the rest of the plumbing, which in your body is called the *cardiovascular system.* Here's a quick look at how it all fits together and functions.

>> **The lungs:** The lungs are composed of an intricate series of air sacs surrounded by a complex, highly branching network of blood vessels. Their sole purpose is to receive the deoxygenated blood from the heart, fill the red corpuscles full of fresh oxygen, and send them back to the heart for delivery to the body. The red blood cells give off waste products such as carbon dioxide at the same time they take on oxygen; the lungs then expel the carbon dioxide. This low-pressure system facilitates the rapid flow and reoxygenation of enormous amounts of blood.

>> **The arteries:** As oxygenated blood returns to the left side of the heart, it's pumped out to the body through the *aorta,* the main artery of the body, and into the rest of the arterial system to feed the entire body with oxygenated blood. Although the heart exerts enough force to push oxygenated blood throughout the body, the arteries also have muscular walls that help push the blood along. The force exerted against resistance of the artery walls creates a high-pressure system that is very *elastic* to allow the arteries to expand or contract to meet the needs of various organs and muscles. Your blood pressure reading results from measuring the pressure in these arteries when contracting and at rest.

>> **The capillaries:** The arterial system divides and redivides into a system of ever smaller branches to distribute nourishing blood to each individual cell, ultimately ending up in a network of microscopic vessels called *capillaries,* which deliver oxygenated blood to the working cells of every organ and muscle in the body.

>> **The veins:** After oxygen leaves the capillary system, the deoxygenated blood and waste products from the cells are carried back through the body in the *veins.* The veins ultimately come together in two very large veins, called the *inferior vena cava* and the *superior vena cava.* The inferior vena cava drains blood from the lower part of the body and superior vena cava drains blood from the upper part of the body. These veins discharge blood into the right atrium of the heart to be pumped into the right ventricle and out to the lungs again to start the whole process over again.

>> **The blood:** Although blood is not considered part of the cardiovascular system, circulating blood to every cell of the body is the reason the cardio-vascular system exists. This red fluid transports oxygen and fuel to the cells and removes waste products. It's also the delivery vehicle for many specialized cells and biochemicals, including those that contribute to the development of heart disease.

Keeping the beat: How the nervous system controls heart rate

In addition to its internal electrical system, the heart has profound linkages to the nervous system that provide additional control of the heart rate. Two main branches of the involuntary nervous system interact with the heart — the sympathetic nervous system and the parasympathetic nervous system. In simple terms, the *sympathetic nervous system* helps the heart speed up, and the *parasympathetic nervous system* helps the heart slow down. They act through direct nerve links to the heart and through the release of chemical substances that reach the heart through the bloodstream.

Breaking Down the Most Common Types of Heart Disease

The human cardiovascular system is wondrously complex. If every element is in balance and working as it should, then the whole system, including the heart and blood vessels, would remain healthy.

Unfortunately, multiple factors related to your biology and lifestyle can tip the system out of balance and trigger the development of heart disease. The earliest changes can silently progress for years before producing changes that can be seen in diagnostic tests or symptoms that you experience.

Exploring coronary heart disease and its root cause

REMEMBER

Coronary heart disease occurs when the major blood vessels supplying the heart can't function as designed because they've become narrowed or blocked.

This narrowing happens when a condition called *atherosclerosis* causes fatty deposits, or *plaque*, to slowly build up inside the walls of medium and large arteries. The disease process starts with small changes in the artery wall and takes years to develop to a point where the narrowing arteries may produce symptoms or negatively affect your health.

Narrowing in the heart's arteries leads to coronary heart disease. CHD gradually starves the heart muscle of the high level of oxygenated blood that it needs to function properly. A lack of adequate blood supply to the heart typically produces symptoms that range from angina and unstable angina (two types of chest pain that are often the first signs of heart disease — see the next section for more) to heart attack or sudden death. Narrowing of the carotid arteries that carry blood to the brain increases your risk of stroke.

These deposits typically start with fatty streaks and grow to large bumps that distort the artery and block its interior where the blood must flow.

Decades of time and the presence of various risk factors are required for the fatty streaks to develop into intermediate (moderate-sized, symptomless) and advanced (larger, symptom-producing) plaques. Figure 15-3 illustrates the typical but gradual development and progression of coronary heart disease.

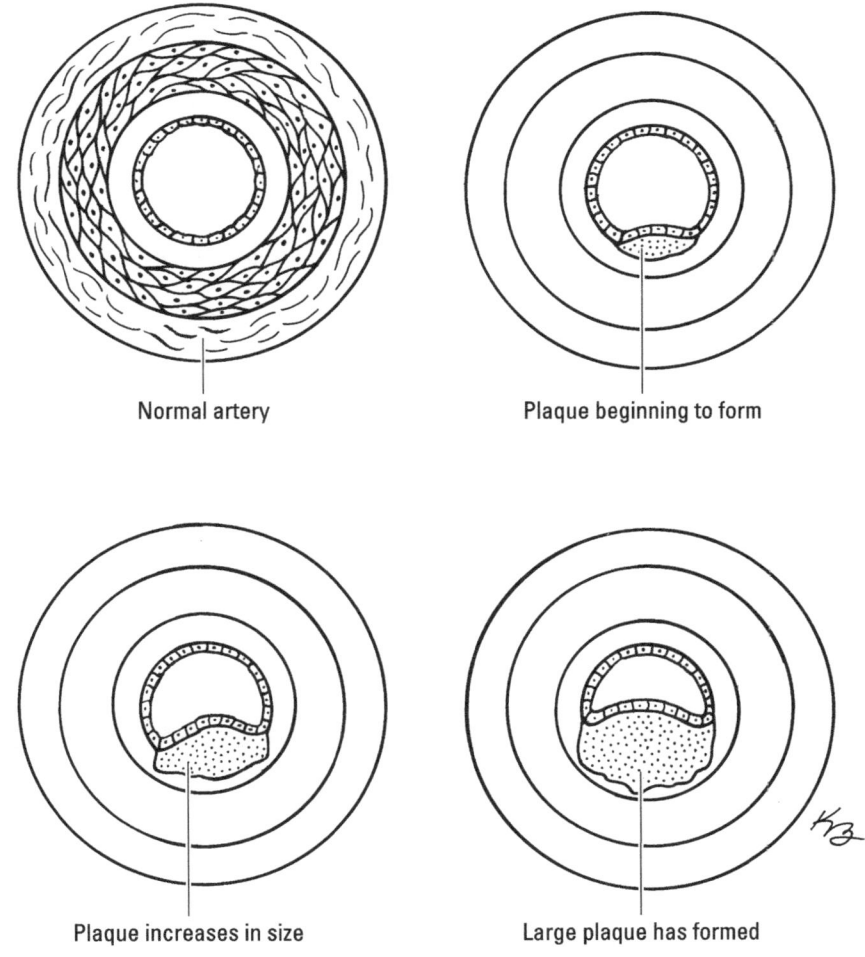

Normal artery

Plaque beginning to form

Plaque increases in size

Large plaque has formed

Illustration by Kathryn Born.

FIGURE 15-3:
The process of coronary artery disease.

Some plaques are stable and others are unstable or vulnerable to cracking or rupturing. The plaques that are more vulnerable to cracking are more likely to form a clot that totally blocks the artery and causes a sudden event such as a heart attack or stroke.

Medical scientists and physicians are particularly interested in ways to accurately identify these types of vulnerable plaques, because they seem to be responsible for the majority of sudden acute cardiovascular events, including heart attack, cardiac arrest, and stroke. Figure 15-4 illustrates the way in which such a process suddenly blocks an artery and causes an acute event.

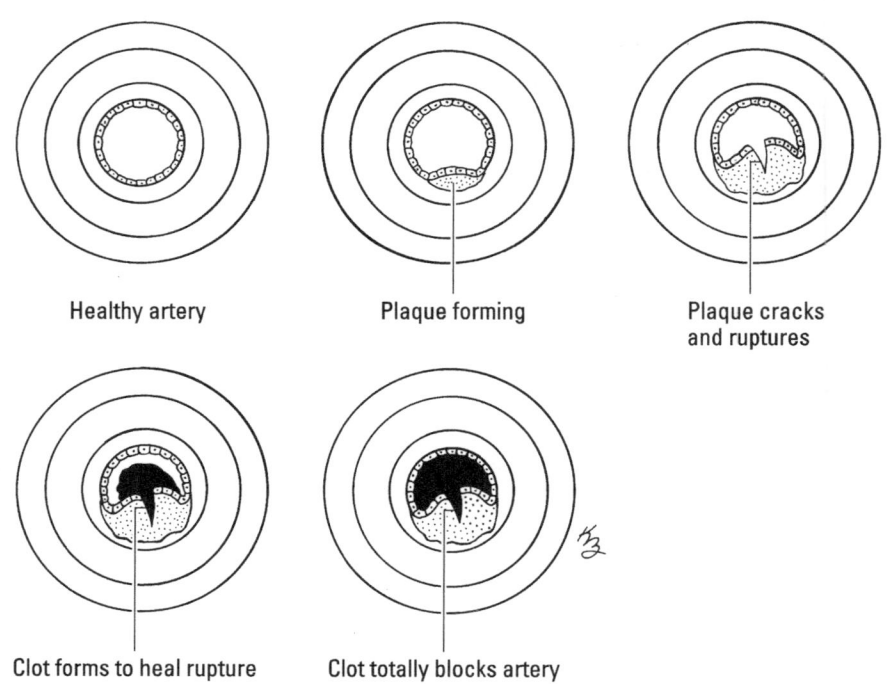

Healthy artery   Plaque forming   Plaque cracks and ruptures

FIGURE 15-4: When the plaque narrowing a coronary artery cracks open or ruptures, a clot forms, which can block the artery entirely, causing a heart attack.

Clot forms to heal rupture   Clot totally blocks artery

Illustration by Kathryn Born.

Spotting the signs of coronary heart disease

Everyone's different, so heart disease doesn't show up the same way in every guy. Not all symptoms happen to everyone, and even common symptoms can feel different from person to person. That said, here's what typically shows up:

>> **Nothing:** Many people can have significant coronary atherosclerosis but experience no discomfort or other sign of the disease; this is called *silent ischemia*. People with diabetes are particularly susceptible to silent ischemia, but others can have it, too.

>> **Angina:** Angina is typified by temporary chest pain, usually during exertion. This pain is usually felt as a tightness or uncomfortable feeling across the chest or up to the neck and jaw, not as a sharp stab. Angina occurs when you ask your heart to work harder, and it therefore demands more blood, but your coronary arteries are so narrowed by atherosclerotic plaques that your blood has a hard time flowing to the heart. Angina episodes resolve with rest or angina medication.

WARNING

>> **Unstable angina:** Unstable angina is when angina gets out of control — the drop in blood and oxygen to the heart becomes sudden and serious, sharply increasing the risk of a heart attack. Symptoms include chest pain that is new, occurs when you're at rest, or suddenly grows more severe. Unstable angina is a medical emergency.

WARNING

>> **Heart attack:** Completely cutting off blood flow to a coronary artery causes an acute heart attack, the most severe result of coronary heart disease. The closure can be gradual or the result of a blood clot. Typical symptoms of a heart attack include uncomfortable pressure, fullness, squeezing, or pain in the center of the chest lasting more than a few minutes; pain spreading to the shoulders, neck, or arms; and chest discomfort with lightheadedness, fainting, sweating, nausea, or shortness of breath.

>> **Sudden death:** For some people, the first sign of CHD is a fatal heart attack or cardiac arrest. Many of these deaths happen to people in their 50s, 40s, or younger.

Looking at other manifestations of heart disease

Atherosclerosis, angina, and heart attack aren't the only types of heart disease. Here's a quick rundown of four other common types:

>> **Arrhythmias** (or *dysrhythmias)* refer to problems with the electrical system that controls the heart's normal rhythm, resulting in a heart rate that isn't normal. They may occur in the context of an acute heart attack or from other causes.

>> **Heart failure** occurs when the heart no longer adequately pumps blood to the lungs and throughout the body. It's usually a slow process that takes place during a period of years. Underlying conditions, such as CHD, leakage from one of the heart valves, an acute heart attack, or various diseases of the heart muscle itself usually cause heart failure.

>> **Stroke** occurs when a blood clot or bleeding suddenly interrupts the flow of blood to an area of the brain. When deprived of blood, brain cells lose their ability to function and, if deprived for too long, die.

>> **Heart value problems** occur when the four heart valves don't open fully and shut tightly, leading to valve leakage (the heart can become overloaded due to the extra strong beat needed to eject extra blood flowing back into it) or narrowing (the heart thickens because it's being asked to pump against much higher pressure).

Assessing Your Risk and Deciding to Make Some Changes

Heart disease takes many forms, and risk factors contribute to each form of heart disease in complex ways. In this section, we discuss the risk factors for atherosclerosis, particularly in the context of coronary heart disease.

What is a risk factor anyway? Just as the name suggests, a *risk factor* is something that increases your chances of developing a chronic condition (that is, an ongoing health condition that you must live with). In the case of cardiac health, a risk factor is a personal habit, practice, or physical characteristic or condition that increases the likelihood that you'll develop heart disease.

Identifying important risk factors and how you can influence them

Your risk of developing heart disease is affected by two things: specific health conditions and your lifestyle choices and habits. Because this chapter is about helping you understand and make changes to live a better and hopefully longer life, we're going to divide the primary risk factors for heart disease into those that you can change and those you can't.

Risk factors you can control

The following are risk factors that increase your chances of developing heart disease but are within your control to change:

>> **High blood pressure:** Elevated blood pressure *(hypertension)* represents a substantial risk for developing CHD and stroke. Reducing high blood pressure by even modest amounts reduces the risk of coronary heart disease, stroke, heart failure, and death from cardiovascular disease.

>> **Unhealthy cholesterol levels:** Simple changes in what you eat can lower total blood cholesterol and LDL-cholesterol, both of which contribute to heart disease.

>> **Obesity:** Obesity contributes to heart disease risk factors, including hypertension, elevated cholesterol levels, and diabetes. Overweight people who lose as little as 5 to 10 percent of their body weight can substantially lower their risk of heart disease. Weight loss can help control cholesterol levels, blood pressure, and diabetes (all found on this list!)

>> **Smoking:** If you smoke, your risk of developing heart disease is tripled. But people who stop smoking cigarettes can return their risk of heart disease and stroke to almost normal levels within five years after stopping. Ceasing smoking can also improve your blood lipids, raising your good cholesterol (HDL) and decreasing the bad (LDL).

>> **Physical inactivity:** A deconditioned heart demands more oxygen and has to pump faster to do its job. Physical activity on a regular basis (just 150 minutes of moderate activity per week) increases cardiac fitness and helps control high blood pressure, elevated blood cholesterol, obesity, and diabetes, and cuts the risk of heart disease in half.

Risk factors you can't control

Here are three risk factors that you can't modify: your age, gender, and family history. If you have one or more of the following risk factors, it's particularly important that you pay close attention to the risk factors that you *can* modify (see preceding section):

>> **Age:** Age is considered a significant risk factor for heart disease for men who are older than 45.

>> **Gender:** Men are more likely to develop coronary heart disease than women. And the onset of symptoms typically occurs ten years earlier in men than women.

>> **Family history and heredity:** If you come from a family in which premature coronary heart disease has occurred (that is, a diagnosed heart condition or the experience of a heart attack or other heart event before age 55 in males), your risk of developing CHD significantly increases. Having a first-degree relative (father, mother, brother, or sister) who fits this description also qualifies as a risk factor.

WARNING

Risk factors don't just add up — they multiply when you've got more than one. If you have only a single major risk factor, you typically double your chance of developing heart disease. When two risk factors are present, the possibility quadruples. And, worse yet, when three risk factors join forces, your chances of developing heart disease increases 8 to 20 times! Sadly, we're not done yet: Having two and three risk factors isn't unusual. In fact, risk factors have a distinct tendency to occur in clusters, particularly in the presence of obesity or diabetes. All the more reason to take control of what's within your control.

Knowing the risks for adults under 65

If you think heart disease is a problem mainly for older adults, that's understandable — the majority of deaths from heart disease do occur in people older than 65. However, the precursors of coronary artery disease are already present in a majority of young adults between the ages of 21 and 39. Here are some other reasons that younger adults should take steps now to prevent heart disease:

>> About half of all sudden cardiac arrests occur in people under age 65, many in people in their 40s and 50s.

>> 38 percent of people hospitalized for stroke are younger than age 65.

>> More than 1 in 5 Americans with heart failure are younger than age 60.

>> An estimated 80 percent of premature heart disease and stroke is preventable.

>> Among U.S. youth and adults aged 12 to 60, almost none meet the seven criteria for ideal heart health established by the American Heart Association (www.heart.org). That figure would be none, except that 0.3 percent of young adults ages 20 to 29 meet the seven ideal criteria.

So if you're younger than 65, there's no time like the present to start taking steps toward better heart health.

Knowing the risks for older adults

Unfortunately, many Americans expect heart trouble to be part of their older years, but it doesn't have to be that way. And if you are older — even if you already have heart disease — you can do plenty to avoid being part of these statistics specific to older adults:

>> Approximately 80 percent of deaths from heart disease occur in people older than 65.

>> More than 77 percent of men aged 60 to 79 have cardiovascular disease. For people age 80 and older, the percentage having heart disease rises to nearly 90 percent of men.

>> After age 55, the incidence of stroke doubles with each decade of life.

>> Two of the most frequent causes of hospitalization for older adults are coronary atherosclerosis and congestive heart failure.

HANDS-ONLY CPR: IT AIN'T AS HARD AS IT LOOKS

Back in the day, learning CPR (*cardiopulmonary resuscitation* — a means of manually pressing on the chest to pump the heart) meant awkward mouth-to-mouth with a plastic doll named Annie — usually starting with, "Annie, Annie, are you OK?" and followed by shaky rescue breaths and chest compressions. Not exactly confidence-inspiring, especially when imagining doing it on a real person. But research by cardiologist and cardiac resuscitation expert Dr. Gordon A. Ewy and others showed that in the first few minutes of cardiac arrest, steady chest compressions alone can be lifesaving. That led to the American Heart Association's Hands-Only CPR guidelines — no mouth-to-mouth required, just solid chest compressions anyone can do.

So how do you teach the masses? Enter the British Heart Foundation's (www.bhf.org.uk) clever ad campaign starring ex-soccer player and movie tough guy Vinnie Jones. He delivers no-nonsense, hands-only CPR instruction to the beat of the Bee Gees' "Stayin' Alive" — gruff, a little menacing, and surprisingly effective. Watch it on YouTube by searching "Vinnie Jones hard and fast CPR".

Managing Your Blood Pressure to Protect Your Heart

High blood pressure is one of the key health risks for developing heart disease. High blood pressure is called the "silent killer" because it typically doesn't cause any noticeable symptoms. Almost 31 percent of adults in the United States have high blood pressure. But what does this actually mean?

Checking out blood pressure basics

As the heart pumps blood through the circulatory system, the blood that's being pumped exerts pressure against the interior walls of the blood vessels. Your *blood pressure* reading consists of two measurements of the pressure exerted and is expressed in millimeters (mm) of mercury (Hg). Two typical readings for *normal blood pressure* include 110/70 mm Hg (read "one hundred-ten over seventy millimeters of mercury") or 120/80 mm Hg. What do these numbers mean?

>> The top or higher number is called the *systolic pressure,* which expresses the pressure exerted as the heart contracts or beats, pumping blood through the circulatory system.

>> The bottom, or lower number, is called *diastolic pressure,* which expresses the pressure exerted when the heart is at rest between beats.

Defining high blood pressure (hypertension)

REMEMBER

Many people mistakenly think that you either have hypertension or you don't. In fact, blood pressure readings span a continuum ranging all the way from *normal* to *severely elevated.* Experiencing one elevated reading doesn't mean that you have hypertension. Everyone's blood pressure tends to spike up in situations that produce anger, pain, fear, high stress, or physical exertion. Blood pressure also varies during the day — it's usually lower when you're resting or sleeping, for example.

Having hypertension doesn't mean you're super tense — even the calmest, most laid-back individuals can have high blood pressure. It means that your blood pressure is consistently elevated above the normal ranges. And knowing whether you have it is no do-it-yourself diagnosis, either. You need to have your blood pressure checked regularly, ideally as part of a regular periodic checkup.

Table 15-1, based on how the American College of Cardiology (www.acc.org) and the American Heart Association categorize blood pressure, shows the range of blood pressure classifications that express the increasing health risks of increasingly higher blood pressure.

TABLE 15-1

Healthy and Unhealthy Blood Pressure Ranges

Category	Systolic (mm Hg)		Diastolic (mm Hg)
Normal blood pressure	Less than 120	and	Less than 80
Elevated blood pressure	120–129	and	Less than 80
Stage 1 hypertension	130–139	or	80–89
Stage 2 hypertension	140 or higher	or	90 or higher

Sources: American College of Cardiology; American Heart Association

Taking charge of your blood pressure

TIP

Controlling many of your daily habits and practices can help you prevent high blood pressure or manage existing hypertension. Taking these lifestyle measures also is an important part of treatment, even if you require medicines to control your blood pressure. We go into detail about these lifestyle habits later in this chapter, but here's a quick rundown to introduce you:

» **Managing your weight:** If you're overweight, even just by 15 or 20 pounds, losing that weight will lower your blood pressure, plain and simple.

» **Becoming more active:** If you're physically active, you reduce your risk of developing high blood pressure by 20 to 50 percent.

» **Eating a low-sodium, heart-healthy diet:** Eating a diet full of fruits and vegetables, whole grains, legumes, lean proteins, low-fat dairy, and healthy oils makes any man healthier. And the best way to lower your sodium intake is to limit the amount of prepackaged, processed, and restaurant foods you eat.

» **Quitting smoking:** Smoking, no matter what type, raises your blood pressure, so if you don't smoke, you're automatically reducing this risk.

» **Limiting alcohol:** If you drink four or more drinks per day and reduce that number to two or fewer, you can demonstrably lower your blood pressure.

» **Managing stress:** Stress can contribute to other risk factors, such as diet and alcohol consumption. Keeping your stress levels in check makes you less likely to overindulge in food or drinks.

Controlling Cholesterol to Cut Heart Disease Risk

Without question, elevated blood cholesterol significantly increases —doubles, in fact — the risk of developing coronary heart disease. And in combination with other risk factors, such as high blood pressure, overweight, or obesity, cholesterol multiplies those risks many times over. So controlling cholesterol is vital to lowering your risk of developing heart disease and to controlling the progression of heart disease if you have it.

The relationship between cholesterol levels and heart disease risk isn't like a light bulb that's either on or off. It's more like the gradual acceleration your car experiences entering a freeway. As cholesterol in the blood gradually rises to a level of about 200 mg/dL and LDL tops 100 mg/dL, the risk of developing heart disease also gradually increases. After your cholesterol goes above those levels, the risk of heart disease and of dying from heart disease increases much more rapidly. By the time your cholesterol level reaches 250, your risk of dying from heart disease grows to more than twice that of individuals whose cholesterol levels are below 200. (Take a look at the upcoming section "Understanding lipoproteins: The good, the bad, and the ugly" for more on HDL and LDL lipoproteins.)

TIP

But good news! The reverse also is true. Lowering your blood cholesterol level by even a smidgen can make a positive difference. And the more you lower it, the greater the benefit. For every one point that your cholesterol drops, estimates indicate your risk of heart disease drops by 2 percent. Thus, a drop of 10 mg/dL in your cholesterol level can decrease your risk of developing heart disease by 20 percent! (Wouldn't you love returns like that on your IRA?)

Comprehending cholesterol

Cholesterol is a naturally occurring waxy substance present in human beings and all other animals. It is an important component of the body's cell walls. The body also requires cholesterol to produce many hormones (including sex hormones) and the bile acids that help it digest food. Because cholesterol plays such important biological roles, having adequate amounts of it is absolutely essential for life itself.

Humans get cholesterol mainly from two sources — your liver (it produces a lot), and animal products that you eat, such as meat, eggs, and dairy products. However, you get into trouble when you have too much cholesterol in your blood, particularly LDL cholesterol. Your level of blood cholesterol grows too high because, usually, you're eating too much saturated fat, trans fat, or very refined, simple carbohydrates (which encourage the liver to manufacture cholesterol) and you're eating too many foods that contain cholesterol (dietary cholesterol).

To get to where it needs to go in your body, cholesterol is carried around in your bloodstream, attached to complicated structures called *lipoproteins*. When cholesterol levels in the blood are too high, excess lipids are deposited on the inside walls of the arteries in the form of *plaque,* which causes arteries to narrow. The result is *atherosclerosis,* which is the basis of CHD and which we dive into in the section "Exploring coronary heart disease and its root cause" earlier in this chapter.

Understanding lipoproteins: The good, the bad, and the ugly

A *lipoprotein* is a cross between a lipid, such as cholesterol or triglycerides, and a protein. Lipoprotein transports cholesterol and other lipids through the bloodstream. Lipoproteins are sort of like a cruise ship steaming across the Atlantic Ocean — think of the ship as the proteins, and all the passengers on board (including the Family Cholesterol) as the lipids. Not a perfect analogy, but you get the point. Lipoproteins can be separated and measured according to their weight and density, and their size.

We want to focus on two of particular importance:

>> **LDL,** or **low-density lipoprotein,** is particularly dangerous because it contains more fat and less protein and easily adheres to artery walls and enters into plaque formation. Because LDL cholesterol plays such a major role in forming atherosclerotic plaque, lowering LDL levels in the blood is an important goal in controlling cholesterol.

>> **HDL,** or **high-density lipoprotein,** is particularly beneficial and can actually help protect your heart from heart disease. HDL doesn't adhere to artery walls. Instead, it helps carry cholesterol away from artery walls. This effect is particularly important for the coronary arteries. Thus, keeping HDL at recommended levels helps control overall cholesterol and its potential negative effects.

When you have a checkup, your doctor may look at the results of your blood tests and say, "Well, you need to work on raising your *good cholesterol* and lowering your *bad cholesterol.*" Wait, which is the good one again? Just look at their names! You want your high-density lipoproteins (HDLs) to be *high* and your low-density lipoproteins (LDLs) to be *low.* High, *high!* Low, *low!*

Testing your cholesterol and other lipid levels

All men should know their respective cholesterol levels. A simple finger-stick blood test is all that's required for testing total cholesterol. You should have such a test at least every five years, or more often if your cholesterol level is elevated or if you have other risk factors for heart disease.

If the simple test shows your cholesterol level is elevated, your physician may recommend that you undergo a fasting blood test called a complete *lipid profile* or *lipid analysis* to determine your levels of LDL, HDL, and triglycerides. Physicians often include this more extensive test as part of your routine physical checkup.

If you take a simple test outside your doctor's office, perhaps at a health fair, and your cholesterol level measures 200 mg/dL or higher, be sure to share this information with your physician so you get proper follow-up.

Understanding the general test results

Here are some general guidelines for interpreting your cholesterol measurements and assessing your risk of developing heart disease (or of experiencing increased complications if you already have it):

>> **"Desirable" cholesterol level —200 mg/dL and lower.** Although 200 mg/dL is considered "desirable," remember that lower is better. Thus, a cholesterol level of 170 mg/dL is better than a cholesterol level of 190 mg/dL.

>> **Borderline high blood cholesterol — 200 mg/dL to 239 mg/dL.** If your cholesterol is within this range, your physician will strongly recommend lifestyle modifications and perhaps medication, depending on your current practices and risk factors.

>> **High blood cholesterol level — 240 mg/dL or greater.** This classification puts you at high risk. Your physician typically will work closely with you to establish an aggressive treatment program that will likely include lifestyle changes and medication.

Understanding LDL and HDL test results

Guidelines from the American Heart Association and American College of Cardiology recommend (in addition to lifestyle therapies) more aggressive treatment with statin medications of certain groups of people:

- **Optimal LDL Cholesterol Level —100 mg/dL and lower.** If your LDL cholesterol levels are optimal and you have no other risk factors for heart disease (such as high blood pressure, diabetes, or overweight), most physicians will recommend using lifestyle measures that keep your LDL as low as possible. It's never too early to pay attention to these bad actors.

- **At-Risk LDL Cholesterol Levels — 100 mg/dL and above.** Although a LDL of 100 to 129 mg/dL has been considered just above optimal, treatment guidelines urge physicians to begin targeting LDL more aggressively, using lifestyle measures and appropriate statin or other medication. So be sure to talk to your doctor about what is right for you. Certainly, LDL levels above 130 mg/dL need lowering.

- **Low HDL Cholesterol Levels — 40 mg/dL and lower.** A low HDL cholesterol level also is considered an independent risk factor for heart disease, over and above total cholesterol and LDL levels. Men whose HDL is below 40 mg/dL should take steps to raise it, usually close to 60 mg/dL.

- **Triglycerides.** If your triglycerides are below 150 mg/dL, they're considered to be *optimal or near optimal.* This recommended classification takes into account the associations between triglycerides and other lipid and nonlipid risk factors. In addition to increasing your risk of CHD, very high levels of triglycerides may also injure the pancreas, a vital organ that's responsible for producing insulin in the body.

Managing your cholesterol with three key lifestyle steps

TIP

How you choose to conduct your daily life in three important areas can help lower your elevated blood cholesterol. The key lifestyle decisions involve committing yourself to proper nutrition, including low saturated fat and low cholesterol consumption, increasing physical activity, and maintaining a healthy weight. Déjà vu? Nope. This "eat right and exercise" refrain is sung all through this book, because a healthy lifestyle reduces your risk of developing many health issues. Here's a quick rundown:

- **Eat a heart-smart diet** full of vegetables, beans, fruits, and whole-grain foods. Choose lean protein like fish, poultry, tofu, and low-fat dairy. Limit foods with cholesterol like eggs, whole milk, and high-fat cuts of meat.

- **Get at least 30 minutes of physical activity** most days. Regular aerobic activity increases HDL cholesterol (remember, HDL, *high*), and strength training builds muscle, which boosts metabolism and helps manage weight.

>> **Maintain a healthy weight.** Weight loss is an important lifestyle intervention for lowering elevated cholesterol if you're overweight. Weight reduction helps lower your LDL cholesterol (remember, you want low LDL), lower triglycerides, and raise HDL cholesterol.

REMEMBER

Many men think that food can't be enjoyable and tasty as part of an eating plan to lower cholesterol (or control high blood pressure). But that's not true. For an entire book full of such tasty, heart-healthy recipes see *The Healthy Heart Cookbook For Dummies* (John Wiley & Sons, Inc., 2000).

Lowering Your Weight to Lighten Your Heart's Load

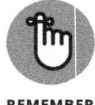

REMEMBER

Being overweight or obese is another key health risk for developing heart disease. If this describes you, one of the best things you can do to reduce multiple risk factors for heart disease is to lose weight. Losing as few as 5 to 10 percent of your body weight can make a significant difference. For many people that's just 10 to 15 pounds.

Most studies indicate that you lose approximately 1 mm Hg from both your systolic and diastolic blood pressure for every two pounds that you lose. So even small amounts of weight loss can make a profound difference in blood-pressure control. Many people who lose 10 to 15 pounds can anticipate a 5 mm Hg to 7 mm Hg reduction in their systolic and diastolic blood pressure levels. For that reason, your doctor is likely to first recommend weight reduction if you're overweight and have high blood pressure. If you're overweight but don't have elevated blood pressure, losing weight is a frontline strategy to keeping your blood pressure where it should be.

Losing weight is easier said than done. Keep reading for some tips that can help you change your habits and lose weight — and reduce your heart disease risk — in the process. Check out Chapter 4 for nutrition basics.

Setting realistic weight-loss goals

Many forces drive us to desire instant satisfaction or accomplishment. But taking an "everything right now or nothing" approach to weight loss (as to so many other things) is a recipe for failure and disappointment. A realistic weight-loss plan should be about discovery, not deprivation. That means that it should help you create new habits that are both enjoyable and healthful.

TIP

To set goals that work, try the following:

>> **Recognize that you're playing the long game.** Losing weight is your measurable objective. But your primary goal is a healthier life, specifically a heart-healthy life. So put less focus on the scale and more focus on developing habits you can sustain — and enjoy — for a lifetime.

>> **Take one step at a time.** Many a man has stumbled on their weight loss journey because they tried to make too many changes at once, which can make you miserable and exhausted. Instead, start with one or two changes — reduce the processed or prepackaged food you eat each day and take a walk after dinner twice weekly. Then you can make some more changes, like filling half your plate with fruits and vegetables, and upping your walking schedule to four times a week. You get the idea.

>> **Track your food intake and daily activities.** Changing the way you eat and adding more physical activity to your day takes a big effort. Stay motivated by keeping track of your daily efforts. Use free apps such as Start Simple with MyPlate or MyFitnessPal, or set up a spreadsheet.

Controlling your portions

TIP

One easy way to reduce calories is to control your portions. Here are some ways you can resize your portions without having to remember a lot of measurement equivalents:

>> **Use smaller plates for meals.** If your plate is 10 inches in diameter rather than 12 inches — or even 8 or 9 inches rather than 10 inches — you'll typically place smaller portions on it.

>> **Use a tall, skinny glass rather than a short, wide glass.** Studies have shown that people pour more and drink more when they use a short, wide glass.

>> **Serve plates in the kitchen, not at the table.** Avoid placing serving bowls on the table to help reduce the chances of second helpings.

>> **Serve a salad before the meal.** Studies show that eating a salad before the main meal reduces overall calorie intake. Two or three cups of salad greens also help you feel full and satisfied.

» **Keep single-serving packets of snacks on hand.** When the munchies hit, having a portion-controlled snack in the pantry can keep you from overeating right out of the box.

Make your own 100 to 120 calorie packets of whole-grain ready-to-eat cereal, trail mix, or nuts. Reusable containers or baggies work fine.

Moving your body to help lose weight

Hundreds of diets pitch "magic" strategies for quick loss. However, there's nothing magic about the basic fact of weight loss: To lose weight, you must burn more energy than you eat. There are two ways to do that — reduce the food calories you eat or burn up more calories than you eat with physical activity.

Extensive research has shown that if you use either of these strategies separately, you'll typically lose more weight with diet alone than with exercise alone. However, the most successful losers in all types of studies with all types of diets have been people who combined a reduced calorie eating plan with regular physical activity or exercise. In fact, adding physical activity or exercise to a reduced calorie diet increases weight loss by about 20 percent over a diet alone.

The activity that's most accessible to most people is walking. All you need to start are good shoes and comfortable clothing. And if you've been sedentary, you're going to start with small sessions of walking and gradually increase both the length of time you walk and the pace at which you walk. Every bit of moderate activity helps you burn more calories than sitting at your computer, or laying on the couch watching TV or playing video games. Take a look at Chapter 5 for additional pointers on moving your body to improve your health.

If you have health issues or are significantly overweight, check with your doctor before beginning an exercise program.

It's important to maintain and even build lean muscle mass when you're trying to lose weight — you'll increase your metabolism (which helps you lose weight faster), your body will more efficiently burn fat, and you'll more easily be able to keep off the weight that you lose. *Aerobic activity* (activity that raises your heart rate — not necessarily aerobics) strengthens muscles to a degree, but actively building muscle requires resistance training.

Most people think of resistance training as weight lifting. However, many other types of exercise also provide resistance and build muscle, like swimming, water aerobics, yoga, and calisthenic exercises such as pushups, squats, and pull-ups (which use the body's weight and opposing muscle groups to provide resistance). Chapter 6 goes into detail about weight training and includes some workouts you can do right now — no gym membership needed.

Quitting Smoking to Strengthen Your Heart's Odds

There's really no upside to smoking and other means of tobacco use, whether cigarettes, cigars, vapes, chewing tobacco, dips, and so on. And with over 65 percent of smokers reporting they want to quit, even most regular nicotine users would like to get off this bandwagon.

WARNING

Cigarette smoking (including breathing secondhand smoke) and the use of other tobacco products increase blood pressure, both in the short term while you're smoking or chewing and in the long term, because components in the smoke or chewing tobacco, such as nicotine, cause your arteries to constrict. Childhood experiments with the nozzle on a garden hose indicate what happens when you force the same volume of liquid through a smaller opening. That higher pressure isn't a happy thing for your arteries.

If you're making lifestyle changes to reduce your chances of getting heart disease and dying earlier than you want to, here are some benefits if you quit smoking too:

>> Your blood pressure stops spiking due to nicotine.

>> The carbon monoxide levels in your blood return to normal, and your circulation and lung function begin to improve. This means oxygen can get to your muscles easier when you work out, increasing your exercise capacity and endurance.

>> You're able to breathe more deeply, you cough less, and you're less often short of breath. Getting 30–45 minutes of moderate activity most days of the week is easier because you don't struggle to breathe or fulfil your minutes.

>> After three to six years of quitting, your risk of developing heart disease goes down by 50 percent.

>> Fifteen years after quitting, your risk of heart disease is almost the same as a non-smoker's.

TIP

Quitting smoking is hard, there's no way around that fact. And the benefits are worth it. Take a look at Chapter 9 for information on stopping.

Breaking Down Other Heart-Healthy Habits

Besides managing your weight and adding regular physical activity to your day-to-day living, you can make some additional lifestyle changes to reduce your risk of developing heart disease — which'll help you live a better life, and quite possibly a longer one.

Building a more active body, not just a lighter one

REMEMBER

Use it (your body) and lose it (your high blood pressure). Physically active people reduce their risk of developing hypertension by 20 percent to 50 percent when compared with their couch potato peers. So getting 30 to 45 minutes of moderate-intensity exercise on most days of the week helps keep your blood pressure normal, which reduces your heart disease risk. This is true even for many older adults.

Even if you feel fine and fit and have no risk factors for heart disease, you can experience several positive changes after just two or three months of regular physical activity:

>> Tasks that previously made you short of breath are easier to perform.

>> Your heart rate when you're resting is lower. Because a more efficient heart pumps more blood on each beat, it requires fewer beats per minute to supply your body with oxygen when you're simply sitting still.

>> Your heart is a stronger muscle. During a lifetime of moderate physical activity, the heart, as a muscle, maintains better condition than the heart of someone who remains or becomes inactive.

>> The coronary arteries, which supply blood to the heart, are more likely to stay large and relatively clean in individuals who exercise on a regular basis. And clean coronary arteries prevent heart attacks.

TIP

The benefits of regular physical activity for controlling blood pressure are added to those of weight loss. Check out Chapters 5 and 6 to learn more about moving your body to make it healthier.

Eating a heart-healthy diet

Here's the first rule of heart-healthy eating: You can eat well in ways that improve your cardiac health without being a food cop. Many aspects of proper nutrition also play significant roles in lowering and maintaining blood pressure and cholesterol levels, so adopting a heart-healthy way of eating is a wise choice.

TIP

Here are some eating-well basics:

>> **Choose a variety of fruits and vegetables daily — at least five servings.** Fruits and vegetables are loaded with fiber, antioxidants, and other phyto-chemicals that lower the risks of heart disease and cancer. In addition, they're low in sodium, and most have no fat. As a result, fruits and vegetables don't increase blood pressure or blood cholesterol. Studies also show that people with high blood pressure who consume a diet containing high levels of fruits and vegetables and low-fat dairy products significantly reduced their blood pressure.

>> **Select a variety of whole-grain foods daily.** Whole-grain foods, such as whole-grain cereals, bread, pasta and brown rice, form a mainstay of heart-healthy eating along with fruits and vegetables, because they're very high in fiber and in complex carbohydrates. In addition to popular whole grains such as oats, wheat, rye, brown rice, and corn, other less familiar whole grains you might try include quinoa, barley, buckwheat, and amaranth.

>> **Choose lean protein foods.** Protein provides the building blocks for the body's cells. If you eat animal protein, select lean cuts of meat and trim visible fat or remove poultry skin before or after cooking. Fish and nonfat or low-fat dairy and eggs also provide protein. You can also get adequate protein from plant sources such as dried beans, tofu and other soy foods, nuts and nut butters, seeds, some whole grains, and nondairy milks (such as soy and nut milks).

>> **Enjoy healthy oils and fats in moderation.** Just as it needs carbs and protein, your body needs the right fats in the right amounts (not too much!) for good heart health. Some healthy oils include olive, canola, peanut, corn, and soybean oils. Healthy fats include fatty fish such as salmon, sardines, herring, lake trout, and canned light tuna, as well as walnuts and flax seeds.

Avoiding too much sodium

On average, most American adults consume about twice the recommended amount of sodium. Guidelines currently recommend that adults consume less than 2,300 milligrams of sodium daily (about 1 teaspoon of table salt, or *sodium chloride*).

And the recommendation is less than 1,500 milligrams daily (just over a half teaspoon) for adults 51 and older, individuals of African American heritage, and anyone with high blood pressure, diabetes, or a diagnosis of heart disease.

Now, we know you don't sprinkle that much salt over your food at the table! But many prepared and convenience foods, plus restaurant foods (whether fast food or haute cuisine), have high levels of sodium. In fact, 70 percent of the sodium Americans eat comes from these items. So a key action you can take to support your heart's health is to limit the amount of packaged, prepared, and restaurant foods you eat.

REMEMBER

The major reason to limit salt/sodium intake has to do with its association with high blood pressure. In societies where less sodium is consumed, the incidence of high blood pressure is dramatically lower than it is in the United States. If people with hypertension pay more attention to strict limitations on salt consumption and control their weight, many can manage blood pressure without medications.

Limiting alcohol

From a cardiovascular point of view, alcohol consumption is a complex issue. Moderate alcohol consumption has been shown to lower the risk of heart attack. Yet alcohol also is loaded with calories and may contribute to weight gain. And importantly, excessive alcohol consumption increases blood pressure and acts in adverse ways on the cardiac muscle itself.

Research and debate continue about the complex mechanisms (including genetic links) and pathways through which alcohol may benefit heart health. Debate also continues about whether red wine in particular is beneficial, or if the lifestyle habits of some red-wine drinkers are as responsible as the wine (or more so) for better health. Chapter 9 explores this a little more.

REMEMBER

Moderate alcohol consumption generally is defined as no more than two drinks per day for men. One drink equals a 1.5 shot of distilled spirits, 5 ounces of wine, or 12 ounces of beer. Higher levels of alcohol consumption carry unacceptable health risks. Fortunately, you can find lots of non-alcoholic options for spirits, wine, and beer, so you can enjoy the flavor without the alcohol risks.

Chilling out to reduce stress

Stress can affect your body in many ways, primarily due to the hormones it causes your body to make. When these stress hormones are present, your heartbeat picks up, your blood vessels narrow, and your blood pressure temporarily spikes. The good news is, when you're no longer stressed, your blood pressure returns to what it was before. But if you get stressed a lot and have a lot of short blood pressure spikes, you could have a heart attack or a stroke. These frequent spikes may also damage your blood vessels and your heart over time, resulting in damage that's like what your body faces from long-term high blood pressure. Take a look at Chapter 7 for more information about how being in this constant state of "fight or flight" hurts your body and contributes to premature death.

Stress and its related hormones can also cause you to try to soothe yourself with food (who hasn't snacked through a bag of potato chips when life feels hard?), or alcohol (exceeding two-drinks-daily by a long shot), or nicotine (that pack of smokes got depleted much quicker than usual).

TIP

If you're in a stressful environment or are feeling high stress frequently, finding ways to de-stress helps lower your blood pressure and reduces your need to self-soothe with habits you're trying to leave behind. Some stress-busting activities include the following:

>> Sticking to (or adopting) a near-daily exercise routine.

>> Practicing yoga or meditation.

>> Fueling your body with good food and sufficient sleep.

>> Making time for your hobbies and activities you enjoy.

>> Spending time in nature.

>> Enjoying time with your favorite people.

You can also figure out what's causing you to be stressed and take steps to reduce or eliminate those causes. Check out Chapter 7 for more information on stress.

Chapter **16**

The Mutants Take Over: Cancer

C ancer is a loaded word if ever there was one — a word incapable of tiptoeing into a conversation. Instead, the word *cancer* storms in, attracting attention much like an oversized neon sign, every letter blinking in brightest red.

Cancer is a disease — more accurately, a group of diseases — and every person's body carries within it the possibility of developing cancer.

Cancer also is a disease on the run. Due to the development of more sophisticated detection methods and improved courses of treatment, the number of people surviving cancer in the United States has more than tripled over the past 30 years — so says the National Cancer Institute and the Centers for Disease Control and Prevention.

In this chapter, we give you an overview of cancer, who's at risk, and how it's treated, and then we focus on the main cancers that men face: prostate, lung, skin, and testicular.

Demystifying the "C" Word

Despite decades of research, there's still much we don't know about cancer. Doctors do know that cancer actually is many different diseases, each one complex in its own way. But they share some behaviors, and that's what this section covers.

Understanding how cancer develops

Cancer is a disease that originates at the cellular level. Cells, you may recall from biology class, grow and divide to make sure that you have all the cells you need when you need them to maintain a healthy body. As you read this, some 10 million of your cells are busy dividing. This is normal.

Usually, cell division is an orderly process, with cells growing, maturing, and then dying off as new cells take their place. Sometimes, for reasons not entirely understood, this routine is interrupted. A single cell that has undergone a mutation — either a spontaneous change as a result of a natural incident or one resulting from exposure to a *carcinogen*, or cancer-causing agent — begins to reproduce and keeps at it, without stopping. These new cells, which never reach maturity, form a growth or mass of tissue, and that mass is called a *tumor*.

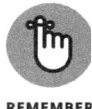

REMEMBER

Tumors come in two types: *benign* (noncancerous) and *malignant:*

>> Generally, benign tumors stay put and do not spread to other parts of the body. If a benign tumor is surgically removed, it usually does not come back.

>> Malignant tumors, on the other hand, contain abnormal cells that continue to divide. Sometimes these cells invade tissue or organs nearby and try to destroy the healthy cells. Sometimes cancerous cells enter the bloodstream or the lymphatic system. When that happens, the cancer cells can spread to sites in the body distant from the site at which the cancer originated.

Figuring out what causes cancer

If only we knew!

Well, actually we know the culprit for some people: genes. About 10 percent of the people who get cancer get it because of abnormalities in their genes. Lots of research is underway to try to pinpoint these abnormalities and find ways to deal with them even before cancer develops.

For the majority of cancers, though, no one yet knows exactly why the switch gets stuck when a particular cell turns "on." We know there are environmental factors that increase your risk, including smoking, an unhealthy diet, and unprotected exposure to the sun's rays. But not all things that *can* lead to cancer (called *carcinogens*) *do* lead to cancer, at least in every instance. Not all carcinogens are created equal, with some being more of a risk in small quantities or smaller durations of exposure, while other carcinogens are dangerous only in higher quantities or with longer exposure.

Research, of course, continues. You can read more about risks in the upcoming section "Getting Real about General Cancer Risks."

Identifying the types of cancer that are most deadly to men

Doctors know that cancer is actually many different diseases, each one complex in its own way. According to the Centers for Disease Control and Prevention in the United States, cancer is the number two killer of men, just behind heart disease. Some of the cancers that are of most concern to men in the United States include the following:

>> **Prostate cancer,** which is the most common cancer men are diagnosed with, excluding skin cancer, and is the second leading cause of cancer death.

>> **Lung cancer** swaps stats with prostate cancer and is the second most common cancer men are diagnosed with and the number one cause of cancer death.

>> **Testicular cancer,** which is the most common cancer in younger men aged 15–35.

Naming cancer based on site of origin

The type of cancer a person is diagnosed with is named for the site where the cancer originates (prostate cancer originates in the prostate, for example). Many of these cancers may spread to other sites — they may *metastasize* or disseminate to other organs. For example, a lung cancer may spread to the bones, brain, or liver.

TECHNICAL
STUFF

If several organs are affected by cancer when a person is diagnosed, a specially trained doctor called a *pathologist* will need to establish the site of the cancer's origin. If you're diagnosed with lung cancer that has metastasized to the adrenal glands, you won't hear the doctors say you have cancer of the adrenal glands. They will say you have lung cancer that has spread, because cancer is always defined according to the primary tumor.

If cancer comes back after treatment, it usually isn't a new cancer; it contains the same cells found in the original tumor, even if the disease now exists in a different part of the body.

Discovering How Treatments Fight Back

Currently, doctors use four different kinds of treatments to fight cancer. These treatments are

>> **Surgery:** Surgery is used to remove a tumor and any tissue around the tumor that may hold cancerous cells. Sometimes, surgery is all the treatment you need.

>> **Chemotherapy:** Also known as *anticancer drugs,* chemotherapy kills cancer cells (see Figure 16-1). When they're dead, these cells can no longer grow or multiply. The body eliminates the dead cells naturally.

Some chemotherapy is administered before surgery to shrink a tumor. Sometimes, the tumor is removed surgically, and chemotherapy is then used to kill any cancer cells that may have spread elsewhere in the body. Some chemotherapy helps relieve symptoms of cancer, so that patients may live with reduced pain.

>> **Radiation therapy:** Radiation therapy stops cancer cells from reproducing. A radiated cell is fried, stopped in its tracks — dead. Again, the body eliminates the dead cells naturally.

REMEMBER

In some cases, doctors use only chemotherapy to fight cancer. In other instances, doctors prescribe radiation therapy, either alone or in addition to chemotherapy.

>> **Biological therapy:** One type of biological therapy called *immunotherapy* helps your immune system destroy cancer cells. Specific drugs are used for specific types of cancers. The drugs you may have heard of include interleukin, interferon, trastuzumab (Herceptin), rituximab (Rituxan), gefitinib (Iressa), erlotonib (Tarceva), and imatinib (Gleevec). One type of immunotherapy drugs are called *checkpoint inhibitors.* Two of note include Durvulumab and Nivolumab, which have revolutionized the treatment of some lung cancers and melanoma, respectively.

A second kind of biological therapy helps control side effects from other cancer treatments. For example, drugs are available that increase your white blood cell count during chemotherapy, make red blood cells if you have anemia, or manufacture platelets. These drugs fall into a general class of medicines called *growth factors* or *colony stimulating factors.*

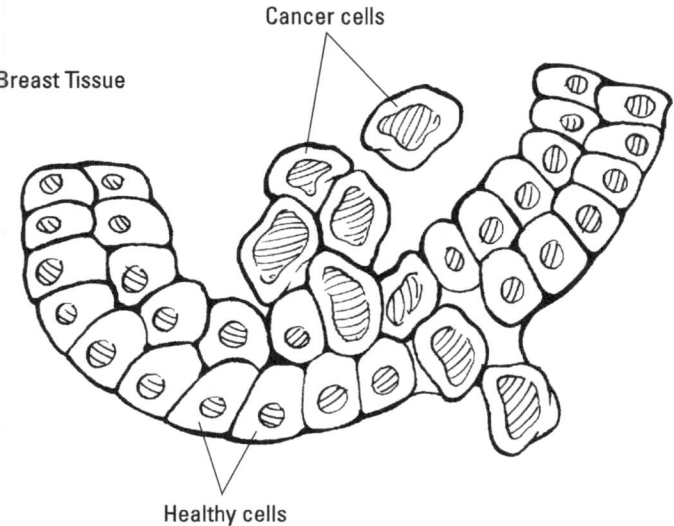

Cancer cells

Breast Tissue

FIGURE 16-1:
Cancer cells differ in appearance considerably from healthy cells.

Healthy cells

Getting Real about General Cancer Risks

What factors contribute to cancer in the other 90 percent of the population? There's no clear-cut answer, but in this section we discuss several well-known factors that may increase the risk of all types of cancer.

TIP

Later in the chapter we talk about who's at risk for the top cancers men face; this section focuses on general risks for all types of cancer. Because if you want to live a better, hopefully longer life, it's important to understand risks so you can make changes to reduce them.

Blaming your genes

We know that for some people genes are the culprits behind cancer. Right now, doctors know that only about 10 percent of all cancers are genetic, or inherited. If you're in that 10 percent — well, you can run, but you can't hide.

TIP

It's a good idea to contact people in your family to figure out your potential risks for developing cancer. Your physician will appreciate this additional family tree information; it will help them determine how aggressive any screenings should be.

WARNING

People may confuse one type of cancer for another, so it's useful to ask some follow-up questions if you find there's a history of cancer in your family. For example, when prostate cancer spreads, it spreads first and mostly to bone. It is this spreading of the cancer that actually kills. In such a case, the man would die from prostate cancer and not bone cancer, because the cancer started in the prostate gland (see "Naming cancer based on site of origin," earlier in this chapter for more on how cancer is named.). However, some of your family members may assume that your relative died of bone cancer. So if your family tree research reveals that an uncle of yours died of cancer, it's worth asking whether your uncle had any other type of cancer before he died.

TIP

If you or your family members have a significant family history of any type of cancer, speak with your doctor about genetic screening, which also can determine other known genetic abnormalities associated with inherited syndromes.

Evaluating environmental factors

Although there's no clear-cut answer about the cause of cancers that aren't genetic, how you live your life and what you're exposed to as you live it (collectively called *environmental factors*) appear to be the main contributors to elevated cancer risk. We said *risk*, not *causes*. It's important to note that although science has proven a correlation between certain environmental factors and cancer, confoundingly, not everyone with a risk factor (or even several) actually gets cancer. In fact, many people with identified risk factors never develop cancer. Conversely, some people who have no known risk factors at all *do* develop cancer.

With all that being said, knowing common risk factors allows you to consider changes you may want to make to your life and habits. So without further ado, here are some of the common risk factors for cancer:

>> **Tobacco:** The National Cancer Institute reports that a third of all cancer deaths each year are due to "smoking tobacco, using smokeless tobacco and being regularly exposed to environmental tobacco smoke." Though smokers are at the highest risk for lung cancer, they also are at higher risk for developing other kinds of cancer. The good news is that soon after a smoker quits, the risk of developing cancer begins to drop. (Check out Chapter 9 for pointers on quitting smoking.)

>> **Alcohol:** The National Institute on Alcohol Abuse and Alcoholism estimates that 2 to 4 percent of all cancer cases are thought to be caused by excessive

consumption of alcohol. What's "excessive"? That depends on many factors — gender, body weight, and family history among them. You probably know better than anyone else when your drinking is out of control (Chapter 9 can help you figure it out).

>> **Diet and exercise:** The American Institute for Cancer Research reports that eating a diet high in vegetables, fruits, whole grains, and beans; maintaining a healthy weight; exercising regularly; and not smoking has "a direct and measurable effect on cancer risk." Chapters 4 and 6 can help you adopt a healthier nutrition and exercise regime.

WARNING

>> **Ultraviolet (UV) radiation:** The Skin Cancer Foundation has declared that skin cancer has reached epidemic proportions. The Foundation's first rule of protection is this: "Do not sunbathe." If you must go out, the Foundation recommends avoiding "unnecessary sun exposure" between 10 a.m. and 4 p.m., which are "the peak hours for harmful ultraviolet radiation."

>> **Chemicals:** *The New England Journal of Medicine* (www.nejm.org) published a report in 2000 by researchers who concluded that "environmental exposures far outweigh the role of heredity in causing cancer." Today, most scientists agree that exposure to some pesticides, metals, and chemicals — such as polychlorinated biphenyls (PCBs) and other mixtures of toxic chemicals, as well as formaldehyde found in some beauty products — may increase the risk of cancer. That also holds true for additives, and for the natural chemicals found in some foods. (That said, some natural chemicals found in fruits and vegetables work in the body to fight cancer.)

>> **X-ray procedures and medical radiation:** The medical journal *The Lancet* (www.thelancet.com), in January 2004, reported that about 700 of the 124,000 cases of cancer diagnosed each year in the United Kingdom "could be attributable to exposure to diagnostic X-rays," which are said to provide "the largest man-made source of radiation exposure to the general population." Radiation therapy treatments, which can damage healthy cells, also carry a slight risk — but, generally, the benefits of treatment are thought to outweigh the risks. If you are considering going through radiation therapy, your radiation oncologist can help you quantify what the risks of damage to healthy cells may be in your case.

Controversy has circled around almost every risk factor listed here — one study shows *this* to be true, the next study shows *that*. But it makes sense to be aware of legitimate dangers to your health, and medical science has proven that changes in some personal behaviors can decrease your cancer risks, even if they can't prevent cancer altogether.

Exploring Prostate Cancer

TECHNICAL STUFF

Before we introduce you to a cancer that many men will be diagnosed with this year, we want to get one thing straight. It's your prosTATE gland, and *not* your prosTRATE gland. *Prostrate* means you're lying down, as in "he was prostrate with grief." You may feel pretty lousy if you worry that you have prostate cancer — or *know* that you have it. And you may feel like lying down. But it's still your prostate.

REMEMBER

More men get prostate cancer than any other type (excluding skin cancer), and behind lung cancer, it's the second leading cause of cancer death in men. Despite its reign near the top of the cancer charts, studies have revealed that most men don't even know that they *have* a prostate gland (unless it gives them trouble). Or, if they know that they have one, many men think of it sort of as a superfluous organ, kind of like your appendix.

Spoiler: your prostate is directly involved in your ability to father children, because it supplies essential nutrients to sperm fluid — hardly superfluous. But if procreation's not in your plans, the prostate gland does nothing but cause trouble; it can interfere with urinating (blocking off urine flow), become infected and cause pain, or develop prostate cancer.

Getting to know your prostate and its neighbors

The healthy prostate gland is a walnut-sized organ that weighs in at about 15 grams, which is a little less than half an ounce, in young men (around age 20 or so) and 30 grams (about an ounce) or more in men who are age 50 or older. Unhealthy prostates can weigh as much as 100 grams or more, resembling the size of an orange or even a small grapefruit. Bigger is not better; in fact, it can be very bad.

REMEMBER

An enlarged prostate doesn't necessarily indicate prostate cancer. Instead, it may indicate a treatable common prostate disease, such as prostatitis or benign prostatic hyperplasia (BPH).

Your prostate sits between your bladder and penis, just above your rectum. Your *urethra,* which is the tube that carries urine from your bladder through your penis and to the outside, runs through your prostate. The prostate gland affects and is affected by the surrounding organs, such as the urinary bladder, the seminal vesicles, and the testicles. (See Figure 16-2 for the location of these organs.)

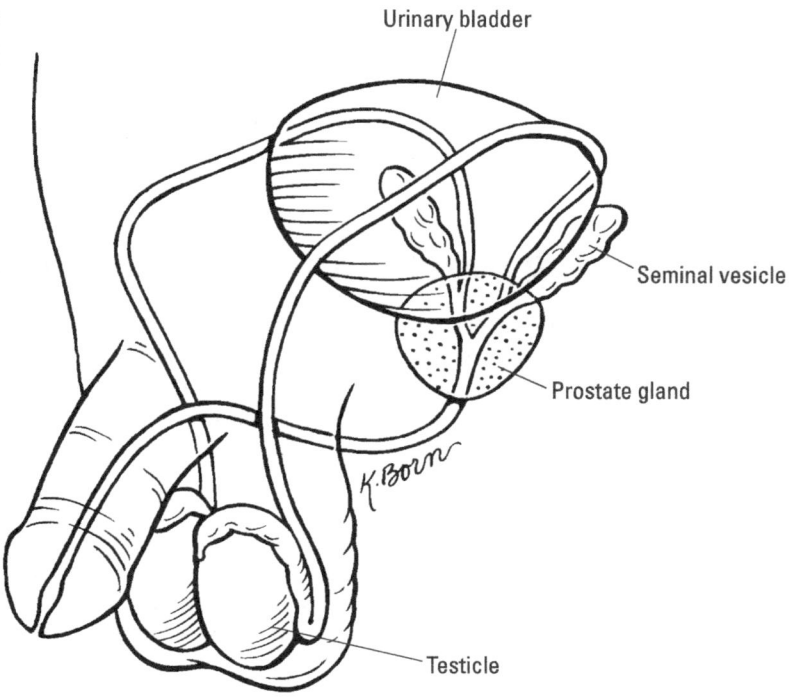

Urinary bladder

Seminal vesicle

Prostate gland

K.Born

Testicle

FIGURE 16-2:
The prostate
gland and other
key reproductive
organs.

>> **Urinary bladder:** A prostate that functions normally doesn't affect the bladder. Consider them neighbors who wave as they pass but don't visit each other's houses. But when the prostate starts having some problems, the neighboring bladder also begins to feel the effects. And the bigger the prostate problem becomes, the greater the impact on the bladder. For example, prostate problems can cause an intense urge to urinate frequently when the prostate is blocking the flow of urine. When the flow of urine is blocked, the bladder has to work harder, causing it to become hyperactive when filling with urine.

>> **Seminal vesicles:** The seminal vesicles supply nutritious fluid to sperm. When the prostate becomes enlarged or infected, it can cause the seminal vesicles to swell up and impede the delivery of seminal fluid. Blocked seminal vesicles can cause pain.

>> **Testicles:** The testicles are sex organs that produce sperm and *testosterone,* a male hormone. The testosterone is sent to the prostate and throughout the bloodstream to the other organs. Testosterone causes male sexual

characteristics, such as a deep voice, body hair, greater muscle tissue than that found in women, and so on.

Prostate cancer thrives and grows when testosterone is around. With advanced prostate cancer, doctors often do things to eliminate testosterone.

Looking more closely at the prostate

In general, the prostate affects two primary functions: reproduction and urination. When you have a problem with your prostate, you may also have a problem with fertility or normal urination. (You can still have prostate cancer and not have any problems with urinating, which we can't emphasize enough.)

Sexually speaking

The prostate is a major player in the production and release of *seminal fluid*, which is the white stuff that's ejaculated, or expelled, when a man has an orgasm. Most of the volume that comprises the seminal fluid comes out of the seminal vesicles (you've got two; see Figure 16-2) and from the prostate. A smaller volume comes from the testicles and contains the sperm.

During orgasm, the fluid from the seminal vesicles and testicles arrives at the prostate and mixes with substances produced by the prostate. One of these substances is *prostate specific antigen (PSA)*. PSA thins out the ejaculate and makes it easier for sperm to travel up a woman's uterus after intercourse in order to reach, penetrate, and fertilize the egg that is released into the upper uterine tube. (See later in this chapter for more information about PSA.)

Your prostate isn't directly involved in your ability to get an erection. However, the nerves that control erections run right next to the prostate, and these nerves can become damaged if the prostate is injured in an accident or if you're treated for prostate cancer with X-rays or surgery.

Urinating matters

The prostate doesn't actually assist the bladder with urination in any way. Instead, it usually just allows it to happen by not interfering with the flow of urine. But a swollen and malfunctioning prostate can impair your urination considerably.

If you look at Figure 16-2, you'll notice that the bladder is right on top of the prostate gland. Narrow tubes called *ureters* carry the urine from your kidneys to your bladder. The urethra travels right through the prostate gland, like a pipeline that cuts through a state. If prostate tissue grows inward and toward your urethra, urinating can become very difficult. If the clog or blockage becomes too severe, you may not be able to urinate at all.

Flagging the symptoms of prostate cancer

Although some men have no symptoms or warnings at all (especially common for men who are in the early stages of prostate cancer that's localized to the gland, with no spread beyond it), most men experience signs that indicate something may be amiss with their prostate.

The following symptoms may be an indication of prostate cancer:

WARNING

>> Problems with urination, including frequent urination (especially at night), painful urination, blood in the urine, a weak urine stream, and a urine stream that stops and starts

If *hematuria* (blood in the urine) is visible to your naked eye, report it to your doctor right away. The blood can indicate a minor or a major problem, so let your doctor determine what is causing it.

>> Trouble getting an erection (erectile dysfunction)

>> Bone pain (may be a symptom of advanced prostate cancer)

>> Constant fatigue

>> An unintended weight loss of ten or fifteen pounds or more

>> Chronic and severe lower back pain

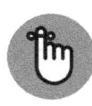

REMEMBER

If you suffer from one or more of the symptoms in this list, you don't necessarily have prostate cancer. But you do need to see your doctor to find out what's actually going on with your body. The section "Working with your doctor to detect prostate cancer" gives more information about testing.

Investigating the risk factors for prostate cancer

Most men have no control over the known risk factors for prostate cancer, primarily age, race/ethnicity, and genetics. (A *risk factor* refers to an increased probability that a health problem may occur because of one or more specific traits.) But other factors that may put you at risk are things you do have control over — such as what you eat and drink, and how much exercise you get.

The known risk factors

The known and accepted risk factors for developing prostate cancer are age, family history, and race. Here's a little more information about each:

>> **Age:** In general, men older than age 50 have a greater risk of developing prostate cancer than younger men, and prostate cancer is very common among men age 65 and older (according to the American Cancer Society, 60 percent of prostate cancers occur in men older than 65). The risk continues to increase with age.

>> **Race/ethnicity:** Men of all races can develop prostate cancer, but the risk is markedly increased for black men. Black men develop prostate cancer at a younger age than white men, and the risk of death from prostate cancer is also greater for black men, followed by the death rates for white men, and then Hispanics, American Indians, and Asians.

If you're a black man, you need to be screened for prostate cancer early (around age 40 or 45). You also need to act aggressively if cancer is detected, because there's some evidence that the cancer can be especially aggressive in black men, although it's not known why this is true.

>> **Genetics:** Your own genetics can affect whether or not you develop prostate cancer. Researchers have determined that if your father and/or brother has had prostate cancer, your risk for developing the disease is approximately double to five times that of other men whose fathers and brothers didn't have the disease. Your risk is higher if your father and/or brother had an early onset of prostate cancer before the age of 55.

The medical histories of the women in your family can also signal a risk for prostate cancer. According to research, men whose mothers or sisters had either breast cancer or ovarian cancer have a greater risk for developing prostate cancer than men whose mothers and sisters have been cancer-free.

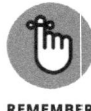

REMEMBER

It's important to keep in mind that you're not doomed to develop prostate cancer merely because you check "yes" in one or more boxes asking you about risk factors. Even if you're black, older than age 50, and have both a brother and a father with prostate cancer, your risk of getting the disease is still low. But your risk is higher than it is for people who don't have all these risk factors, so it's important for you to be diligent in obtaining annual screenings and receive prompt treatment if your doctor does find prostate cancer.

Other risk factors

Although you can't control your age or your race or your family history, you should also consider other health habits that may be risk factors, such as drinking alcoholic beverages and smoking tobacco (wait, have we heard this song before?). Adopting healthy habits is a good preventive strategy against prostate cancer.

TIP

Here's a list of other potential risk factors for prostate cancer — consider if you can make changes to any of these to improve your well-being and reduce your prostate cancer risk:

>> **Physically inactive lifestyles:** If you're physically inactive, you're more likely to be overweight or obese. Together, these factors may contribute to your risk of developing prostate cancer (although research has not definitively proven this connection). Doctors do know that obesity can impair treatment when cancer is diagnosed. For example, obese men may be ordered by their surgeons to lose weight, simply because it's dangerous to cut through a lot of fat tissue during surgery.

>> **Heavy consumption of red meat and fatty foods:** According to clinical studies in the United States and other countries, chowing down on too many overly generous portions of steak and roast beef, and skimping on your intake of vegetables and fruits may lead to prostate cancer. Don't worry, you don't have to subsist entirely on a diet of just tofu and bean sprouts. But if you're addicted to milk shakes and burgers, you may want to seriously rethink your diet — or at least make some changes to it.

>> **High stress levels:** Studies indicate that very high levels of stress can raise your levels of PSA. It's not known if this may cause prostate cancer to occur (or recur), but to be on the safe side, try to minimize your stress levels as much as possible. Check out Chapter 7 for some ideas on how to do that.

>> **Excessive smoking and drinking:** Some studies indicate that smoking and heavy drinking may contribute to the development of prostate cancer, although it is not known by what mechanism this occurs. You can improve your health and lower your chances for developing prostate cancer by ending these problem health habits as soon as possible; Chapter 9 has information that may help.

Working with your doctor to detect prostate cancer

Because prostate cancer frequently causes few symptoms — or no symptoms at all — it's often first detected during routine testing by primary-care physicians (PCP) Your PCP may be an *internist* (a physician who specializes in medical illnesses of the internal organs), a *family practitioner* (a generalist who treats routine medical problems that are found both inside and outside your body), or a *specialist* (a doctor who specializes in treating certain areas of the body).

Your doctor may discover a possible problem during your annual exam or note red flags raised by the results of annual blood tests. This section covers both.

Reporting your medical history

When you meet with the doctor, you'll start by talking about you. Here's what you can expect you'll do:

>> **Talk about your medical history.** You might fill out some forms prior to the appointment or while you're waiting to see the doctor, but the doctor will go over your history with you as well. To receive the best medical analysis, answer your doctor's questions honestly. Be truthful about the amount of alcohol you drink per week, if you smoke, and how often you exercise, and so on.

>> **Discuss your past illnesses.** A review of your general health and medical history is important, because medical problems that you experienced in the past can have a direct effect on the medical problems you're having right now.

If anyone in your family has had prostate cancer, make sure to share this. Cancer isn't contagious, but it may be hereditary. If your father and brother had prostate cancer — and now you're age 50 and you're having urinary problems — you definitely need to be screened for prostate cancer.

>> **Go over how you're feeling right now.** This is relevant, even if you're feeling just fine. Prostate cancer usually doesn't come with early symptoms. And if you've noticed a problem that seems pretty minor, report it to your doctor and let them decide whether it's significant. For example, if you have any problems with urination, share that, whether the problem is frequent urination, a slow stream, trouble with stopping and starting, pain with urination, or all of the above.

>> **Discuss medications you take.** Be sure to leave nothing out! Tell your doctor about any prescriptions you take, any other-the-counter medicine you use frequently (think pain relievers, heartburn chewables, and so on), and any alternative or natural remedies you regularly use.

When you see a doctor for the first time, bring a printed list of all your medications, along with the dosages. If you don't have time to do that, put all your medicines in a bag and bring them with you!

>> **Talk about any allergies you have.** Always tell any new doctor about any drug allergies you may have, such as an allergy to penicillin, sulfa, or any other drug. Allergies can affect what medication your doctor will consider prescribing for you. It can't hurt to remind your regular doctor about any drug allergies, as well.

When talking with your doctor, be sure to volunteer important information even if your doctor doesn't ask you for it. In particular, share

>> Any symptoms pertaining to the urinary tract (pain, difficulty, frequency, or any other trouble with urination)

>> Significant changes in your weight, changes in your overall sleep habits or energy levels

>> Instances of cancer in your family (especially your parents and siblings)

>> Any pain you have, especially significant pain that's getting worse (when prostate cancer spreads, it mostly goes to the bone — in rare cases, the first sign of prostate cancer can be bone pain)

Getting screened with a digital rectal exam and PSA test

In addition to the information your doctor can learn from your health history, two prostate-specific screenings can give them important information about your prostate health — the digital rectal exam and the PSA test.

All men who are 50 years old and older should be screened with both a rectal exam and an annual PSA test as part of their routine physical exam.

REMEMBER

If you have risk factors for the disease, such as being a black man and/or having a family history of prostate cancer, you should start annual testing around age 40 or 45. The more risk factors you have, the greater your need for annual screenings beginning at age 40.

Should older men (age 70 and older) be screened for prostate cancer? We don't like age cutoffs for screening, so we vote yes, on a case-by-case basis. We primarily consider the man's life expectancy, and whether a man is likely to live for ten or more years from now. Some men who are 70 years old have the physical health and stamina of a man who's 60 or younger. Other men are age 70, and they're severely ill with heart disease, diabetes, and other serious medical problems, and they're unlikely to live for ten more years, whether or not they have prostate cancer.

TIP

If you're _under_ age 50, you're in one or more of the high-risk groups discussed in this section on prostate cancer, and your doctor or insurance company doesn't recognize your need for an annual screening for prostate cancer, seriously consider paying for it yourself. The PSA test usually costs less than $80 and is a small price to pay for the valuable information you get.

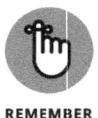

REMEMBER

PSA tests are good at screening for prostate cancer, but sometimes cancer can still be present with a normal PSA. So make sure you share with your doctor any unusual symptoms you may find. Check out the section "Reporting your medical history" for specific pointers.

Having a digital rectal exam

Your doctor may want to perform a digital rectal exam, particularly if you have any symptoms that may be prostate related (although some doctors include this as a routine screening test). The *digital rectal examination* (DRE), typically provided annually after age 50, is a physical examination of your rectal area and prostate gland; it takes a maximum of 15 seconds to perform. When your doctor performs this test, they look for any deviations from the way your prostate should normally feel, which is fairly smooth and pliant.

UNDERSTANDING HOW THE DRE IS PERFORMED

Doctors perform digital rectal examinations in a variety of ways. Some doctors have you stand up, spread your legs, bend over, and lean against the examining table. Others have you lie on your side on the examination table. Still others have you get up on the table on your elbows and knees. Your doctor will ask you to assume a position that they find works best for the exam — try to work with them on this one.

The doctor uses a lubricated gloved finger to probe the area for possible problems. (Check out Figure 16-3 to see how the rectal exam is performed.) When your doctor performs the exam, you may feel brief, slightly cold pressure in the area of your prostate. The doctor feels for bumps and lumps that shouldn't be there. Suspicious bumps and lumps can tell them if you have a problem that should be evaluated further.

TIP

For the best and fastest results with a rectal examination, try not to tense up. Of course, it isn't easy to relax when your doctor is probing a private part of your body. But the more you tense up, the harder you make it on yourself, and the longer the exam will last. And the doctor's experience can speed things up — usually, the more rectal exams a doctor has performed, the better they are at doing them fast and efficiently with little discomfort.

If your doctor thinks that your prostate may be infected, they'll press on it during the rectal exam, which can hurt a bit. The doctor may press long enough to generate some prostatic fluid, which will come out of the tip of your penis. This fluid is checked for infection, either under the microscope or in a culture.

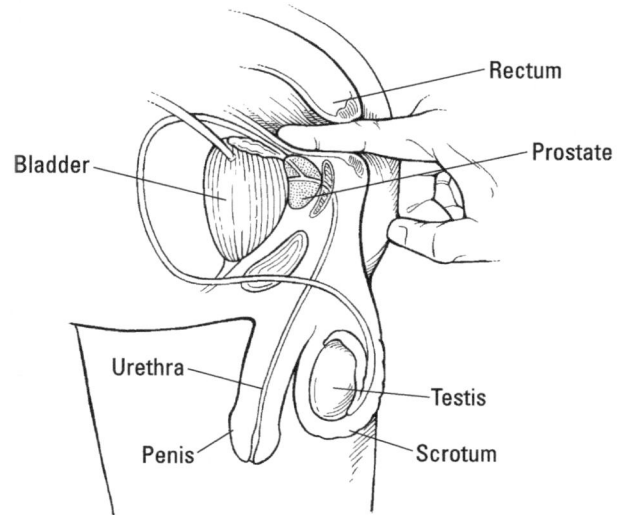

FIGURE 16-3:
The digital rectal
examination. This
drawing shows
the relationship
of the prostate to
other nearby
organs, as well as
how the doctor's
gloved finger
can probe the
prostate through
the rectum.

Rectum

Bladder

Prostate

Urethra

Testis

Penis

Scrotum

Illustration by Kathryn Born.

INTERPRETING THE RESULTS OF YOUR DRE

Your doctor may suspect the presence of prostate cancer based on the findings from your digital rectal examination. When cancer is present, the prostate gland may feel different than normal. It may feel uneven, lumpy, or bumpy, rather than its normal smooth self. If your doctor has performed rectal exams on you before, they have a general feel for what your prostate usually feels like and can tell if something is potentially wrong. If your doctor detects any deviations, they may refer you to a specialist (usually a urologist) for further evaluation.

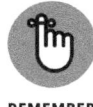

REMEMBER

If your doctor feels some lumps or bumps on your prostate, it doesn't necessarily mean that you have cancer. Your doctor won't know if it's cancer for sure until a biopsy test confirms that cancer is present. The lumps may be a result of prostatitis or some other problem, so don't panic if your doctor sends you to a urologist for a further check of your prostate gland.

Pondering the PSA test

The PSA test is a relatively painless blood test, and it helps your doctor identify the possible presence of prostate cancer by checking for *prostate specific antigen* (a protein substance produced by the prostate gland), which is present in high levels in many people who have prostate cancer. We consider the PSA test to be as important a screening device for detecting prostate cancer among men as the mammogram is for detecting breast cancer among women.

Deciphering your test results

PSA levels can be anywhere from zero to a thousand or more. But generally, in men who still have their prostate gland, a normal value is considered to be 4 nanograms per milliliter or lower.

TECHNICAL STUFF

Your PSA levels may affect whether the doctor chooses to order a biopsy. Even if your prostate feels okay to your doctor during your rectal exam, they may still order a biopsy if they consider your PSA level to be high. Because some men with PSA levels under 4 have prostate cancer (more typical of men under age 60), some doctors argue that the normal level of PSA (and the point at which doctors should consider doing biopsies of the prostate) should be *lowered* to 2.5 or 3 so that even more cases of cancer can be caught before they advance further.

Your doctor may also take into account your *PSA velocity,* which is how fast your PSA levels go up over time. If your PSA level was 1 last year, and now it's 2.4, your doctor has cause for concern, and more frequent testing (and even a biopsy) may be advised. To determine the frequency of the screening needed to diagnose prostate cancer, your doctor may consider the size of your prostate gland compared to your PSA level. This comparison is called *PSA density.* Generally, a high PSA level in a man with a small prostate is more disturbing than the same PSA level in a man with a large prostate.

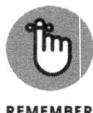

REMEMBER

An above-normal PSA test result may indicate cancer. It may also indicate *prostatitis* (inflammation of the prostate) or *benign prostatic hyperplasia* (BPH, an overgrowth of noncancerous cells that causes an enlargement of the prostate gland, and present to some extent in all men as they age). Make sure you tell your doctor if you're being treated for BPH, as the drugs to treat it may lower your PSA result, and prostate cancer could be missed. Frequently, above-normal PSA tests indicate "none of the above." Men can be healthy and well despite an elevated PSA.

Considering additional lab work

In addition to the DRE and the PSA test (LMK if you're following), your doctor may also request general laboratory tests to go along with the rectal exam and PSA test. For example, they may want to request a *complete blood count (CBC)*, a determination of the number of white and red blood cells in your blood, or a *blood urea nitrogen (BUN)* test, a blood test that may be abnormal in the presence of prostate cancer blocking the urine flow. The doctor may also order a urinalysis or urine culture to check your urine for possible infection. These tests aren't markers for cancer, but they're important because they can provide your doctor with information on your overall health.

TECHNICAL STUFF

Some doctors may also order a blood test of your prostatic acid phosphatase (PAP), which is a tumor marker, because elevated levels of PAP are sometimes found in men with prostate cancer. However, the PSA is a far more effective and targeted test for prostate cancer.

Coming to Terms with Lung Cancer

Behind prostate cancer, lung cancer is the most common cancer men are diagnosed with (excluding skin cancer), and it's the number one cause of male cancer deaths. The American Cancer Society estimates that in the United States in 2025, about 111,000 new cases of lung cancer will be diagnosed in men; they estimate that about 64,000 men will die of lung cancer. The good news is, those numbers are shrinking — the number of men diagnosed with lung cancer is going down, and so is the number of men who die from it.

You probably know that smoking is the biggest contributor to getting lung cancer. In this section, we seek to give you information about this disease, who's at risk, and what you can do to reduce your risk and live more of your good life.

Recognizing that lungs are not just bags of hot air

Your lungs are important organs that have two main jobs — to take in oxygen as you breathe in and deliver that oxygen to your blood, and to remove carbon dioxide from your blood and expel it from your body as you breathe out. They can't perform this important function as needed if they're not in top-notch shape.

WARNING

It's no secret that long-term exposure to smoke from cigarettes causes lung cancer. According to the American Cancer Society, about 80 percent of lung cancer deaths are caused by smoking. Fifteen percent of lung cancer deaths occur in people who don't smoke; some factors responsible for their cancer include environmental exposure to radon gas, asbestos, secondhand smoke, and air pollution. Changes to their genes are also to blame.

A takeaway here is that men have a significant opportunity to support the health of their lungs, and to reduce their chances of being diagnosed with or dying from lung cancer by ceasing to smoke and better yet, never starting.

Getting the lung cancer lowdown

Lung cancer is classified according to the type of cell involved. Two major types make up 97 percent of all lung cancers:

>> Most lung cancers (80–85 percent) are *non-small cell lung cancers* (NSCLCs). Non-small cell lung cancer develops slowly compared to small cell lung cancers, but even though they aren't rapid growers, someone with NSCLC may not show symptoms, which means NSCLC can metastasize to other parts of your body before you even know you have cancer.

>> About 10–15 percent are *small cell lung cancers* (SCLCs), which, despite being made up of small cells, produce a large tumor. Like NSCLC, small cell lung cancers may not reveal themselves via symptoms until after they've spread to other parts of your body.

REMEMBER

Normally, the first sign of lung cancer is a cough that doesn't go away. Some other signs and symptoms follow:

>> Cough that produces blood

>> Difficulty swallowing

>> Hoarse voice

>> Pain in the chest or abdomen

>> Pneumonia

>> Shortness of breath

>> Unexplained weight loss and loss of appetite

TIP

Early detection greatly improves survival rates, so if you notice any of these symptoms, make sure to share them with your doctor. You probably don't have lung cancer, but giving your doctor a chance to check you out means any cancer that does exist can be found and treated more quickly.

Discovering who's at risk for developing lung cancer

If you're a tobacco smoker, you're by far more at risk of developing lung cancer than non-smokers. The risk is greater based on the number of years you've smoked and the number of packs a day you smoked during those years. Cigar and pipe smoke has about the same risk as cigarette smoking.

Exposure to secondhand smoke and to *radon* (a naturally occurring radioactive gas that can be dangerous when concentrated inside homes, where radon is often found) also increases your risk of developing lung cancer. In fact, behind smoking tobacco, these two factors are the second and third most common causes of lung cancer in the United States.

Also at higher risk are people exposed to other environmental factors such as asbestos (encountered when working in mines, mills, and textile plants), and people who are frequently exposed to diesel exhaust.

Some risk factors you have little or no control over are outdoor air pollution and a family history of lung cancer. Neither contributes significantly to lung cancer deaths, so time you spend considering how you might reduce your risk is best spent on minimizing exposure to smoke (yours or someone else's) and, to a much lesser extent, exposure to environmental factors listed in this section.

Older adults are more at risk of developing lung cancer than younger adults — the median age for a lung cancer diagnosis is 71. This can be attributed at least in part to the longer duration of exposure to the various risk factors.

Diagnosing and treating lung cancer

A chest X-ray is the first study done to look for lung cancer. It may show the tumor and/or widening of the structures in the middle of the chest from the cancer's spread to the lymph nodes there. The tumor then is biopsied to make a definitive diagnosis.

Treatment depends on the type of cell, the amount of spread, and the physical fitness of the patient. A key treatment includes immunotherapy, specifically *checkpoint inhibitors,* which help the immune system kill cancer cells (Durvulumab has revolutionized the treatment of some lung cancers). Other treatments include surgical removal (if possible), chemotherapy, and radiation therapy. Surgery can involve anything from removing part of the lobe of the lung in which the tumor is found, to removing an entire lung. As with other cancers, the tumor is staged based on how much spread has occurred at the time of diagnosis.

REMEMBER

Prognosis for either non-small cell lung cancer or small cell lung cancer is poor. By the time the diagnosis is made, the cancer is usually advanced. It makes good sense to try to prevent lung cancer instead of treating it after it has occurred.

Reducing your risks of lung cancer

TIP

You won't be surprised when we tell you the best thing you can do to reduce your lung cancer risk is to stop smoking, or to never start. Chapter 9 can help you quit if you're a smoker and want support.

You can also limit your exposure to radon (have your home tested, and if needed, install a radon mitigation system) and your exposure to secondhand smoke. Fortunately, most public places now ban smoking indoors and within a specific distance of buildings and entryways, so it's easier than it's ever been to avoid exposure to secondhand smoke.

The nutrition pointers found in Chapter 4 apply here. In particular a healthy diet with lots of fruits and vegetables can help reduce your risk, even if you currently smoke or used to.

Spotting Skin Cancer

We all go outside, which means we're all at risk for developing skin cancer. Fortunately, skin cancer is usually successfully treated when it's found in its early stages. Along with making sure a skin cancer screening is part of your annual checkup, a key to early detection is monthly self-exam.

By knowing what your skin normally looks like, and how to spot the various types of skin cancer, you'll be able to alert your doctor at the first sign of a skin abnormality so you can get the treatment you need.

TIP

Skin cancer can grow on parts of your body where the sun doesn't shine. Be sure to look at every inch of your skin, from your scalp, to your genitals, to the soles of your feet. Make a note of any scars, moles, freckles, or other marks so you know what's ordinary for you. Use a full-length mirror, a hand-held mirror, and a magnifying glass to make sure you don't miss a mark. And regularly take photos of the back of your body (or enlist a partner or friend if needed) so you can be as diligent about monitoring your back as you are your front.

The four most prevalent skin cancers are basal cell, squamous cell, melanoma, and merkel cell. Each carries its own set of symptoms.

Basal cell carcinoma

This is the most common and easily treatable skin cancer. Although it's the least likely to spread, if you've had one basal cell growth, you have a high likelihood of developing another one within five years. Basal cell carcinoma has a multi-faceted appearance. Here's what to look for:

>> A pearly white, firm bump that gradually gets larger. It may bleed, crust over or develop a depression in the middle. The bump may be brown or black in darker-skinned people. Tiny blood vessels might be visible on the surface of the bump.

>> A bleeding sore that scabs and heals but then comes back and starts bleeding again.

>> Pink or red lesions that have a rough appearance and bleed easily.

>> A flat area that looks brown and crusty but can also be flesh colored.

>> A waxy scar that is skin colored, white, or yellow.

Squamous cell carcinoma

This is the second most common form of skin cancer. Like melanoma and merkel cancers, it will spread if left untreated. However, the survival rate is 95 percent if found early. Here are signs of squamous cell growth:

>> A scab-like or scaly area.

>> An area that's red, raised, and firm.

>> An ulcerated sore that won't close and heal.

Melanoma

Melanoma is the most-deadly form of skin cancer because it's the most likely to invade other parts of your body. Even so, with early detection and proper treatment, it too is highly curable. The 5-year survival rate for localized melanoma is 95 percent.

Melanomas can develop on any part of your skin, including moles you've had since childhood. Moles are the starting place for 20 to 40 percent of all melanomas. To help you remember what to look for when examining your moles, the medical community has developed an easy technique called the ABCDE rule.

>> A is for asymmetry. One half of your mole looks different from the other half.

>> B is for border. The edges of your mole are uneven, notched or not well defined.

>> C is for color. Healthy moles have consistent color throughout. Melanoma moles have a mixture of colors, including brown, black, red, blue, tan, and/or white.

>> D is for diameter. If your mole has grown by a quarter-inch or more, melanoma may be present.

>> E is for evolving. Moles should stay the same color, shape, and size throughout our adult lives. If yours has changed or suddenly starts bleeding or itching, it's time to see your doctor.

Other melanoma warning signs include:

>> The area around the mole assumes the same color and appearance as the mole or becomes red and swollen; the mole seems to spread.

>> Any new growth on your skin (although most melanomas are pigmented black, gray, deep blue, or brown, some are not).

>> Any sore that won't heal.

>> Itchiness, tenderness, scaling, or pain in one particular area of your skin.

>> A black streak or bruised appearance under your fingernail or toenail that won't go away.

Merkel cell carcinoma

Although this is still a rare form of cancer, affecting only 1,500 Americans a year, its numbers are increasing. It develops mostly in fair-skinned people over the age of 50. Merkel cell cancer can spread quickly, but if treated early, the survival rate is 90 percent.

It develops as a shiny, firm nodule or nodules on your skin. The painless growths are flesh-colored, red, blue, or purple. They may look like a pimple, cyst, stye, or bug bite.

Testing for Testicular Cancer

Even though the testicles are easily accessible, most men don't pay all that much attention to them (apart from trying to protect them from getting kicked — something fathers of toddlers who love slamming into Dad are well aware of). That can prove unfortunate, because testicular cancer can be deadly if you don't find it in time.

WARNING

Testicular cancer most often appears in men from ages 15 to 35 — the average age a man is when diagnosed is 33 (in comparison to the average age a man is when diagnosed with lung cancer, which is 71). In fact, testicular cancer is the most common form of cancer in men in their 20s and 30s.

Because testicular cancer is the number one cancer in younger men, and because the disease is also easily curable, this section focuses primarily on self-examination that can help you identify any issues you need to bring to your doctor's attention right away.

Checking for lumps

Because the testicles are outside the body and can be examined, men can easily feel testicular cancer if it's present. And because the testicles are so accessible, men can spare themselves the trouble of going to a doctor for the examination (as women must do with cervical cancer) by examining their testicles themselves.

Testicular cancer usually begins as a painless lump. The sooner you find such a lump, the better your chances of having it treated without any serious medical consequences. Begin checking for lumps in your teen years.

TIP

The best time to perform a self-exam is after a hot shower or bath because the warm water allows the scrotum to relax and the testicles to drop down. You can do the check while you're sitting, standing, or lying down.

To check for lumps:

1. **Gently take each testicle and roll it between your thumb and forefinger to see if you detect anything different about how it feels compared with last time.**

   Your testicle should feel smooth and firm with a slight softness, a lot like a hard-boiled egg without the shell.

2. **As a guide, compare your two testicles to each other.**

   Remember, it's normal for one testicle to be slightly larger than the other and/or one to hang lower than the other.

3. **If you do find something that feels different, pick up the phone right away and make an appointment to see a urologist.**

4. **Do this test around the same time each month to get into the habit.**

As we mention in Chapter 11, the epididymis sits on top of the testicle. Some men examining themselves for testicular cancer mistake it for a strange lump. They get a real fright before a doctor explains to them what it is. So what you need to have clear in your mind is that you are checking your testicle — the hard-boiled egg. The lumpy epididymis, which lies on top of the testicle, belongs there and is supposed to be lumpy but not tender.

TIP

Testicular cancer can hit any man, but men who had one or both undescended testicles at birth (Chapter 11 contains more info) are at higher risk. So if either or both of your testicles had not descended when you were born, make doubly sure that you perform this exam every month.

Sometimes a minor injury to the groin area may cause some swelling. This swelling can mask the presence of an undetected cancerous growth. This is why a monthly checkup is necessary — so you know what's normal for you from month to month, and what's not.

REMEMBER

We know that many men are squeamish about medical things, particularly when it comes to something in the genital area. But this testing is important, so please don't be lax about it. Early detection and immediate medical attention are the keys for successful treatment.

If you really don't like the idea of examining yourself, and if you have a partner, maybe you can ask them to complete this exercise. We don't know if they'll like doing it any better than you would, but you both may profit from the side effects.

Feeling testicular pain

Many men prefer to keep certain matters private (especially when the matter pertains to anything hanging between their legs), but feeling a twinge of pain from time to time in the scrotum is quite common. If you experience this sort of pain and it disappears after a minute or two, you don't have to worry. The testicles are very sensitive, and in all probability, one got bumped or twisted a bit, which caused this momentary pain.

WARNING

If you experience continuous pain, then you should go to see a doctor immediately. One of the more severe conditions that may be causing the pain is *testicular torsion*, where the testicle gets twisted around inside the scrotum and blood no longer flows into it. This is an emergency condition that needs to be treated very quickly.

A more common cause of pain is *epididymitis*, which is an infection of the epididymis gland. The infection is easily diagnosed by a doctor and treated with antibiotics.

Chapter **17**

Risky Business: Dying by Accident

M any health conditions that shorten men's lives have a genetic component — something you can't change. Healthy habits such as eating well, exercising, and getting enough sleep can lower the odds, but they can't always prevent you from getting a serious disease.

Accidents, however, are a different story. They play a big role in premature male deaths — much more than in females — and most are preventable. Sure, some risks are hard to dodge (like working a dangerous job to pay the bills), but for the most part, avoiding "death by accident" is squarely in men's control. In other words, it's your move if you want to cross off that square on your Live Longer bingo card.

Getting Acquainted with Accidents

Unintentional injuries, better known as accidents, aren't just mishaps — they're one of the biggest silent killers for guys. These are injuries that don't occur on purpose (which means they're preventable) and happen without intent to harm. According to the United States Centers for Disease Control and Prevention

(CDC, www.cdc.gov), unintentional injuries include motor vehicle crashes, unintentional drowning, unintentional falls, and unintentional poisoning (including opioid overdoses — detailed later in this chapter).

REMEMBER

Men are dramatically overrepresented in injury death stats. In the United States, accidents are the third leading cause of premature death in men. And accidental deaths aren't a risk just for Americans — according to the World Health Organization (WHO, www.who.int), about 75 percent of the world's 4.4 million injury-related deaths each year are due to accidents.

WARNING

These accidental deaths affect young people more significantly than their silver-haired counterparts by a landslide. Not only are accidents the leading cause of death in Americans under age 45, but in 2023, people under 45 were over four times more likely to die from accidents than cancer. And don't think you're getting off the hook, Mr. Turning-Silver Fox — unintentional injury deaths are still very high until you hit your early 60s, when this cause declines meaningfully.

The good news is, accidents can usually be prevented, so you can skip the "sudden, tragic ending" chapter in your life story.

Preventing Killers: Premature Deaths You Can Avoid

Accidents that result in premature death fall into four main causes — overdoses, transportation, drowning, and banana peels, er, falling. Keep reading for more.

Dodging deadly doses: Unintentional poisoning

According to the National Safety Council (www.nsc.org), unintentional poisoning is by far the number one cause of preventable injuries in men. In the United States, 75 percent of those deaths were from drug overdoses, synthetic opioids specifically (heavy-hitters like fentanyl and tramadol). Other opioids, like oxycodone (such as OxyContin), hydrocodone (such as Vicodin), morphine, and heroin, also contributed to overdose deaths, but to a much lesser extent.

TECHNICAL STUFF

Opioids work by reducing the perception of pain and producing euphoria. When opioids first came on the market, they offered a doctor-prescribed pain-management lifeline to many people who struggled with severe or chronic pain. They've since gained fame for their effectiveness and notoriety for their risk.

What makes opioids both life-saving and dangerous is their potent, quick-acting results. Their ability to trigger intense pleasure makes them highly addictive, especially when misused or taken longer than prescribed.

WARNING

This misuse can easily lead to accidental overdose because taking too much — whether by misjudging a dose, mixing with alcohol or other depressants, or using a batch with unexpected potency (common with illicit fentanyl) — can cause your breathing and heart rate to slow and then stop before help arrives.

Increased access to naloxone (a life-saving injection), wider availability of treatment programs, including medication-assisted treatments (such as methadone or buprenorphine), and tighter prescription monitoring have reduced the number of unintended deaths and have helped more guys stay alive in the face of a potential overdose.

Crashing cars and taking risks

Unintentional vehicle deaths of men look like a steep ski slope on CDC line graphs. Under age 16, boys face fewer than 150 deaths a year. Then the graph blasts off, peaking around age 20–22, before gradually sliding down through the 30s and leveling off for decades. Men don't see a real drop in vehicle-related accidents until their early 60s. (For women, deaths stay steady — about a third of men's — until men's rates dip in their late 40s, narrowing the gap.) Worldwide, the WHO reports men make up 75 percent of the roughly 1 million annual road traffic deaths.

WARNING

Some reasons men face fatal vehicle crashes more often than women, particularly males aged 18-22, focus on their willingness to tolerate risky driving:

>> **Men are more likely to ignore traffic rules.** If you don't behave as other drivers expect, the risk of accidents increases.

>> **Men are more willing to exceed the speed limit.** It's easier to lose control of a vehicle at higher speeds. And the consequences of a high-speed accident are more significant than a slow-speed fender-bender.

>> **Men are more likely to drink or do drugs and operate a vehicle.** Impaired drivers are less able to gauge their speeds, they don't make decisions as well as their sober counterparts, and they have lower response times when a driving incident occurs. Simply put, impaired drivers are more likely to get into accidents than those who are sober.

>> **Men are less likely to wear seat belts.** Using a seat belt while driving or riding in a passenger vehicle reduces the risk of fatal injury by 45 percent, but a belt can't help you if you're not wearing it.

Taking a tumble

Globally, falls are the second leading cause of accident-related deaths, with over 600,000 deaths per year. Nearly 50,000 Americans die from falls annually, with men facing no greater risk than women do. This includes falls from one level to another as well as falling to the ground you're standing on.

Most of the time, in the United States at least, falls are most dangerous to men over age 65 versus their younger counterparts, but young pups need to be careful, too.

Falls in the workplace

WARNING

Most falls occur outside of work, but some professions in particular put guys at higher risk. The reasons include the following:

>> Men may have jobs with higher risk of falling due to the heights they work at, the heaviness of the machinery they use, or both. Some of the jobs with the highest risk of falling include jobs within the transportation or moving industries as well as jobs in construction and extraction occupations, where workers use machinery to mine minerals (such as coal), oil, gas, or other natural resources from the earth.

>> Construction workers often use ladders or scaffolding while they're building or repairing buildings, including roof work, which in and of itself is a higher risk.

Falls at home

Fall risk isn't isolated to the workplace — weekend warriors need to be careful, too, making sure to follow ladder safety protocols, removing all hazards from the work area, and wearing clothing that won't get caught on equipment or tools.

TIP

And if you're an older guy, 65 or over and especially over age 75, even just day-to-day living can present fall risks. Maybe you keep the spare batteries on a second shelf, you cover your cold hardwood floors with rugs, or your spouse prefers cozy mood lighting over more illuminating light bulbs. Stay on top of fall risks, even if your home has no steps inside or out.

Fighting for breath: Unintentional drowning

Fatal drowning happens when your nose and mouth are underwater long enough to stop you from breathing — and ultimately, to die. An estimated 300,000 people drown to death across the world each year (two times as many males as females), and in the United States, boys and men (especially young men) drown to death three times more often than girls and women.

WARNING

Similar to vehicle accidents, a main reason behind men's unintentional drowning includes risky behavior, including swimming and boating while under the influence of alcohol or drugs, swimming at night, and swimming alone. Globally, men who fish for a living are (not surprisingly) also at greater risk, as are men who rely on water transportation, which isn't well-regulated in many countries.

Understanding Risks and Root Causes

In this section, we dig into men's brain health and its effects on behavior — starting with the hard truth that men's brains are wired a bit differently. Hormones such as testosterone don't just shape bodies; they can nudge decision-making, risk-taking, and impulse control in ways that set up men for both bold achievements and unnecessary hazards.

A primer on male sex hormones

Testosterone is the star sex hormone for males, but it's not just about strong bones, big muscles, and masculinity. Testosterone plays a crucial role in shaping the male brain, influencing everything from mood regulation to cognitive function.

In young men, healthy testosterone levels are associated with good mental health, sharp cognitive abilities, and robust physical health. As men age, starting by age 40, testosterone levels naturally decline slightly. This decline can impact mood, leading to symptoms such as irritability and depression, and affect cognitive functions such as memory and concentration.

Youthful misadventure

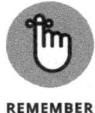

REMEMBER

As so many cringe-worthy (our development editor calls them "classic") movies from the 1980s illustrate, adolescence and young adulthood is a time marked by heightened thrill-seeking and risk-taking. Sensation-seeking, defined as the pursuit of high-intensity and stimulating experiences, increases significantly during adolescence due to a combination of rising reproductive hormones and social pressures. This drive often leads to behaviors such as experimenting with drugs, engaging in unprotected sex, and other impulsive actions like driving too fast.

This dual pattern of heightened sensation-seeking and still-developing impulse control during adolescence helps explain why teenagers are particularly prone to risky behaviors, even when they're cognitively aware of potential negative outcomes. And the behaviors don't necessarily stop when puberty ends. As we discuss in the sections within "Preventing Killers: Premature Deaths You Can Avoid," young males continue to participate in risky behaviors like excessive alcohol consumption and unsafe driving.

Whether it's drug use that goes too far, careless or thrill-seeking driving (and the late-teen/early-20s car insurance rates that accompany it!), or goofing around while on a job site, a young man's willingness to take risks can sometimes result in an unintentional end.

The brain and occupational risks

When you consider occupational risks and their effects on men's brain health, you'll find significant differences between the sexes, particularly outside Western, Educated, Industrialized, Rich, and Democratic (WEIRD) societies. We mention this to recognize that men and women often occupy different roles especially in the developing world, which exposes them to varying risks.

Compared to women, men are more likely to work in places that put their brain health at risk, such as construction sites, factories, or military settings. These occupations can expose men to the risks of falls, toxin exposure, and high levels of stress or potential for trauma, all of which can negatively affect brain health and its long-term ability to function as well as designed.

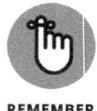

REMEMBER

It's easy to roll your eyes at occupational health and safety measures, but proper safety equipment, regular health screenings, and workplace mental health support can mitigate these risks. Governments, employers, and employees alike must be proactive in creating safer work environments that prioritize men's physical and mental health.

From heart health to brain health

As you age, you experience changes in cognitive function, which can range from those tip-of-the-tongue moments, to sound decision-making, to more serious issues such as dementia. Interestingly, men's cognitive decline is closely linked to cardiovascular health. If you want to keep your processing and decision-making skills in tip-top shape to help you avoid unintentional fatal accidents, then take a look at Chapter 15 for good heart health habits. (And check out Chapter 20 for more on Alzheimer's disease and dementia.)

Not hormones, but mental health

Mental health symptoms sometimes manifest differently in men, which can cause mental health problems to go under-recognized and under-treated. Rather than the stereotypical symptoms of sadness or withdrawal, sometimes these symptoms show as feeling angry or irritable, drinking too much, or behaving recklessly.

No matter where in the world you live, there's still stigma associated with men seeking help for mental health issues, which can prevent many from accessing the support they need and, in the process, potentially minimizing risks for accident-related deaths. It's vital to watch out for your friends and maintain relationships. Men's health organizations the world over promote the mental health benefits of community and relationships, such as sports teams, social organizations, and the like. You can find more information on keeping your mental health in good shape, and supportive resources if you need them, in Chapter 7.

Changing Your Behavior to Change Your Destiny

The good news is that many accidents are preventable. You can take steps that will significantly reduce your risk of dying early from unintended injuries.

Here are some actions you can take:

>> **Take medications as prescribed.** When your doctor prescribes medication, especially pain meds, take them as directed. Take them on time, don't double up, don't take them more frequently than prescribed, and follow any restrictions on the bottle related to alcohol consumption or driving or operating heavy machinery. Don't share them with friends!

Most people don't overdose on purpose, and sometimes an overdose occurs not because of excessive dosage but because the meds have been mixed with alcohol in a dangerous way. If you have any questions about taking prescribed medicines, make sure to talk to your doctor or a registered pharmacist.

>> **Get help if you suspect you have a problem.** If you have trouble staying on your prescribed dose schedule and feel you need to take prescription meds more frequently than directed, or if you need to take more than the prescribed dose to get the results they were prescribed for, you may be treading in dangerous waters. Talk to your doctor as soon as possible. You can also call or text 988 (in the United States) or contact Narcotics Anonymous (na.com in the United States, 0300 999 1212 or ukna.org in the U.K.) for substance use support.

>> **Get help for illicit drug use.** If you're using heroin or other illicit drugs, contact the resources in the preceding bullet for help.

>> **Obey traffic rules.** Stick to the speed limit, obey traffic lights, and follow all other guidelines you learned when you got licensed.

>> **Secure your body and your head.** Wear your seat belt when in a car or truck, whether you're the driver or passenger, and wear a helmet when driving or riding on a motorcycle, scooter, or other motorized vehicle requiring one.

>> **Drive sober and boat sober.** Enough said.

>> **Operate equipment correctly.** When operating heavy machinery, know how to do so correctly, and have a safety plan at the ready.

>> **Don't take risks with ladders.** Set them up on level ground, make sure they're locked in place before you step on one, don't climb above the third-highest rung, and have a spotter nearby in case you need additional support.

Use the *4-to-1 rule* to place a ladder a safe distance from a building or other structure (place the ladder's base one foot from the wall for every four feet of height).

>> **Avoid fall risks.** Keep your workspace and your home free of trip risks. Wear supportive shoes. When working on projects, avoid loose clothing that could get caught in tools or equipment. Install and use handrails and grab bars on stairways and in bathrooms, and get somebody's help when you need to reach something higher than your upstretched arms.

>> **Enjoy water safely.** Learn to swim or wear a life jacket if you're an inexperienced or weak swimmer. Wear a life jacket when boating and participating in water-based activities. Swim only in daylight. Don't swim alone. Stay sober when having fun on the water.

Chapter **18**

Stroke: A Brain Attack

ere's the hard truth: Stroke doesn't mess around. It kills, it disables, and it doesn't care how strong or smart you are. For men in the United States, stroke is the fifth leading cause of death — and the number one reason people end up with serious long-term disabilities. One year after the most common kind of stroke, about 30 percent of guys won't have made it. Another 30 percent are living with moderate to severe disability.

Now for some better news: Of those who experience the most common type of stroke, approximately 40 percent are left with only a mild disability, or none, one year later. And each year more people survive and recover from stroke as medical research continues to advance effective treatment. Today, recovery with improvement is the rule rather than the exception.

Sobering, for sure. But here's some good news — the way you live your life can make your stroke risk less. If you take care of your body, it will be better able to take care of you. Although you can't definitively prevent a stroke, there's much you can do to reduce your chances of having one.

Attacking Out of the Blue, Racing Against the Clock

Stroke is sometimes called a *brain attack*. We wish this label would catch on, because people might better understand that stroke is an emergency — like a heart attack — and call 911 right away! A heart attack threatens your heart; a stroke threatens your brain. In truth, most stroke *is* like a heart attack: It's a problem with blood vessels, and time is really important. However, heart attack is a little easier to recognize. First of all, the pain tells you something is wrong — and it is usually near your heart. Most strokes are painless, and the symptoms, a paralyzed arm or leg for instance, are not obviously related to the brain.

REMEMBER

The more you know about stroke — its symptoms, causes, risks, and prevention — the better your chances of living a full and productive life without stroke. And the first lesson is to learn what stroke is and how and why stroke occurs.

Stroke is nothing if not *fast.* Each year, as many as 795,000 people in the United States suffer a sudden and unexpected attack of the brain. When part of the brain is deprived of oxygen — which is what's happening when stroke hits — it doesn't take long for the catastrophe to make itself evident. A minute or less.

Whether it's a sudden inability to speak, the crash of a dish from a hand that can no longer grasp, or loss of consciousness, a brain attack strikes its victims quickly and powerfully and without warning.

Or does it? Although your stroke may occur in a lightning flash, it has most likely been years in the making, with conditions such as high blood pressure, high cholesterol, obesity, and diabetes possibly serving as warning signs that the brain is in danger. Basically, as these conditions cause wear and tear on your blood vessels, your risks increase of suffering either a blockage or rupture of a brain artery. And — suddenly — you're in stroke mode.

So how does it happen? It starts with the brain.

REAL-LIFE EXAMPLES

A 57-year-old man, Alan, arrives early at work to prepare for an important presentation he has to make at 10 a.m. At about 9:15 he notices a headache. He thinks this is unusual, because he doesn't have many headaches. He remembers that he did forget his blood pressure medication. Alan continues to work for a few minutes and then notices his right hand is not working and he can't concentrate. He calls for his assistant who finds him looking very unusual. His mouth is twisted. He starts to talk but his speech is difficult to understand. She asks if he is okay. He says no. He starts to get up but his right arm gives way and he almost falls. His assistant calls 911.

A 68-year-old man, Ben, is preparing breakfast for himself and his partner. His partner has made the coffee and is reading the newspaper, then hears a plate drop and looks up to see Ben standing and looking at his left hand. He asks Ben what's wrong. Ben says he doesn't know. Ben's face — particularly the way he is holding his mouth — looks unusual. He keeps looking at his hand. "My hand is numb," he says. His partner asks Ben to sit down. Ben seems confused as he is led to a chair, and when asked if it hurts, says no. "I think you're having a stroke," his partner says, and dials 911.

A 38-year-old lawyer, Christopher, is out jogging on a canal towpath. He starts to feel pain in his head that gets worse and worse. Christopher stops, puts his hand to his head, and falls to the ground. A woman walking ahead of him sees him fall. She runs to him but he is unconscious. She pulls out her phone and dials 911.

Going to the source: Stroke is in the brain

Because of a number of possible causes, part of your brain may be deprived of blood. When that happens, it doesn't take long for your brain to suffer. In a nutshell, the glucose and oxygen transported by one of the brain's arteries are not reaching some part of the brain, which in less than a minute will begin to shut down. And you will show signs of stroke.

WARNING

The 16 professional groups forming the Brain Attack Coalition describe the signs of stroke as follows:

>> Sudden numbness or weakness of face, arm, or leg, especially on one side of the body

>> Sudden confusion, trouble speaking or understanding speech

>> Sudden trouble seeing in one or both eyes

>> Sudden trouble walking, dizziness, loss of balance or coordination

>> Sudden severe headache with no known cause

Most of the time, a stroke victim feels no pain as the stroke is occurring — so there is not much evidence to clue you in that the reason your hand looks funny and doesn't move when you want is because there's something wrong in your head.

Most people who have a stroke don't know what is happening to them. Most people who see someone who's had a stroke don't know what is happening.

A stroke doesn't hurt (except if a headache accompanies it), and its most obvious effects are far from the brain where the problem is located. This means a lot of people don't recognize they're having a stroke and can't use the opportunities they have to get into the hospital quickly and be treated.

Damage in your brain, symptoms someplace else

So, why is it that a blocked artery in your brain causes you to lose control of your legs and fall to the floor? Suppose a small blood clot forms in your heart and flows with the blood up into your brain and plugs an artery that feeds a part of your brain near the top of your head. Normally, that part of the brain sends nerve impulses down threadlike fibers through the base of your brain and along your spinal cord down to a point a couple of inches below your lowest rib. There those nerve fibers connect to other nerve fibers that extend down to muscles in your legs.

But without blood flow, the affected part of the brain stops sending messages. Your leg muscles only work when they receive messages, so they stop working. But the other parts of your brain that *are* getting oxygen and glucose don't understand that the whole team's not on board and look at the leg in confusion, trying to comprehend why it's not cooperating, not realizing that the problem is right upstairs.

The brain is sensitive to the slightest touch of your skin, but completely insensitive to serious injury to itself. As remarkable as it may seem, the brain is very poor at recognizing when it has been injured. This makes it hard for you to figure out what is going on when you have a stroke.

Responding quickly: Time is brain

Your brain is completely unprepared when blood flow is cut off. The organ is so packed full of knowledge and memories that there is no room in the design for storing sugars and fats that could keep brain cells alive in hard times when blood stops flowing.

Most other cells in the body can survive for up to an hour without blood flow. The brain cells stop working in a matter of seconds and start dying after five minutes.

The brain counts on the heart to do its job. That's why when you have cardiac arrest (when the heart stops, as opposed to a heart attack, when the heart muscle dies) it is so important to get the heart restarted quickly. Within seconds of your heart stopping, your brain stops working. Within minutes of the heart stopping, the brain is permanently injured and can't recover even if the heart gets going again.

REMEMBER

In stroke, you have a *little* more time than when you have cardiac arrest. Because the heart keeps pumping, some blood can often get around the obstruction or broken portion of the blood vessels, or seep in from areas of the brain that are still getting blood. *But get yourself to a hospital right away. Call 911.* If you are going to get the best treatment, you need to get to a hospital within 60 minutes.

Recognizing Types of Stroke: Same Symptoms, Different Causes

Doctors can typically identify stroke when a patient comes in with symptoms — they're even pretty good at knowing what part of your brain may be damaged by the stroke just by looking at you. With some scenarios, such as a bursting *aneurysm,* a doctor can guess what caused the stroke. With other cases, it is almost impossible to tell what caused the stroke, although there is little doubt that a stroke is in progress.

Sometimes, with severe headache, for example, it's hard to tell whether a stroke is happening at all because the symptoms are similar to those of a migraine headache. A stroke might cause dizziness that is difficult to distinguish from an inner-ear infection.

Fortunately, testing instruments such as CT or MRI scans can indicate if there is a stroke and what its cause might be.

TIP

Blood clots and bleeding aren't the only causes of stroke — but about 99 percent of strokes can be attributed to one of these reasons. For information about the causes of the other 1 percent, and more detail about the most common stroke scenarios that we introduce in the following sections, check out *Stroke For Dummies* (John Wiley & Sons, Inc, 2005).

Color-coding stroke types: Red or white

A cardiologist once told us that neurologists make stroke too complicated with their jargon and classification. He said he just thinks of stroke like wine: There's red wine and white wine — and red stroke and white stroke.

What did he mean by this? Basically, some strokes are caused by *broken* blood vessels — which results in blood in the brain or brain area (thus, the *red*); other strokes are caused by the *blockage* of vessels to the brain, so no blood gets there (hence, *white*).

We liked his use of the color-coding and have found that when we talk to patients and their families, this explanation helps them better understand the cause of the stroke and what is happening in the brain. So you'll see that we classify the five major types of stroke into two general categories based on whether they're caused by bleeding (red) or blockage (white).

TIP

We give you the complex, hard-to-pronounce terminology, as well! If you're ready now to track it down in a medical textbook, you'll find out more about red stroke under the term *hemorrhagic* stroke or *intracerebral hemorrhage.* White stroke is covered under the term *ischemic* stroke, *embolic* stroke, or *thrombotic* stroke.

A STROKE BY ANY OTHER NAME

Stroke means that part of your brain has suddenly stopped working because of a problem with its blood supply. As we mention, it may help to think of strokes caused by blockage as *white* strokes; they're most typically referred to as *ischemic* strokes by doctors. But here are some other names for this type of stroke:

- occlusive stroke

- cerebrovascular accident (CVA)

- acute ischemic stroke

- atherothrombotic stroke

- embolic stroke

- small vessel stroke

- lacunar stroke

- large vessel stroke

- cardioembolic stroke

Ischemic stroke and *CVA* are probably the most common terms used. Doctors usually know what all these terms mean and use them each in different situations to mean virtually the same thing. "Little white stroke" and "big white stroke" could probably replace all these fine technical terms just as well, and everyone would know exactly what they meant.

We refer to strokes caused by bleeding in or around the brain as *red* strokes. Names for these types of stroke are equally varied:

- subarachnoid hemorrhage (SAH)

- intracranial hemorrhage

- intracerebral hemorrhage (ICH)

- brain bleeding

- brain hemorrhage

Understanding white stroke

As you age, your blood pressure, diet, and the ravages of time roughen the fragile lining of your blood vessels and heart.

REMEMBER

Your blood-vessel lining is like the coating on your best cookware — it keeps your blood from sticking and clotting. However, as you approach senior status, that Teflon-like protection starts breaking down, and your vessels develop spots where blood and other buildup stick to them.

Blood clots block blood to the brain

The most common sign of blood-vessel damage is *atherosclerosis,* also known as *hardening of the arteries,* the condition in which a rough, scarred area called a *plaque* forms because of high blood pressure and high fat content in your blood. (There is more about atherosclerosis in Chapter 15.) The roughness makes it more likely that blood inside your arteries will form clots that can block arteries in the brain or break up into smaller pieces that are carried downstream to lodge in small brain arteries. Sometimes blood clots can break off and flow downstream to form a blockage somewhere else, called an *embolism* (see Figure 18-1 for illustrations of atherosclerosis, blood clots, and embolism).

If the clot blocks blood to a part of your brain, you have a stroke. If the clot stays in place for even a short time, part of your brain dies, leaving a hole called a brain *infarction.* The affected area of brain turns from pink to white because there is no red blood flowing (another good reason to refer to this type of stroke as *white*).

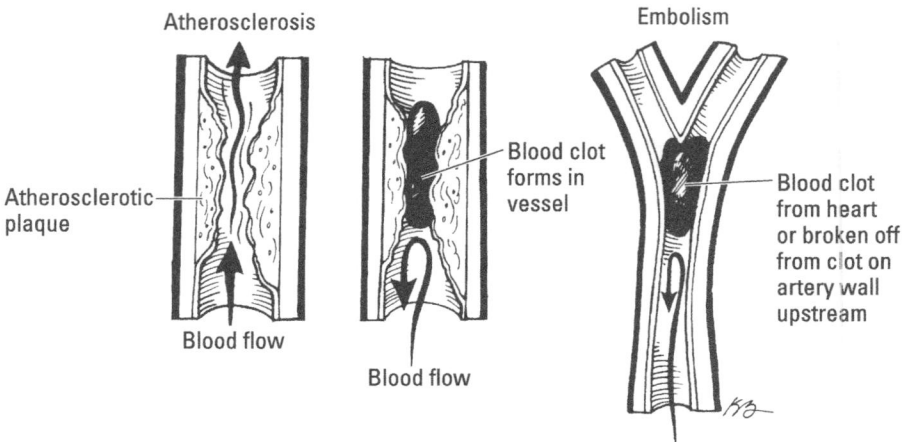

FIGURE 18-1:
Plaque building up in the blood vessel causes a blood clot to form, which can block an artery and end up causing a stroke. Clots can also travel and block vessels at points downstream.

Atherosclerosis

Embolism

Atherosclerotic plaque

Blood flow

Blood clot forms in vessel

Blood flow

Blood clot from heart or broken off from clot on artery wall upstream

Illustration by Kathryn Born.

Dissection: Blood vessel lining splits

White ischemic strokes are also caused by *dissection.* No, this doesn't mean somebody is practicing brain surgery on you. *Dissection* refers to the splitting of the blood vessel lining, typically occurring at a place where the blood vessel bends back and forth, such as in your neck. It can also happen where *atherosclerotic plaque* has built up in a brain artery. At the bend point or at the rough surface of atherosclerosis, a little flap of the vessel lining peels off and catches the blood as it flows quickly past. The blood dives under the flap and keeps tearing it. Eventually the blood can pack the lining against the other side of the vessel and stop blood flow completely. When the blood stops flowing, a white stroke occurs. Figure 18-2 shows how dissection causes stroke.

Transient strokes: Just as serious

White ischemic strokes may last just a couple of minutes and then clear completely. If the blood clot breaks up right away, the stroke is *transient* — so fleeting that no permanent tissue death occurred. These transient strokes are officially called *transient ischemic attacks.* Try to say that ten times fast. Doctors abbreviate it as *TIA.*

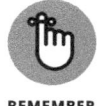

REMEMBER

We don't like the term TIA or what it stands for because it doesn't tell you plainly that you had a stroke. A stroke is very serious even if it is transient, and you still need to consider it a medical emergency requiring a rapid response. After a TIA stroke, your next stroke may *not* be transient, and you need to get busy to prevent it from happening. It could happen tomorrow.

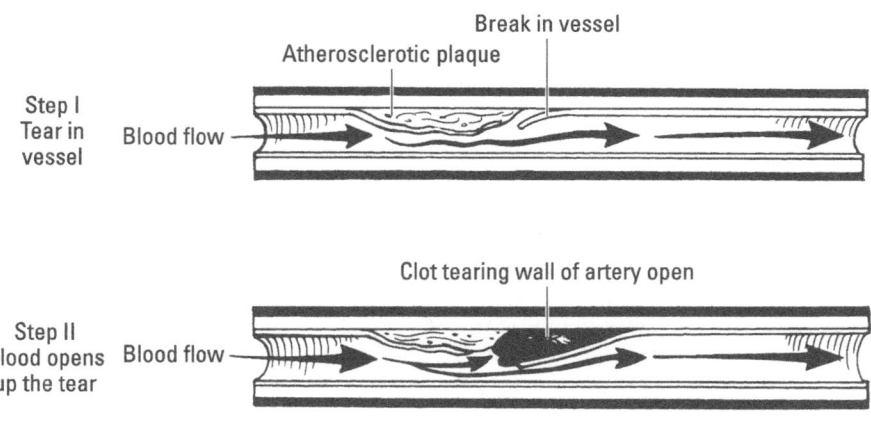

Step I
Tear in
vessel

Blood flow

Atherosclerotic plaque

Break in vessel

Step II
Blood opens
up the tear

Blood flow

Clot tearing wall of artery open

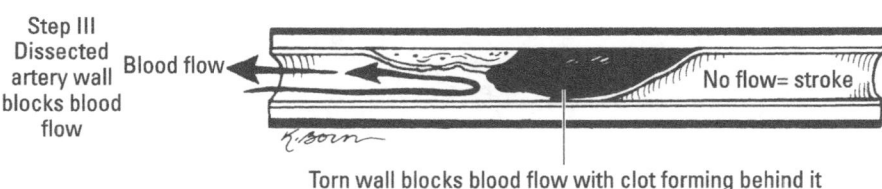

Step III
Dissected
artery wall
blocks blood
flow

Blood flow

No flow= stroke

Torn wall blocks blood flow with clot forming behind it

Illustration by Kathryn Born.

You can have more than one transient ischemic stroke. As the number of these small strokes add up, your brain can just slow down generally, and you can suffer from dementia, as each small stroke erodes away more of your brain. Small white ischemic stroke dementia is often called *vascular dementia* or *vascular cognitive impairment.* This is the death of the brain by a thousand cuts.

Getting a handle on red stroke

Blood vessels can break and bleed into or around the brain, causing some of the most serious and deadly strokes. These strokes may result in similar symptoms to white stokes — although some are unique to red stroke — but in many cases, they should be treated differently.

Bleeding within the brain

A stroke caused by a blood vessel that breaks inside the substance of the brain is called *intracerebral hemorrhage, brain hemorrhage,* or *brain bleeding.* The brain goes from pink to red. Hence, the term *red stroke.* The vessels that bleed are often damaged extensively by high blood pressure or diabetes (Figure 18-3). The blood vessels have thick, fibrous, but weak walls. They form little *blebs* — bubble-like growths — from time to time. These brain vessels are very prone to break, especially when blood pressure is high.

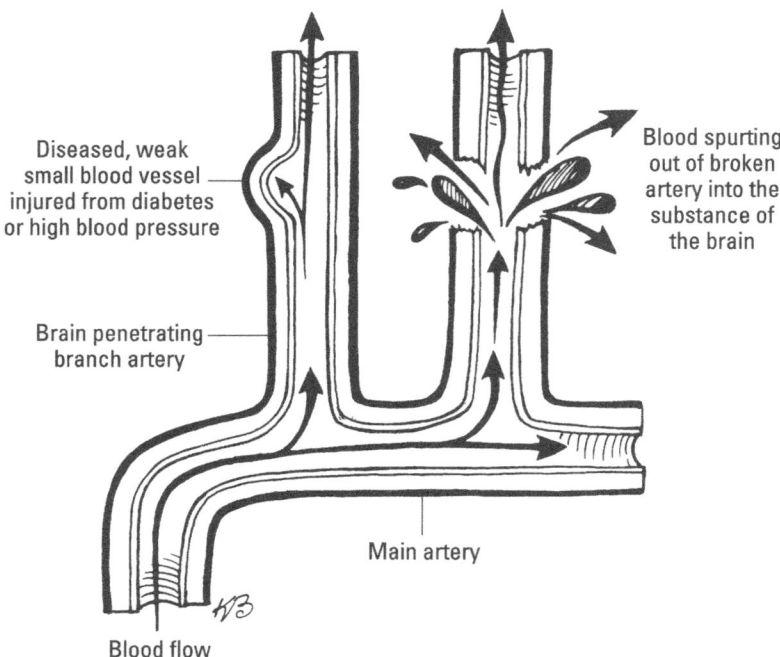

Diseased, weak small blood vessel injured from diabetes or high blood pressure

Blood spurting out of broken artery into the substance of the brain

Brain penetrating branch artery

Main artery

Blood flow

Illustration by Kathryn Born.

FIGURE 18-3:
When a weakened blood vessel bursts inside the brain, an intracerebral hemorrhage is the result.

Bleeding around the brain

Sometimes red — or hemorrhagic — strokes are caused by bleeding just outside the brain, but still inside the skull (Figure 18-4). This type of red stroke is known as *subarachnoid hemorrhage.* The most common cause in this case is a little peanut or marble-sized bubble or pouch that forms at a Y-junction in a brain-bound artery. This bubble is called an *aneurysm.* It has tough, thin, rubbery walls and may actually be present for years before it starts causing trouble. Some never do cause trouble. But aneurysms may get larger as time passes and, as they do, doctors believe they're more likely to burst.

The result can be devastating as high-pressure blood from larger brain arteries floods into the space around the brain. If you aren't killed immediately, you have to survive weeks of recovery as your body tries to clean up the resulting mess. Further injury to your brain and rebleeding are likely, unless you get immediate medical attention.

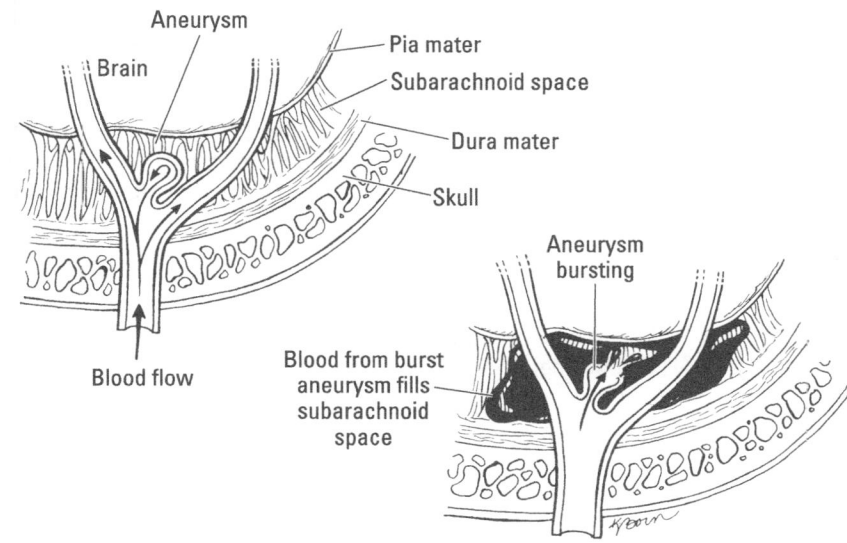

FIGURE 18-4:
When a vessel bleeds into the space surrounding the brain, the result is a stroke called a subarachnoid hemorrhage.

Aneurysm

Brain

Pia mater

Subarachnoid space

Dura mater

Skull

Blood flow

Aneurysm bursting

Blood from burst aneurysm fills subarachnoid space

Illustration by Kathryn Born.

WARNING

This type of red subarachnoid hemorrhage stroke is usually accompanied by severe headache. Many people also fall down unconscious when the stroke first hits. The pain and loss of consciousness are both strong warnings that something serious is happening.

Combining colors: When red and white stroke occur together

White ischemic strokes can turn red if a blood vessel is injured and breaks in the area where lack of blood flow caused a brain infarction. The bleeding can become a major intracranial hemorrhage or it may just be a small leak that doesn't do much more damage than has already been done by the ischemia.

In a stroke that starts out as subarachnoid hemorrhage caused by an aneurysm, white ischemic strokes can occur 4 to 14 days after the aneurysm bursts. This is a time when the blood around the brain irritates the brain's blood vessels and they clamp shut. Blood flow stops and ischemic stroke can result. This is of course bad news for someone who has just started to recover from the bleeding.

Sizing Up Stroke Risk and Scaling It Down

TECHNICAL STUFF

If you've suffered a stroke, let us assure you of one thing: You are not alone. In the United States, 795,000 people experience a stroke each year. Of these three-quarters of a million strokes, here's how they break down in our red and white categories:

>> Eighty-seven percent are white ischemic strokes, including TIA and dementia.

>> Thirteen percent are red intracerebral hemorrhages and red subarachnoid hemorrhages.

Survival rates for stroke vary greatly, and are influenced by (among other things) the type of stroke a guy has, whether it's their first or they've had one or more strokes previously, and how quickly they get medical care — that is, whether they or others recognize a potential stroke and get treatment asap, as well as their proximity to a hospital or stroke center when a stroke is suspected.

Fact is, neither you nor your doctor knows for certain whether a stroke is in your future. It's not really possible to predict with any certainty exactly who will suffer a stroke. To some extent, having a stroke is a matter of bad luck.

Researchers have identified a number of indicators that can help predict the likelihood of stroke. Some you can't influence, unfortunately, such as your heredity. But the good news is, many of these risk factors are within your control, which means you can make some changes in how you live and how you take care of your body, and in doing so reduce the possibility of having a stroke.

Risk factors beyond your control

Unfortunately, some of the factors that increase your likelihood of having a stroke are those you can't affect. You may be carrying some genetic, hereditary, sex, or age baggage that you simply can't change, such as:

>> You've already had a stroke.

>> You are 65 or older.

>> You are African American.

>> You are Hispanic.

>> Stroke runs in your family.

>> You are a man.

>> You have diabetes.

But take heart — some of the key risk factors are certainly within your control to change, as outlined in the next section.

Risk factors you can control

You can't change your age (don't we all wish we could?), your sex, your past, or your forebears' genetic makeup. But we can offer you plenty of ways to make changes in your life that'll significantly reduce your risk of stroke.

TIP

Some of the steps you can take to improve your outlook for a stroke-free future include the following:

>> Treat high blood pressure with medication, if necessary.

>> Reduce sodium in your diet to help control high blood pressure.

>> Stop smoking.

>> Lower "bad" cholesterol and raise "good" cholesterol through medication and diet.

>> Maintain a healthy weight, which may reduce blood pressure and improve cholesterol levels.

Heart disease and stroke share many of the same underlying causes, so check out Chapter 15 for a deeper dive into steps you can take to lower your chances of both.

Chapter **19**

Struggling to Breathe: Chronic Lower Respiratory Diseases

A mong the many things we take for granted every day, breathing is near the top of the list. You might think about your breath when you're working out, when you're trying to calm your nerves, or when you're competing to see who can stay underwater the longest during your family's annual Reunion Olympics. But most of the time, most of us just inhale and exhale without thinking about it, until it becomes a struggle.

Chronic lower respiratory diseases might sound like something you'd hear in a medical school lecture, but they're a major player when it comes to long-term health issues — especially for men. We're not talking about your garden-variety dry cough. These conditions involve persistent inflammation or obstruction of the airways, making it hard for your lungs to do their job. The two main chronic lower respiratory diseases that contribute to death and disability are *chronic obstructive pulmonary disease* (COPD) and *asthma.* Neither is curable, so your best options are to minimize your risks of developing them and to take advantage of treatments and behaviors that help make life more manageable.

Grasping COPD: The Essentials in One Breath

Chronic obstructive pulmonary disease, or COPD, is an umbrella term covering any long-term, irreversible damage to the lungs that interferes with breathing, specifically with getting air out of the lungs. You have trouble getting air out of your lungs because your airways are continually blocked.

Not being able to get air out is a problem because, when that air is trapped in your lungs, you can't inhale enough air to supply your body with oxygen. Your body senses that you aren't getting enough oxygen and sends signals telling you to breathe faster to correct the problem. This process is what makes you feel like you can't catch your breath.

COPD in the United States primarily involves chronic bronchitis, emphysema, or both, and is the fifth leading cause of death for American men. Some 16 million American adults have been diagnosed with COPD, and evidence suggests another 15 million may have it but don't know it.

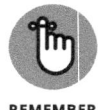

REMEMBER

COPD is a progressive disease, meaning it develops and gets worse over time. You don't just wake up one morning and realize you have COPD. Instead, you find that activities that used to be easy for you are harder now. You may become breathless walking upstairs, or you may have trouble carrying groceries into the house. You may not have the energy to eat at night, and this may lead to weight loss and a feeling of overall weakness; you may also have weight loss due to the additional energy your body needs to expend in order to breathe. Even when you're sitting quietly, you may feel like you can't catch your breath.

And you may attribute all these symptoms to age, because COPD usually doesn't begin to make itself noticed until you're in your 40s, 50s, or 60s.

Smoking is the number one risk factor for COPD, but it is by no means the only one. Long-term exposure to dust, chemical fumes, secondhand smoke, and other pollutants can lead to COPD, and there's even a genetic condition that, though rare, can cause the disease.

Part of the reason COPD is so severely under-diagnosed is that many physicians mistake its symptoms for other illnesses, particularly asthma. But effective treatments for asthma and COPD differ, and if you're being treated for asthma when you really suffer from COPD, chances are, your symptoms won't improve much.

New treatments and better understanding have improved management of its symptoms, but there is no cure. The earlier you get diagnosed, the better — after damage is done to your lungs by smoking or other factors, that damage can't be reversed, so unsurprisingly, the average life expectancy after diagnosis is longer the earlier COPD is spotted.

Attacking Airways: COPD's Deadly Combo

In the vast majority of patients, at least in the United States, COPD refers to a combination of chronic bronchitis and emphysema. (Other countries have higher incidences of other lung diseases that can fall under the definition of COPD.) Most COPD patients have both conditions, although one may be more advanced than the other.

Chronic bronchitis

Bronchitis is a condition in which the airways in your lungs are inflamed, making them narrower. Inflammation is usually a response to an irritant, like cigarette smoke, dust, or pollen. When your airways are irritated, they create more mucus in an effort to rid your lungs of the irritants. But this extra mucus, combined with the narrowing of the airways themselves, can end up blocking your airways. Air then gets trapped in your lungs, and you feel short of breath.

In chronic bronchitis, your airways become scarred, and the partial blockage is permanent. Extra mucus is produced all the time, which can make you feel congested and prompt continual coughing. You become more susceptible to respiratory infections because the extra mucus in your airways provides an admirable breeding ground for bacteria and viruses. Figure 19-1 shows how chronic bronchitis affects your airways.

Chronic bronchitis develops over several years. It can affect people of any age, but it's most common in smokers who are in their 40s or older. About 3 million American men have been diagnosed with chronic bronchitis.

Symptoms include chronic coughing and throat clearing, increased mucus, and shortness of breath. To meet the clinical definition of chronic bronchitis, you must cough up mucus most days for at least three months of the year for two consecutive years.

WARNING

Many people ignore their chronic bronchitis symptoms because they mistakenly believe it isn't serious. The earlier you see your doctor, the better your chances of preventing serious damage to your lungs.

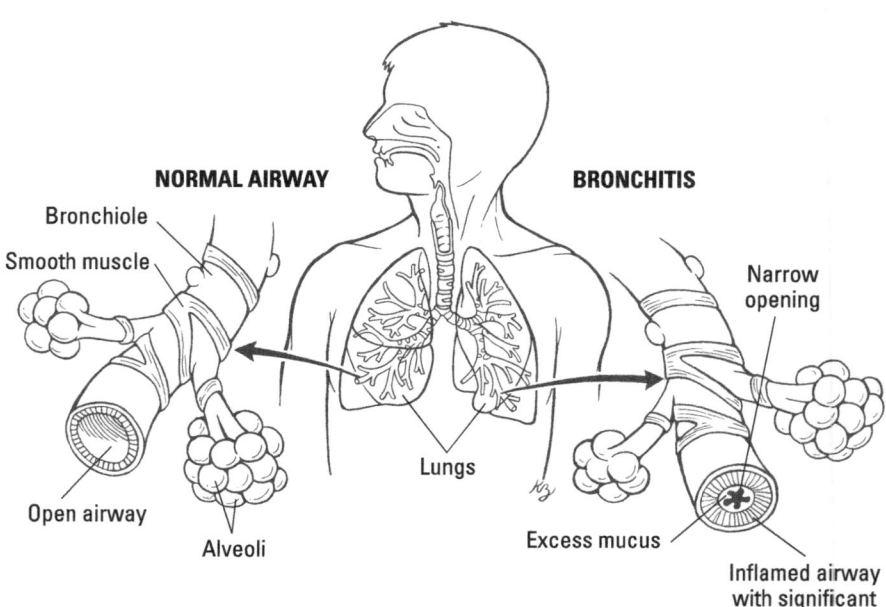

FIGURE 19-1: Chronic bronchitis inflames and narrows your airways.

Emphysema

Chronic bronchitis affects your airways, the tubes that branch out into your lungs. *Emphysema* affects the tiny air sacs at the ends of your airways. This is where the oxygen in the air you inhale is exchanged for carbon dioxide and other waste material in your blood. To facilitate this exchange, the walls of your air sacs naturally are quite thin and fragile. In emphysema, the walls of the air sacs are stretched, distended, and eventually destroyed, leaving permanent holes in your lungs. The fewer air sacs there are, the more difficult the *gas exchange* — trading oxygen from inhaled air for carbon dioxide in your blood — becomes, and this can contribute to you feeling short of breath. Figure 19-2 shows how emphysema affects your lungs.

Emphysema takes time to develop; nine out of ten people diagnosed with it are 45 or older. Early symptoms of emphysema are vague and often attributed to age rather than to any lung problem. Most people figure their cough is from smoking and their shortness of breath is from the infamous "middle-age spread," so they don't consider it worth mentioning to their doctors. By the time symptoms begin to cause concern — like feeling short of breath even while sitting or lying down — emphysema has caused quite a bit of damage.

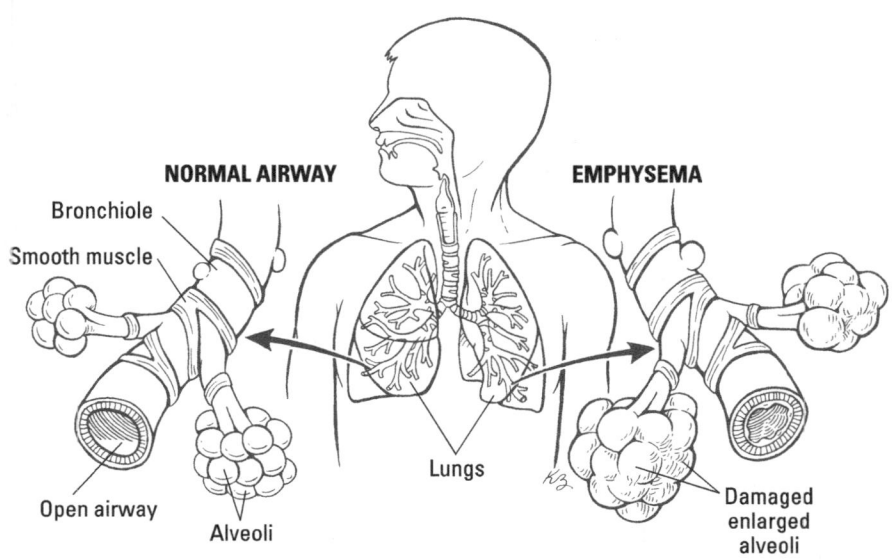

FIGURE 19-2:
Emphysema
harms the tiny air
sacs in your
lungs, eventually
destroying them.

**TECHNICAL
STUFF**

Emphysema also robs your lungs of their elasticity, which can cause smaller airways to collapse, thus trapping more air in the lower lungs. This can make it difficult to bring in new air for gas exchanges, which worsens the function of your respiratory muscles, which makes you work harder at breathing, which makes you feel short of breath.

Knowing How COPD Affects Your Body

COPD steals your energy, which has a cascade effect through the rest of your body. It's a gradual loss, which is why early COPD symptoms are so often ignored — if they're noticed at all. Many people with mild COPD don't have any symptoms beyond a vague tendency to get tired more quickly than they used to. But, as the disease progresses, they face the following:

>> **The lack of energy becomes far more pronounced.** Healthy people only use energy to breathe in, when they inflate the lungs; exhaling is a mostly passive activity because healthy lungs are elastic and push air out on their own. With COPD, the lungs lose that elastic quality, so you have to use extra energy to force air out of your lungs. You also have to breathe more often when you have COPD, because the air that's trapped in your lungs reduces the volume of air you can take in with your next breath.

>> **Overall physical weakness increases.** Many COPD patients find that they're too tired to prepare or eat meals, so their caloric intake drops, giving them less fuel for their bodies at a time when they're using more energy to breathe than healthy people need. The lack of oxygen and the insufficient calorie intake leads to loss of muscle mass and strength.

>> **Even the smallest of tasks drains them of whatever energy they have**. As COPD progresses, patients find that it takes more energy to do less. Even relatively passive activities like reaching for something on a shelf or bending over to pick up something from the floor can leave people with severe COPD feeling exhausted. So much of the body's resources are diverted to the task of breathing that, eventually, there's next to nothing left over for other activities.

TIP

EXERCISE IS GOOD MEDICINE

Exercise is a critical component of a comprehensive treatment plan for COPD. Aerobic exercise like walking or riding a stationary bike helps bring more oxygen into your body and tone your muscles, including the muscles involved in breathing. This kind of conditioning has been shown to reduce symptoms of being short of breath and improve overall quality of life for COPD patients, no matter how far their illness has progressed.

Exercise has other benefits of particular importance to COPD patients, too. COPD is often accompanied by heart disease or circulatory problems, and exercise can help make your heart and circulatory system stronger; exercise is known to help control blood pressure and improve the heart's ability to pump blood efficiently. A regular exercise regimen improves sleep quality, which helps you feel more energetic, and it promotes better posture, balance, and flexibility.

Exercise also is effective in counteracting many of the emotional effects of the disease. Forced inactivity can lead to a sense of isolation and depression; exercise is a proven mood brightener and self-confidence booster. Take a look at Chapter 5 for more exercise basics, including how to get started on a walking program.

The goal of virtually every COPD treatment plan is to fend off the energy-stealing stage of the disease for as long as possible. The right combination of medications, nutrition, exercise, and emotional and social support is far more effective in achieving this goal than any individual element can be.

Identifying What Raises Your Risk for COPD

Risk factors for COPD come under three main headings: behavior, demographics, and medical history. Some of these things you can control; others you just have to accept are beyond your control. Either way, knowing your COPD risk factors helps you and your doctor evaluate and properly identify any lung problems you may have.

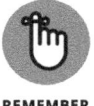

REMEMBER

You aren't necessarily doomed to COPD just because some of these risk factors apply to you. Individuals vary widely in their tolerance for and response to all kinds of risks. But even if you don't have any COPD symptoms, knowing how your behavior and background may affect your lung health can help you take preventive steps now. And because there is no cure for COPD, an ounce of prevention is absolutely priceless.

Risks from behaviors

When we talk about risky behaviors, we're not talking about things like forgetting to wear your seat belt or spending your weekends skydiving. When it comes to the health of your lungs, risky behaviors are activities that expose your lungs to harmful gases, fumes, and dust — things that, over the course of many years, can cause permanent damage to your lungs.

Some of these behaviors are matters of personal choice, like smoking. Some are not; if you're a miner or construction worker or nurse, for example, some exposure to noxious elements is virtually inevitable. Even if you can't avoid all potentially risky behaviors, you can take steps to minimize your risk, when you know where the risk lies.

Cigarette smoke: The number one risk

The correlation between smoking and COPD is exceptionally strong. As many as 90 percent of all COPD cases occur in people who currently smoke or who are former smokers. This doesn't mean you'll definitely develop COPD if you are or once were a smoker. But because so many cases of COPD are linked to smoking, it's considered the single biggest risk factor for the disease.

WARNING

Exposure to secondhand smoke can be just as harmful to you as if you were an active smoker. Even if you've never smoked a single cigarette, you may be at risk if you're around smokers a lot.

On-the-job risks

Occupational hazards have been linked to many lung diseases, including COPD. Workers who are exposed to high levels of so-called *nuisance dust* (dust that the U.S. Occupational Safety and Health Administration defines as containing less than 1 percent silica and that, therefore, is not harmful to the lungs) are almost one and a half times more likely to suffer impaired lung function, and those who are exposed to high levels of dust are more than three and a half times more likely to develop symptoms of asthma or COPD.

Even if you're a nonsmoker (meaning you've never smoked), if you're exposed to dust, fumes, or other pollutants at your job, you have a higher risk of developing COPD; the effects of inhaling dust are fully half the effects of smoking.

WARNING

COPD has been linked with several specific occupations, including:

>> Construction

>> Factory work, especially leather, rubber, and plastics

>> Textiles, such as cotton workers and weavers

>> Food products (processing and manufacturing)

>> Spray painting

>> Welding

>> Concrete manufacturing

>> Non-mining air quality

Risks due to gender, age, and economic status

Researchers have linked demographic factors to the risk of developing COPD, although the reasons for these links aren't always clear. Some of these include:

>> **Being a woman:** Recent research indicates that merely being female puts you at higher risk for COPD. So being a guy gives you a slightly lesser risk of developing COPD.

>> **Being older than age 40:** COPD is the result of years of exposure to smoke, industrial pollutants, and other irritants that cause repeated damage to the lungs, so it makes sense that COPD is more common in people who are older.

>> **Having low income:** Worldwide, COPD is more common among low-income patients, potentially because they're more likely to be smokers; they're more often exposed to environment hazards at home (through use of fuels like wood, the presence of mold in poorly maintained housing, and more neighborhood air pollution); and they may delay medical care due to constraints with insurance, work time off, or transportation.

Risks from the wayback machine: Heredity and medical history

Genetics, your family's medical history, and your own medical history all can influence your overall risk for developing COPD. Not all of these are fully understood, and some of the potential risks may be canceled out by protective factors — and some of those protective factors you and your doctor may never be aware of, especially if they're genetic. There's very little you can do about your hereditary risk. However, knowing the possible risks in your broad medical history should motivate you to do what you can to minimize the risk factors you can control.

>> **Genetic link to COPD.** COPD risk may be influenced by multiple genetic factors, although most remain poorly understood. A known genetic risk is *alpha-1 antitrypsin (ATT)* deficiency, a rare condition that significantly increases emphysema risk, especially in smokers.

>> **Family history risk.** Having a first-degree relative (parent or sibling) with COPD, chronic bronchitis, or emphysema increases your risk of developing COPD; your familial risk is less if the relative is more distant (grandparent or cousin, for example).

>> **Your medical history.** Factors from your childhood and your lifestyle as an adult can influence your COPD risk. For example, severe respiratory infections during childhood or exposure to secondhand smoke or mold and mildew during childhood may make COPD more likely.

>> **Other possible risk factors.** Gum disease may signal higher COPD risk; inflammation may be the link. Skin wrinkles in smokers are associated with undiagnosed COPD, regardless of sun exposure or smoking level. Poor diet (high in fat, sugar, processed grains) increases your COPD risk; a healthy diet cuts it dramatically.

Assessing how high your risk is

TIP

All this information about risk factors can be overwhelming, especially if several factors apply to you to one degree or another. Before you get too worked up, read the following questions and answer yes or no. This will give you a quick idea of whether you just need to be aware of your risks, or whether it's time to make an appointment with your doctor.

>> Are you a current or former smoker?

>> Have you smoked (or did you smoke) for more than ten years?

>> Do you cough nearly every day?

>> Do you cough up mucus most of the time?

>> Do you expect to get bronchitis at least once every winter?

>> Do you get colds that last several weeks instead of seven to ten days?

>> Are you 40 or older?

If you answered yes to three or more of these questions, make an appointment with your doctor to discuss your concerns about COPD and set up the appropriate tests.

Dodging a COPD Diagnosis (or Living Well with It)

TIP

Although you can't control all of the risk factors for developing COPD, you can make some behavioral changes that'll make a difference in living a COPD-free life. And if you already have COPD, making the following changes will make it easier to manage your condition:

>> **Quit smoking.** As many as nine out of ten COPD cases are attributed to smoking, and the surest way to reduce your risk is to toss the cigarettes (see Chapter 9 for help doing just that). Although you can't reverse the damage to your lungs, quitting smoking means you aren't adding to that damage.

And smoking affects more than just your lungs; it also affects your heart and circulatory system, your digestive system, your sleep, and even your cognitive function. The health benefits of quitting kick in as early as 20 minutes after you take that last drag, and they just get better the longer you're smoke-free.

>> **Limit exposure to secondhand smoke and other lung irritants.**
Secondhand smoke can damage your lungs just as much as active smoking
can. Indeed, some research indicates that secondhand smoke is more
dangerous to your lungs because there is no filter to block out any of the
harmful gases. And dust from the environment (whether at work or at home)
is nearly as dangerous as cigarette smoke.

So when you can't avoid dust, fumes, or other pollutants, make sure you're
working in a well-ventilated space, and consider wearing a face covering to
offer extra lung protection.

>> **Stay current on vaccines for respiratory viruses.** These include COVID-19,
pneumonia, and flu vaccines. Doing so helps keep your lungs healthy and less
susceptible to the negative effects of lung irritants when you can't avoid them.

Breaking Down Asthma Types and Triggers

Along with COPD, asthma is the other top condition that falls under the umbrella
of chronic lower respiratory disease. According to many experts, asthma is now a
global epidemic, and its prevalence and severity continue to grow in many
parts of the world, including the United States, Western Europe, Australia,
and New Zealand. The American Academy of Allergy, Asthma, & Immunology
(www.aaaai.org) estimates that 9 percent of adults have asthma, and more than
25 million people in the United States alone and more than 330 million globally
have some form of asthma. So you can understand why it's one of the top conditions resulting in a man's death. Taking care of asthma means taking care of your
whole body — from your brain to your nose to your lungs.

We start with the basics of asthma: what it is and how it affects you. Although
much of this may seem like high-school biology, it's helpful to understand the
contributing factors of asthma, as well as how to live a full life with the condition.
And because the causes of asthma aren't known, you can't necessarily prevent its
onset — but you can live your life aware of and, if needed, avoiding triggers.

Airflow, interrupted: Understanding asthma basics

Asthma is a chronic condition where your lung's airways become inflamed and
narrowed, making it harder to breathe. A wide range of factors can trigger an
asthma attack or flare: exercise, cold air, a virus, pollution, smoke, and, for many,
a host of allergens.

Your lung airways are vital to your health. This network of bronchial tubes enables your lungs to absorb oxygen into the blood and get rid of carbon dioxide; the process is called *respiration* or breathing. Most guys take breathing for granted; you usually don't need to even think about it unless something interferes with the process by obstructing your airways.

How normal breathing works

TECHNICAL STUFF

To better understand how asthma adversely affects your airways, consider what happens in normal breathing:

>> The air you inhale flows into your nose and/or mouth and into your *trachea,* or windpipe.

>> Your trachea then divides in the lung into right and left main *bronchi,* or branches, funneling the air into each of your lungs.

>> The main bronchi branch into smaller airways called *bronchial tubes*, which are wrapped in muscles that tighten and relax as you breathe.

>> Your airways end in tiny air sacs called *alveoli* — little grape-like clusters — which contain blood vessels that enable vital respiratory exchange. Oxygen from the air you breathe is absorbed into the bloodstream, while carbon dioxide gas from your blood exits your body as you exhale.

How airway obstruction develops

Here's an overview of how the mechanisms of asthma interact. Although we've itemized these processes to explain them, keep in mind that they're often ongoing events that can occur simultaneously in your lungs. As you read these descriptions, take a look at Figure 19-3, which compares a normal airway with an asthmatic airway.

>> **Airway constriction:** When a trigger or precipitating factor irritates your airways, causing the release of chemical mediators, the muscles around your bronchial tubes can tighten, leading to *airway constriction.* This process results in narrowing airways and breathing difficulty.

>> **Airway hyperresponsiveness:** The underlying airway inflammation in asthma can cause *airway hyperresponsiveness* as the muscles around your bronchial tubes twitch or feel ticklish. This twitchy or ticklish feeling indicates that your muscles overreact and tighten, causing acute bronchoconstriction or bronchospasms even if you're exposed only to otherwise harmless substances.

- **Airway congestion:** Mucus and fluids are released as part of the inflammatory process and can accumulate in your airways, overwhelming the *cilia* (tiny hairlike projections from certain cells that sweep debris-laden mucus through your airways) and leading to *airway congestion.* This accumulation of mucus and fluids may make you feel the urge to cough up phlegm to relieve your chest congestion.

- **Airway edema:** The long-term release of inflammatory fluids in constricted, hyperresponsive, and congested airways can lead to *airway edema* (swelling of the airway), causing bronchial tubes to become more rigid and further interfering with airflow.

- **Airway remodeling:** If airway inflammation is left untreated or poorly managed for many years, the constant injury to your bronchial tubes due to ongoing airway constriction, airway hyperresponsiveness, and airway congestion can lead to *airway remodeling,* as scar tissue permanently replaces your normal airway tissue, leading to the eventual loss of your airway function as well as potentially irreversible lung damage.

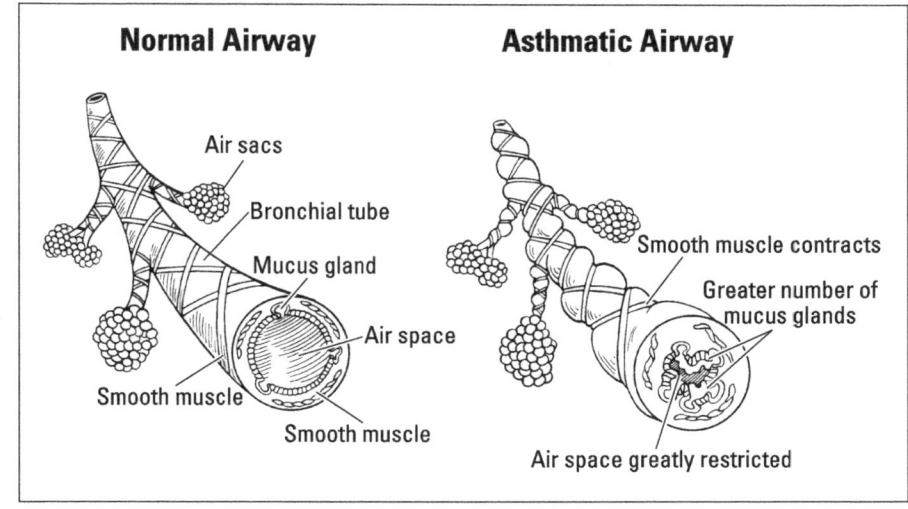

FIGURE 19-3:
A normal airway and an asthmatic airway. Note the muscle contractions (*bronchospasms*) and airway inflammation.

© PSQUAD.

REMEMBER

This cycle of asthma can develop gradually, over hours or even days following exposure to triggers or precipitating factors. After this cycle is set in motion, you can suffer severe and long-lasting consequences.

Sorting asthma by its triggers

Asthma can show up in various ways. The underlying mechanism causing many of the symptoms of asthma is due to a complex series of events involving many types of cells and tissue that reside in your lungs.

REMEMBER

Because such a wide range of factors can precipitate asthma symptoms, and because certain triggers can cause stronger reactions in some asthma patients than in others, doctors often classify asthma according to the triggers that instigate your symptoms. Classifying asthma in this way can help you and your doctor understand the cause of your symptoms.

>> **Allergic (or *atopic*) asthma** is asthma that's triggered by allergens like pollen, pets, and dust mites. About 80 percent of people with allergic asthma have a related condition like hay fever, eczema, or food allergies.

   If you have allergic asthma, your doctor is likely to prescribe a *preventer inhaler* to take every day and a *reliever inhaler* to use when you have asthma symptoms. It's also important to avoid your asthma triggers as much as possible.

>> **Nonallergic asthma, or *nonatopic* asthma,** is a type of asthma that isn't related to an allergy trigger like pollen or dust and is less common than allergic asthma. The causes are not well understood, but it often develops later in life and can be more severe than other types of asthma.

>> **Occupational asthma** is usually a type of allergic asthma and is caused directly by the work you do. For example, if you work in a bakery, you may be allergic to flour dust, or if you work in healthcare, the dust from latex gloves can trigger symptoms. You may have occupational asthma if

   ● Your asthma symptoms started in adulthood.

   ● Your asthma symptoms improve on the days you're not at work.

>> **Exercise-induced asthma** is when you experience asthma-like symptoms triggered only by exercise. A better term is *exercise-induced bronchoconstriction* (EIB) because the tightening and narrowing of the airways (bronchoconstriction) isn't caused by already having asthma. EIB commonly affects elite athletes or people doing strenuous exercise in very cold conditions.

>> **Aspirin-induced asthma** (AIA) is a condition in which asthma symptoms can develop after taking aspirin or other nonsteroidal anti-inflammatory drugs (NSAIDs). The American Academy of Allergy, Asthma, & Immunology estimates that 30 percent of adults who have asthma and nasal polyps may also have AIA.

>> **Food and food allergies** Food and food allergies may create an indirect connection to asthma for some people. Although food isn't a common asthma trigger, your asthma can be affected by eating. Asthma can also affect how you react if you have food allergies. Staying away from the food(s) that trigger your reactions is the only way to prevent problems.

Understanding Who Gets Asthma and Why

The strongest predictor that an individual may develop asthma is a family history of allergies and asthma and/or *atopy*, an inherited tendency to develop hyper-sensitivities to allergic triggers. This tendency is almost always due to an over-active immune system that produces elevated levels of immunoglobulin E (IgE) antibodies to allergens.

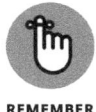

REMEMBER

The predisposition to asthma is inherited. This genetic inheritance can be a sig-nificant factor in developing the condition: Two-thirds of asthma patients have a family member who also has the disease.

Most cases of asthma are of an allergic nature (known as *allergic asthma*), and usually begin to manifest during childhood, affecting boys more often than girls. In fact, asthma is the most common chronic disease of childhood. Other allergic disorders, such as food allergies, *atopic dermatitis* (allergic eczema), or *allergic rhinitis* (hay fever), which are also indicators of atopy in young children, can pre-cede this form of the ailment, often referred to as *childhood-onset asthma*.

Adult-onset asthma, which is less common than childhood-onset asthma, devel-ops in adults older than 40, more often in women (but guys aren't off the hook). Atopy doesn't appear to play a role in these cases. Rather, adult-onset asthma more often seems to be triggered by various nonallergic factors, including sinus-itis, upper respiratory infections, nasal polyps, gastroesophageal reflux disease (GERD), sensitivities to aspirin and related NSAIDs, as well as occupational exposures to chemicals, such as those found in fumes, gases, resins, dust, and insecticides. However, many episodes seem to occur spontaneously without known triggers.

REMEMBER

Keep in mind these points about asthma:

>> Important symptoms of asthma in infancy and early childhood include persistent coughing, wheezing, and recurring or lingering chest colds.

>> Inflammation of the airways is the single most important underlying factor in asthma. If you have asthma, your symptoms may come and go, but the underlying inflammation usually persists. Episodes of asthma symptoms can vary in length from minutes to hours and even from days to weeks, depending on your medical treatment, the severity of your symptoms, and the character of the triggering mechanism.

>> Although no cure for asthma exists, in most cases you can manage and even reverse the effects of the disease. However, poorly managed or undertreated asthma may lead to loss of airway functions and, in some cases, irreversible lung damage as a result of airway remodeling.

>> Early, aggressive treatment with appropriate medication is vital to effectively managing your asthma.

Preventing Asthma . . . or Can You?

Unfortunately, totally preventing asthma isn't yet possible. Your genetics are your genetics, and you can't change them. And aside from genetics, we don't know the exact causes of asthma yet, so we can't give you any hard-and-fast tips for preventing the development of asthma.

But you can take control of your life and make decisions that minimize your chances for an asthma attack and support a healthier you.

Creating an asthma action plan

You may have heard the terms *asthma action plan* or *asthma self-management plan*. Both terms refer to how you take care of or manage your asthma, and it's something you create in conjunction with your doctor. An asthma action plan is a written document, based on your goals, that details how you manage your asthma to feel well, what needs to happen if you start to show asthma symptoms, and what actions need to take place if you're having severe symptoms and may need medical treatment. Having and following this plan helps you stay in the "green" or "feel well" zone as much as possible, and helps you and others know what to do if you start feeling unwell.

Avoiding triggers

TIP

Careful planning and avoiding asthma triggers are the best ways to prevent asthma attacks; see the following tips. And if you don't have asthma (that you know of) and just want to minimize the chances of having an unexpected asthma attack, the following are some behaviors you can adopt:

>> **Limit exposure to asthma triggers.** High pollen counts in spring and fall can cause asthma symptoms to flare. Dust mites and pet dander are allergens commonly found inside the home that can worsen asthma. Food and medicine can also cause asthma attacks. Know your allergens by getting tested and then avoid the things that trigger asthma symptoms.

>> **Don't smoke, and don't allow smoking around you.** Exposure to tobacco smoke is a common trigger of asthma attacks for people of any age. Avoid secondhand smoke or find ways to limit your exposure if you live with a smoker. Steer clear of campfires, wood-burning fireplaces, and outdoor bonfires if they trigger your symptoms.

>> **Avoid respiratory infections:** A common cold, the flu or even a sinus infection can make your asthma flare. Wash your hands often and completely, get your flu and COVID vaccines (unless your doctor advises you not to), and avoid people who may be contagious.

>> **Manage your exposure to animals:** Your furry and feathery friends shed dander and saliva that can trigger your asthma. Vacuuming and damp dusting weekly and keeping pets out of your bedroom can help you manage exposure.

Taking care of yourself

TIP

Have you noticed that most self-care advice involves taking a deep breath? That may seem simple to most people, but it's not always easy if you have asthma. Living with asthma can sometimes feel unpredictable. Taking time to focus on self-care can help you manage your symptoms, take control of your condition, and feel prepared for whatever comes next. Here are some suggestions:

>> **Eat a well-balanced diet.** The right nutrients in your diet can help you breathe easier, and in some cases, help minimize asthma symptoms. Some people feel that eating a diet with fewer carbohydrates and more healthy fats helps them breathe easier. Avoid foods with sulfites, which can worsen your asthma (including pickles, shrimp, bottled lemon or lime juice, and alcohol). Avoid foods that cause gas or bloating (such as beans, carbonated drinks, onions, garlic, and fried foods). Chapter 4 gives a good introduction to nutrition basics.

>> **Get enough sleep.** Eliminate allergens and potential asthma triggers from your bedroom. If you suffer from acid reflux at night, avoid overeating at dinner, reduce reflux triggers like spicy food or chocolate, and sleep with your head slightly elevated. Work with your doctor to manage sleep apnea (a disorder where you have repeated pauses in breathing throughout the night) if you suspect you have it. We provide further sleep tips in Chapter 8.

>> **Be active.** As long as your asthma is well controlled, regular physical activity can help your lungs work more efficiently. Yoga, for example, is a great way to move your body while also focusing on breathwork, which we think gives you two benefits in one. Flip to Chapters 5 and 6 for more information on physical activity and weight training. And if you have exercise-induced asthma, make a plan with your doctor to prevent and manage your symptoms so you can enjoy exercising safely.

>> **Maintain a healthy weight.** Being overweight can worsen asthma symptoms, and it puts you at risk of other health problems. Chapter 4 can help you create a solid nutrition plan that, combined with regular exercise (Chapter 5), will help you lose weight or keep within a recommended range.

>> **Understand how to take your medications and do so consistently.** Medications can be an integral part of a successful treatment plan. And with asthma, your medications — particularly inhalers — may need to be taken preventively or they may be intended for reactive use, as needed, so understanding when to take them and how to use them is important.

>> **See the doctor regularly.** At least twice a year, even if you're feeling well. And don't ignore signs that your asthma may not be under control, such as needing to use a quick-relief inhaler too often. Asthma changes over time. Consulting your doctor can help you make needed treatment adjustments to keep symptoms under control. Take a look at Chapter 10 for pointers on having a successful doctor's visit.

REMEMBER

Asthma doesn't need to contribute to a shorter lifespan for men. With consistent care and healthy habits, it can be something you successfully manage for a lifetime.

Chapter **20**

Two Silent Threats: Diabetes and Alzheimer's Disease

Today, 415 million people worldwide are living with diabetes. In the United States, it's estimated that one in two adults currently have either diabetes or prediabetes. If you don't already have a diagnosis, chances are good you'll develop one or the other in your lifetime. And diabetes is one of the top ten contributors to men's deaths, so this is a chapter worth reading.

Wait; what? Hold up. Simmer down now. Are we saying between you and your best friend, one of you will almost certainly develop diabetes or prediabetes if you don't already have it? Well, yes . . . if you don't make essential lifestyle changes that can significantly reduce your risk. Because the very good news is that diabetes, especially type 2 diabetes, as well as prediabetes, can often be prevented, and if you already have diabetes, it can be reversed. The body can heal itself with the proper treatment. A delicious and diabetes-friendly diet, pleasurable physical activity, lifestyle enhancements, and (at times) pharmaceutical drugs can help a man avoid being diagnosed with diabetes or feel better than before if already diagnosed.

Diabetes isn't the only condition to round out the top ten contributors to men's deaths. Another is Alzheimer's disease. Whether you're 18 or 80, you've undoubtedly encountered a blip in your memory. The name of the classic rock anthem that vanishes the second its iconic riff hits the speakers, the car keys you swore you put *right there* but are nowhere to be found, or the name of your middle child when you're trying to get their attention (Michaelbrianfido*jonathan* — even the dog got a mention before you finally landed). Most of the time, these little lapses are nothing to worry about, but sometimes they could be early signs of something more serious. Unfortunately Alzheimer's disease isn't as definitively preventable or reversable as diabetes, but it's another one where how you take care of your body and your mind can make a difference to your long-term risks.

Deciphering Diabetes: What's Happening in Your Body

Diabetes is a condition that affects how the body uses blood sugar (*glucose*) to make energy. Diabetes occurs when the pancreas isn't able to properly regulate the amount of glucose in the blood — either because the body doesn't produce enough of the hormone *insulin* to handle the amount of glucose, or when the body can't effectively use the insulin it produces. Either way, glucose builds up in your bloodstream and becomes too much of a good thing.

WARNING

If you consistently have too much of this good thing — your glucose is consistently too high — you can develop serious complications, including life-threatening health issues such as heart disease as well as damage to your nerves and eyes.

Understanding your body's engine and its fuel

Although "living to eat" can make life more enjoyable — is there anything more sublime than a summer caprese salad with perfectly ripe tomatoes, garden-grown basil, and delicate fresh mozzarella, topped with a peppery Spanish olive oil — ultimately food is what fuels our bodies as it's converted to energy.

REMEMBER

Nearly all of the food we consume falls into one of three categories: carbohydrates, fats, and proteins. And of these, carbohydrates are the go-to nutrients for easily accessed fuel for living. Carbohydrates exist in two forms:

>> **Simple,** readily available small molecular forms called *sugars*. Simple sugars are present naturally in varying amounts in fruits, milk, and honey, for example, and they taste sweet.

>> **Complex** forms where multiple different sugar molecules are bound together and need to be broken down before they can release the simpler molecules for energy. Examples of complex carbs include starchy veggies like potatoes and corn, whole grains like oatmeal and brown rice, as well as legumes, nuts, seeds, and some fruits. Complex carbohydrates may taste sweet but usually don't.

So whether the carbs you eat start simple or end up that way after being broken down, simple sugars are what fuel your body (including that weekend warrior activity). *Glucose* is the most common type of simple sugar.

Digging deeper: Insulin as fuel injector

The hormone *insulin* finely controls the level of glucose in your blood by acting like a key to open a cell (such as a muscle, fat, or liver cell) so that glucose can enter. If glucose can't enter the cell, it can't provide energy to the body.

Insulin is the major player in regulating your sugar level. Especially when you eat, your body responds with insulin to control the amount of circulating glucose, keeping things in balance as you consume food and utilize energy to live. When there's extra glucose, insulin helps store it as fat. When your body needs energy, it helps release that stored glucose.

Getting to know your pancreas and its role in diabetes

We know insulin is the Great Glucose Regulator (see the preceding section). Where does insulin come from? Cue Heywood Banks's witty and inimitable song *Pancreas,* while we sing this organ's praises. (Seriously, look it up on YouTube.) It's amazing to think of the impact that a tiny organ like the pancreas can play in your health. Most people aren't as familiar with the pancreas as they are with other organs, such as the heart, liver, and lungs.

TECHNICAL
STUFF

Most of the time, your pancreas hides behind your stomach, quietly doing its work. One of its major functions, albeit unrelated to diabetes, is to produce digestive enzymes, which help break down food.

Your pancreas's other function, which *does* pertain to diabetes, is to produce insulin and to secrete it directly into the blood. In a matter of speaking, it turns on the flow of insulin.

What's turned on eventually must be turned off. After glucose leaves your blood and enters your cells, your blood glucose level falls. Your pancreas can tell when your glucose is falling, and it turns off the release of insulin to prevent *hypoglycemia,* an unhealthy low level of blood glucose. At the same time, your liver begins to release glucose from storage and makes new glucose from amino acids in your blood.

This balance is key. Doctors have proven that high blood glucose is bad for you and that keeping the blood glucose as normal as possible prevents the complications of diabetes. Most treatments for diabetes are directed at restoring the blood glucose to normal.

Knowing the Differences Between Type 1 and Type 2 Diabetes

REMEMBER

When you have diabetes, you have high blood glucose, and this overabundance is due to one of two causes:

>> Your pancreas doesn't make enough (or any) insulin

>> Your body isn't acting the way it's supposed to when your pancreas releases insulin

Although there are several types of diabetes, men overwhelmingly face one of two types, plus a condition that can be a harbinger of bigger issues to come. Take a look at the following sections for more on the two main types of diabetes men face (and the upcoming section "Monitoring Prediabetes: Your Body's Yellow Warning Light" for information on that important wake-up call).

Type 1: When your body attacks itself

Type 1 diabetes is an *autoimmune disease,* meaning that your body is unkind enough to react against — and in this case, destroy — a vital part of itself, namely the insulin-producing beta (B) cells of the pancreas. If the cells are destroyed, your body can't produce (enough) insulin, so someone with type 1 diabetes needs to take insulin shots every day for their entire lives to make sure their blood sugar stays at the correct levels.

Symptoms of type 1 diabetes

Following are some of the major signs and symptoms of type 1 diabetes:

» Frequent urination

» Increase in thirst

» Weight loss

» Increase in hunger

» Weakness

Type 1 diabetes is usually diagnosed in children and young adults (although adults can be diagnosed as well) and in the past was commonly known as *juvenile diabetes.*

Who gets type 1 diabetes

People who get type 1 diabetes more frequently have certain abnormal characteristics on their genetic material (their *chromosomes)* that aren't present in people who don't get type 1 diabetes.

TECHNICAL STUFF

UNDERSTANDING HBA1C — YOUR PERSONAL MONITOR

Your *blood glucose level* is the level of sugar in your blood, a key measure of diabetes. There are a couple of ways to measure your blood glucose level:

• Individual blood glucose tests are great for determining how you're doing at a particular moment and what to do to make it better. They capture a moment in time versus the big picture.

• The *hemoglobin A1C* (often shortened to HBA1C or simply A1C) is the test that gives an integrated picture of many days, weeks, or even months of blood glucose levels. This test is particularly important in seeing the big picture, as glucose can change a great deal even in 30 minutes, especially before or after meals.

Hemoglobin A1C can be used to identify the presence of diabetes in people who may be unaware they have the condition. According to one study, in the United States, hemoglobin A1C detects that diabetes is present in one in every five people who don't already have a diagnosis of diabetes, regardless of the reason they're admitted to a hospital.

Another essential factor in predicting whether you'll develop type 1 diabetes is your exposure to something in the environment, most likely a virus. A particular virus may cause diabetes by attacking your pancreas directly and diminishing your ability to produce insulin, which quickly creates the diabetic condition in your body. Alternatively, the virus may look similar to parts of insulin-producing cells in the pancreas, resulting in the immune system mistakenly attacking the cells.

Also, some research shows that the naturally occurring bacteria in the gut — *microbiome* — may have a role to play in the development of type 1 diabetes, but more research is needed in this field.

Although genetics plays a role in developing type 1 diabetes, the connection is relatively minor. An identical twin has only a 20 percent chance of developing type 1 diabetes if the other twin (who has the exact same genetic material) has it.

Type 2: When your lifestyle is a contributing culprit

People with type 2 diabetes have plenty of insulin in their bodies (unlike people with type 1 diabetes), but their bodies respond to the insulin in abnormal ways. Their bodies need to make extra insulin just to keep their blood glucose normal, because their insulin is less effective than it should be. This is called having *insulin resistance.*

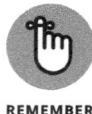

REMEMBER

Insulin resistance isn't a one-way street. We now know that genes, diet, a healthy gut microbiome, exercise, and even better-quality sleep can work the other way and support insulin to work more efficiently, decreasing insulin resistance. This is described as increasing insulin *sensitivity.* So, the good news is that you can counter even genetic predisposition to insulin resistance through lifestyle changes.

Type 2 diabetes is much more common than type 1; recent statistics show that among those who were diagnosed with diabetes, 91.2 percent had type 2 diabetes and 5.6 percent had type 1 diabetes. Although type 2 is much more prevalent, those with type 2 diabetes seem in general to have milder complications (such as eye disease and kidney disease) from diabetes.

Type 2 diabetes is often a result of lifestyle habits, including being overweight and not being active enough; it's often preventable by eating healthfully, maintaining a healthy weight, and exercising regularly.

Symptoms of type 2 diabetes

The symptoms of type 2 diabetes can be subtle and easy to overlook at first. If you experience two or more of the following symptoms and haven't already been diagnosed with diabetes, call your doctor:

>> **Fatigue:** Type 2 diabetes makes you tired because your body's cells aren't getting the glucose fuel that they need. Even though your blood has plenty of insulin, your body is resistant to its actions.

>> **Frequent urination and thirst:** As with type 1 diabetes, you find yourself urinating more frequently than usual, which dehydrates your body and leaves you thirsty.

>> **Blurred vision:** The lenses of your eyes swell and shrink as your blood glucose levels rise and fall. Your vision blurs because your eyes can't adjust quickly enough to these lens changes.

>> **Slow healing of skin, gum, and urinary infections:** Your white blood cells, which help with healing and defend your body against infections, don't function correctly in the high-glucose environment present in your body when it has diabetes.

>> **Numbness in the feet or legs:** You experience numbness because of a common long-term complication of diabetes called *neuropathy,* a type of nerve damage.

>> **Heart disease, stroke, and peripheral vascular disease:** Heart disease, stroke, and peripheral vascular disease (blockage of arteries in the legs) occur much more often in people with type 2 diabetes.

How type 2 and type 1 symptoms differ

TECHNICAL
STUFF

The signs and symptoms of type 2 diabetes are similar in some cases to the symptoms of type 1 diabetes, but in many ways, they're different. The following list shows some of the differences between symptoms in type 1 and type 2 diabetes:

>> **Age of onset:** People with type 2 diabetes are usually older than those with type 1 diabetes. However, the increasing incidence of type 2 diabetes in overweight children is making this difference less useful for separating type 1 and type 2 diabetes.

>> **Body weight:** Obesity is a common characteristic of people with type 2 diabetes, whereas people with type 1 diabetes are usually thin or normal in weight.

>> **Level of glucose:** People with type 2 diabetes have lower glucose levels at the onset of the disease.

>> **Severity of onset:** Type 2 diabetes gradually shows its symptoms, whereas type 1 diabetes usually has a much more severe onset.

IS TYPE 2 DIABETES GENETIC?

Usually, people with type 2 diabetes can find a relative who has had the disease. Therefore, doctors consider type 2 diabetes to have much more of a genetic component than type 1 diabetes. However, we now know that it's possible to prevent or even reverse conditions despite a genetic predisposition. You may not be able to change your genes, but with diet and lifestyle changes, you can certainly influence your tendency to develop some gene-related diseases.

Who gets type 2 diabetes

Most people with type 2 diabetes are over the age of 40, and your chances of getting type 2 diabetes increase as you get older. People who are overweight, don't get much physical activity, and have a family history of type 2 diabetes are more likely to develop it. Type 2 diabetes is a disease of gradual onset rather than the severe emergency that can herald type 1 diabetes. Because the symptoms are so mild at first, you may not notice them. You may ignore these symptoms for years before they become bothersome enough to consult your doctor. Doctors believe that no virus is involved in the onset of type 2 diabetes.

Monitoring Prediabetes: Your Body's Yellow Warning Light

Diabetes doesn't suddenly appear one day without your body having raised some red flags. For a period of time, which may last up to ten years, you may have elevated blood glucose levels — they may not reach the threshold for a diagnosis of diabetes, but they're still elevated above normal. These not-normal-yet-not-diabetes blood glucose levels indicate *prediabetes.*

In such situations, your body is making extra insulin just to keep your blood glucose normal, but your insulin is less effective than it should be and isn't quite doing the job — this is called *insulin resistance.* If your insulin resistance worsens to the point that your body just can't produce enough insulin to keep your blood glucose normal, or if your pancreas starts to get "tired" of making so much extra insulin, your blood sugars become abnormal, and the yellow warning light of prediabetes turns on.

Other contributors that hinder your pancreas from keeping up with your insulin demands include overweight, a sedentary lifestyle, certain medications, and aging. After prediabetes develops, approximately 25 percent of people will develop diabetes within three to five years, with as many as 70 percent of those diagnosed with prediabetes progressing to diabetes in their lifetime

TIP

Adopting lifestyle changes can significantly improve a person with prediabetes's chances of not developing diabetes. So if you're diagnosed with prediabetes, consider that information a golden ticket to better health, if you're willing to make some changes.

Symptoms of prediabetes

A person with prediabetes doesn't usually have any symptoms or develop eye disease, kidney disease, or nerve damage (all potential complications of diabetes). But as we mentioned earlier, if you have prediabetes, you're probably overweight and don't get much exercise.

Who gets prediabetes

Because so many people have prediabetes (or diabetes) without knowing it or showing symptoms, testing for prediabetes is a good idea for everyone over the age of 45. It also may be recommended to get tested if you're under 45 and overweight or eat more than ten teaspoons of added sugar daily and have one or more of the following risk factors:

>> You're in a high-risk group: African-American, Latino, Asian, or Native American.

>> You have high blood pressure.

>> You have low HDL ("good" cholesterol).

>> You have high triglycerides.

>> You have a family history of diabetes.

Implementing Diabetes Prevention Strategies

Although there's not a lot you can do to reduce your risk of developing type 1 diabetes, you can make numerous adjustments in your life to help minimize your chances of developing type 2 diabetes. And if you haven't already made lifestyle changes and get a prediabetes diagnosis, well, use the diagnosis as a signal that you might be running out of time on the free-of-diabetes clock, so now's the time to get serious about living a healthier life and reducing your risk in the process.

TIP

If you recognize any of the following factors in your body or lifestyle, correcting them in time can help you avoid a diabetes diagnosis or control the disease if you already have it:

>> **Maintain a healthy body-mass index.** The *body-mass index* (BMI) is the way that doctors look at weight in relation to height. BMI is a better indicator of a healthy weight than just weight alone because taller people tend to weigh more. (Although it's not without its flaws — muscle weighs more than fat, so a very muscular person would be considered obese based on BMI. BMI isn't perfect, but it gives a decent indication of healthy body mass for most people.) Current guidelines state that a BMI between 18.5 and 25 is considered

normal; if your BMI is higher than this range, you're predisposed to type 2 diabetes. (A BMI from 25 to 29.9 is considered overweight, and a BMI of 30 or greater is considered obese.) Go to www.nhlbi.nih.gov/calculate-your-bmi to figure out yours.

>> **Get enough physical activity.** Physical inactivity has a high association with diabetes. Most adults and those with type1 and type 2 diabetes should perform at least 150 minutes of moderate-intensity *aerobic* (meaning it gets your heart rate moving) physical activity each week, spread over at least three days per week, with no more than two consecutive days without exercise. Check out Chapters 5 and 6 for information on aerobic exercise and weight training.

>> **Don't cop a squat for too long.** Prolonged sitting should be interrupted every 30 minutes for blood glucose benefits. So get up from your desk or your comfy lounge chair regularly to help maintain balanced blood sugar levels. Similarly, taking a short walk after meals can help regulate blood glucose and avoid excessive glucose spikes.

>> **Shrink your waistline.** Extra weight carried around your midsection is known as *visceral fat*. Visceral fat seems to cause more insulin resistance than fat in other areas. A person with visceral fat is more apple-shaped than pear-shaped. If you have a lot of visceral fat, losing just 5 to 10 percent of your weight may dramatically reduce your chance of diabetes or a heart attack.

>> **Adopt a high-quality diet.** Populations with a high prevalence of diabetes often have poor eating habits, which lead to higher BMI and more belly fat, both of which are factors that increase the likelihood of developing diabetes. Take a look at Chapter 4 for healthy-eating pointers.

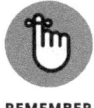

REMEMBER

When many people decide to make healthier lifestyle commitments, they often take on an "all or nothing" attitude, which can be difficult to maintain. When scheduling good-for-you activities, make sure that you're being realistic with your calendar. On the days that you work longer, you may need shorter workouts, time outdoors, or naps. Try to think in intervals of 10 minutes and in getting the most bang for your buck. If you can schedule only 30 minutes a day to work toward a healthier life, you could spend 10 minutes walking outdoors, 10 minutes meditating or napping, and another 10 minutes whipping up something satisfying to eat. In the course of a month, those 10-minute interludes will have already begun to make a difference. Use your days off to enjoy more physical exercise, relaxation, and meal prep for busier days.

Cutting Through the Confusion about Alzheimer's

Dementia and Alzheimer's disease with prediabetes — are they interchangeable terms? Is Alzheimer's disease just a fancy word for dementia? No, they aren't exactly the same.

REMEMBER

Alzheimer's disease is a *type* of dementia. Many types of dementia exist, with Alzheimer's disease being the most common. Currently 55 million people worldwide live with dementia, and approximately 60-70 percent of them have Alzheimer's disease. Approximately one in ten American men aged 65 and older will be diagnosed with Alzheimer's disease in their lifetimes (making it one of the ten leading causes of death for men in the United States). And Alzheimer's disease isn't an "old person's disease" — globally over 70,000 people are currently living with *young onset dementia* (dementia that develops before age 65).

In this section we demystify Alzheimer's disease and its connection to dementia.

Untangling the terms: Dementia versus Alzheimer's disease

Dementia is a general term for a decline in mental ability (including impaired memory, language, reasoning, judgment, visuospatial skills, and orientation) severe enough to interfere with daily life. Dementia is chronic and progressive, meaning it is ongoing long term and gets steadily worse over time.

Dementia isn't normal aging. It's not something you get from using deodorant or cooking in aluminum pans. Dementia is caused by several brain diseases that gradually worsen and affect how a person thinks, feels, and behaves; eventually, the person loses the ability to carry out the basic tasks of daily living.

REMEMBER

Alzheimer's disease (AD) is a type of dementia. This type of brain disease slowly destroys memory and thinking skills, and eventually someone with AD becomes unable to carry out even simple tasks. When you have AD, abnormal deposits of specific proteins inside the brain disrupt normal brain function and cause the cognitive and functional problems typically associated with AD. Eventually, as these deposits spread throughout the brain, brain tissue starts dying, which leads to further cognitive impairment. The resulting brain shrinkage can be seen in CT scans and MRI scans. There is no cure for AD.

ALZHEIMER'S DISEASE AND ITS COUSINS: THE BIG FOUR

One of the most common misconceptions about dementia is that it means AD. Alzheimer's disease certainly does mean dementia, but numerous other causes of dementia also exist. If you have dementia, you don't necessarily have AD.

Dementia can be broken down into four primary conditions; here's a quick field guide:

- **Alzheimer's disease** is the most common cause of dementia worldwide. In the United States, it's the cause of dementia in 62 to 80 percent of cases. Alzheimer's disease is one of the top causes of men's death in the United States and is the seventh leading cause of death in Americans age 65 and older.

- **Vascular dementia** occurs when the oxygen supply to the brain is limited by blood vessel blockage or bleeding from strokes. Vascular dementia symptoms can look a lot like Alzheimer's, but they vary depending on which parts of the brain were affected by strokes and how much damage was done.

- **Lewy body disease** is rarer. *Lewy bodies* are protein deposits that damage brain cells (and are also seen in Parkinson's disease, which is why the two share symptoms). Like Alzheimer's, Lewy body dementia affects memory and thinking — but it also causes muscle stiffness, tremors, shakiness, and slower movement.

- **Frontotemporal dementia** is the least common of the "big four" but is the most likely to be diagnosed in people under the age of 65. This type of dementia targets the brain's frontal and temporal lobes — areas tied to memory and personality, and brings symptoms like disinhibited or odd behavior, lack of empathy, and repetitive speech or actions.

Scientists don't fully understand what causes Alzheimer's disease in most people. Although certain forms of AD run in families, these forms are extremely rare, accounting for less than 5 percent of all cases. Most of the time, the causes appear to be a combination of age, overall health, and lifestyle.

Mild cognitive impairment: Precursor to Alzheimer's disease?

Dementia isn't just about memory loss — it also affects how you think, feel, and handle everyday tasks. Like dementia, *mild cognitive impairment* (MCI) can affect a variety of normal thought processes including memory, planning, and judgment, but it doesn't impact mood or a person's ability to perform day-to-day functions.

MCI goes beyond normal age-related forgetfulness, but it's not severe enough to qualify as AD or dementia. Long-term studies suggest that 10 to 20 percent of adults over 65 may have it.

For some people, mild cognitive impairment can be a sign of future dementia, most likely Alzheimer's disease. Fortunately, around 60 percent of people who develop mild cognitive impairment don't get any worse and some even get better. (And as an aside, many times MCI is due to causes other than AD, including depression and medication side effects. If you feel you're showing symptoms of MCI, talk to your doctor so you can rule out — and address — reversible causes.)

TIP

No specific treatment for MCI exists and, in particular, no evidence suggests that the drugs used to treat Alzheimer's disease are of any use. You can gain some mileage, however, by addressing risk factors for poor circulation by controlling your blood pressure, eating a low-carbohydrate and high-fiber diet, quitting smoking, drinking alcohol within the limits of recommended guidelines (that's two drinks per day for guys), and getting regular exercise. Now where have you heard that before (clue: throughout this book)? It's remarkable how making some lifestyle changes reduces your risks for so many diseases that may shorten your life and make your living less enjoyable.

Brushing Up on Brain Basics and Dementia Disruption

Before we go any further, we want to give you a quick overview of how your brain and memory work normally, when they're not affected by disease. Understanding a normal brain function can help you better understand what goes wrong in dementia and Alzheimer's disease.

Knowing about neurons and your noggin

TECHNICAL
STUFF

An adult brain weighs around 3.3 pounds and has the consistency of tofu. It's made up of around 86 billion nerve cells, called *neurons*, arranged into two halves, called *hemispheres*, which are each divided further into four lobes: *frontal, parietal, temporal,* and *occipital.*

Neurons are the brain's main messengers, sending electrical signals to help different parts of the brain communicate. These signals jump from one neuron to the next at tiny gaps called *synapses*, using chemical messengers to keep the conversation going. Of these chemicals, called *neurotransmitters*, dopamine, glutamate, and acetylcholine have the most relevance to dementia.

Understanding the memory-making process

REMEMBER

Memory is obviously vital to normal functioning, hence the disability that results when it starts to fail. Without memory, you can't learn from or make links to the past, so you can't plan for the future. You can also get lost, not only geographically but also emotionally, while carrying out tasks or in the middle of conversations. Lack of memory prevents you from being able to follow instructions and even to recognize those you love.

Humans have two main types of memory: short term and long term.

>> *Short-term memory* (sometimes called *working memory)* allows you to remember things such as telephone numbers or drink orders at the bar. It has limited storage capacity and empties quickly so new items can be remembered.

>> *Long-term memory* allows you to lay down your memories for keeps. Examples include the address of your first home, the recipe for Grandpa's dill pickles, the Super Bowl final score in 1969 (New York Jets 16, Baltimore Colts 7, in case you're interested), or Pythagoras's theorem. Memories aren't stored in one particular part of the brain but involve the interaction and cooperation of a few different regions.

For memory to work, your brain has to go through three stages: encoding (taking in information), storage, and retrieval. A failure of all or any of these individual processes can cause memory impairment. For example, encoding and storage may be fine, but with no capacity for retrieval you won't recall what you've stored. Likewise, encoded information won't be retrieved if it wasn't stored.

Realizing what goes wrong in dementia and Alzheimer's disease

Dementia interferes with the functioning of brain cells, which stops them communicating between each other and therefore carrying out their normal business. The process of dementia inflicts two major types of damage on nerve cells, which then produces symptoms:

>> The cells can be killed off or rendered largely inactive because they receive insufficient oxygen in the bloodstream, as in vascular dementia.

>> Protein deposits, such as plaques and tangles in Alzheimer's disease and Lewy bodies in Lewy body dementia, form within and mess up the internal workings of the cells.

Obviously, this view is simplistic. However, it gives you an idea of what can go wrong in an individual brain cell; these changes have to then occur in many cells to impair how the whole brain works. This loss of function, coupled with a reduction in levels of some of the neurotransmitters that let cells "talk" to each other, can cause large parts of a person's central nervous system to fail.

In dementia, both the type of brain damage and where it happens matter—they work together to shape the symptoms a person experiences. In Alzheimer's disease, the main area of the brain that's affected is the *hippocampus*, which is involved in converting short-term memories into long-term memories (cue the initial classic symptom where a person has difficulty remembering what's just happened, although memories already stored long term can sometimes still be recalled).

Spotting the Signs: When "Senior Moments" Become Something More

Dementia doesn't look the same for everyone, but certain common signs often sound the alarm. In the early stages, though, it's important not to panic and see dementia lurking behind every forgetful or confused moment, because these types of memory lapses are often a normal part of aging.

Identifying normal forgetfulness versus red flags

We all forget where we put our cellphone sometimes. Many things can make most people absentminded, from simple tiredness and poor concentration to a period of low mood or actual depression. How many men, caught up in an engrossing task or conversation, forget to leave for a dental appointment or accidentally burn dinner?

WARNING

When forgetting becomes a regular part of your behavior, though, you may be seeing signs of something more serious. And it's rare for memory issues alone to suggest you might be showing signs of dementia. If you're having problems with finding the right words, confusion over using money, or uncertainty in how to follow a favorite recipe, and you're noticing changes in mood and loss of confidence in social situations, then you may be facing issues that exceed normal forgetfulness.

Recognizing early symptoms when they appear

WARNING

Here's a run-down of some important early symptoms to look out for if you suspect your forgetfulness is a concern. To get a diagnosis, someone needs to show at least two of these ten warning signs — often subtle at first, but more obvious as the disease progresses:

>> **Memory problems that affect daily life.** You struggle to remember important dates and events, the route taken on well-traveled journeys, where you've left important paperwork, or names and faces of familiar friends, neighbors, and work colleagues. You notice a pattern of steadily worsening memory loss.

>> **Difficulty with planning and problem-solving.** You become confused using a debit card, credit card, or checking account. You lose track of what your bank statement or credit card statement shows, or you have difficulty paying bills or filing taxes. You become confused while trying to put gas in the car.

>> **Problems finding the right word.** Words may regularly become elusive, and you find it difficult to communicate effectively, leading to huge amounts of frustration. When you can't find the word you're after, you may substitute something similar, such as a football becoming a *kick ball,* or a wristwatch becoming a *hand clock.*

>> **Confusion about time and place.** You often lose track of time or become muddled about the date. You may forget where you are or how you got there.

>> **Poor judgment.** Your ability to make good judgment declines. Your normally frugal self may end up spending money on things you don't need, or you may dress yourself in clothes not appropriate for the activity (wearing a coat and hat to the beach, for example).

>> **Visuospatial difficulties.** You may find yourself becoming increasingly clumsy. You lose your ability to judge widths and distances, and you suffer more falls and breaks, or more dings (or worse) when parking or driving a car.

>> **Misplacing things.** You increasingly leave things in the wrong place (slippers in the refrigerator). When you forget where you've put your keys or cellphone, you can't retrace your steps to find them.

>> **Changes in mood.** Mood swings can return with puberty-like intensity, with rapid switches between extremes of sadness, fear, and anger. Low moods and depression become extremely common.

>> **Loss of initiative.** You may lose interest in taking part in your usual activities; you may need repeated prompting before participating in group settings.

>> **Personality changes.** Your normal behavior changes. If you're usually reserved and quiet, you may become flirty and disinhibited, or if you're usually extroverted and lively, you may become withdrawn and reclusive. You may increasingly become confused, suspicious, withdrawn, angry, or sexually disinhibited.

Assessing Your Alzheimer's Risks and Picking Prevention

As the adage goes, an ounce of prevention is better than a pound of cure. And with Alzheimer's disease, for which no cure exists and the symptoms are so devastatingly awful, surely anything is worth trying to prevent it.

Unfortunately, doctors can't put their fingers on a single trigger for dementia, so there's not necessarily one thing you can do (or cease doing) to substantially reduce your risk of developing this condition. The good news, however, is that some scientific evidence suggests that changing diet and lifestyle — keeping mentally and physically active — can help you avoid developing dementia. (You're definitely getting a lotta preventive bang for your buck when making changes to how you eat and take care of your body!)

This section explains who's at greatest risk for developing AD or dementia and how you might reduce those risks.

Taking age into account

If you had a dollar for every senior who has said, "I'm just getting old," you'd have more money than Warren Buffett. Although dementia isn't a part of normal aging, human brains and bodies do undergo changes as a person grows older. You may need bifocals to both read and drive without constantly changing eyeglasses, it becomes harder to hear high-pitched tones, and your hair turns gray (or white) and may desert you altogether. Contrary to popular belief, not everyone develops dementia, but the reality is that advancing age increases your likelihood of developing AD.

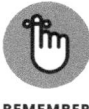

REMEMBER

Although dementia does become a more common occurrence with advancing years, dementia isn't limited to the aging generation. Some younger people can fall victim to it, too. Although the Alzheimer's Association (www.alz.org) estimates that 1 in 14 people older than the age of 65 will develop dementia, its statistics also show that 200,000 of the 5.3 million people with dementia in the United States are younger than 65. And given that the Alzheimer's Association also estimates that less than 50 percent of people with dementia in the United States have actually been diagnosed, this number is likely to rise as pick-up rates improve.

Over the age of 75 most people diagnosed with dementia are diagnosed with Alzheimer's disease or vascular dementia, with some cases of mixed dementia thrown in as well.

Understanding your genetic risk

Unlike many health conditions, the genetic risks for dementia aren't substantial. Although certain forms of Alzheimer's disease run in families, these forms are extremely rare, accounting for less than 5 percent of all cases. So just because your mother or your brother was diagnosed with AD doesn't automatically mean that you're going to be as well.

Reducing your lifestyle risks

Some factors have been proven to increase your risk for Alzheimer's disease and dementia, so modifying those factors naturally reduces your risk. We know no one lives a completely healthy lifestyle all the time — we don't! (We may run marathons and take part in 100-mile bike rides, but we still enjoy a pizza and a beer.) But changing what you eat and how you live most of the time will still reap benefits.

TIP

A healthy lifestyle that helps reduce risk for AD includes

>> Refraining from using illicit drugs

>> Drinking caffeinated beverages in moderation

>> Drinking alcohol responsibly, if at all

>> Not smoking

>> Eating more fruit and fiber

>> Eating fewer burgers and other fast food

>> Exercising more

» Keeping your brain active (learn new skills, try out different hobbies, do puzzles like crosswords and sudoku)

» Getting seven to eight hours of sleep per night

» Socializing with others, such as clubs and hobbies you can do together

» Managing stress with twice-daily meditation or taking up yoga

Take a look at the chapters in Part 2 for a deeper dive into lifestyle decisions that can reduce your risk of developing Alzheimer's and other diseases.

5

The Part of Tens

IN THIS PART . . .

Get tips on making smart food choices that boost your brain.

Make sure your immune system is as strong as it can be so you can live the longer life you deserve.

Discover quick workouts that help your heart and reduce your risk of developing a fatal disease.

Chapter **21**

Ten Food Choices to Benefit Your Brain

The average, 175-pound adult male's brain weighs about 3.5 pounds, about 2 percent of their body weight. But that 2 percent uses nearly 20 percent of the calories a guy consumes each day to power more than 100 billion neurons (nerve cells) that, working at top speed, convert those calories into enough energy to turn on a 25-watt incandescent light bulb.

What you eat and *when* you eat it can influence how your brain functions. Take a look at these tips to use food to help your brain work better for you. Maybe you'll even overhear someone say, "Check out the big brain on Brad."

Putting Brain-Boosting Plants on Your Plate

Plants are deceptive. On the outside, they're mostly green and calm. On the inside, they're busy little chemical factories churning out multitudinous compounds, many of which have properties that protect the plant — and various parts of your body, including, of course, your brain.

One class of these natural chemicals is the *polyphenols.* Polyphenols are widely distributed in fruits and vegetables as well as in nuts, seeds, and grains. Some have antioxidant, antiallergic, anti-inflammatory, antiviral, or antiproliferative (prevents cell from irregular reproduction, an anticancer trait) effects.

One group of important antioxidant and anti-inflammatory polyphenols are the *flavonoids*, the pigments that color plants yellow, red, orange, green, or white. Some flavonoids may also be antiviral and antiproliferative. So eat those dark- and vibrant-colored veggies often.

Minding Your MIND Diet to Minimize Dementia

If there is one — no, two — diets on whose virtues every reputable expert agrees, it's the Mediterranean diet (see Chapter 4) and DASH (also known as *Dietary Approaches to Stop Hypertension*). Both the Med and DASH diets, built on a base of plant foods plus low-fat, protein-rich foods, such as fish and poultry, are known to reduce the risk of cardiovascular disease.

A team of nutritional epidemiologists at Harvard University and Rush University Medical Center in Chicago put them together to create the MIND diet (short for *Mediterranean-DASH Intervention for Neurodegenerative Delay*, a mouthful in itself). The MIND diet has 15 food categories: 10 are brain-healthy; 5, not so much:

>> **The ten "good" foods** are berries, beans, fish, nuts, olive oil, poultry, vegetables (green leafy), vegetables (everything else), whole grains, and wine.

>> **The five "not so good" foods** are butter and stick margarine, cheese, fried or fast food, pastries and sweets, and red meats.

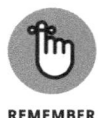

The principles of the MIND diet are:

>> Three servings of whole grains, one salad, and one or more vegetables a day

>> Beans every other day

>> Poultry and berries at least twice a week

>> Fish at least once a week

>> Eat nuts for your snacks

- » Have a glass of wine to top off every day's delights

- » Less than a tablespoon of butter or stick margarine a day

- » Less than one serving of fried or fast food a week

Research has shown that the MIND diet, when followed to the letter, reduced the risk of Alzheimer's by as much as 53 percent. And good news for those of us who fall on the, shall we say, less rigorous end of the stickler scale, the research revealed that even following the diet imperfectly reduced risk by about 35 percent.

Sipping Smart for a Moment of Mellow

Alcohol is man's most widely used natural relaxant. Contrary to common belief, alcohol is a depressant, not a mood elevator. If you feel relaxed or, conversely, exuberant after one drink, the reason isn't that the alcohol is speeding up your brain; it's that alcohol loosens your *controls,* the brain signals that normally tell you not to put a lampshade on your head or take off your clothes in public.

For more about alcohol's effects on the body, turn to Chapter 9. Right here, it's enough to say that many people find that, taken with food and in moderation — defined as a maximum of two drinks a day for a man — alcohol can comfortably change a mood from tense to mellow.

Reducing Stress with a Little Dark Chocolate

In 2009, a team of nutrition scientists at the Nestle Research Center in Lausanne (Switzerland) produced the still-classic study of the beneficial effects of chocolate. Their results revealed that 40 grams (about 1.5 ounces) of dark chocolate a day helped reduce the body's production of stress hormones.

TIP

Use chocolate with 74 percent cocoa, and give yourself two servings per day, 20 grams in the morning and 20 grams in the afternoon. You may feel your stress melt away, or maybe you'll just add a bright spot to your AM and PM. Sounds like win/win either way.

Thinking Quicker with a Cuppa Joe

Caffeine is a mild stimulant that not only increases your level of *serotonin* (the calming neurotransmitter), but also helps your brain cells become more reactive to stimulants such as noise and light, making you talk faster and think faster. One cup of coffee in the morning is a pleasant push into alertness and can increase your effectiveness at certain tasks. But keep in mind balance — too many cups of coffee a day can make your hands shake.

Getting Energy from Protein or Calm from Carbs

No food will change your personality or alter the course of a mood disorder. But some may add a little lift or a small moment of calm to your day, make you more alert, or give you a neat little push over the finish line.

A grilled chicken breast (white meat, no skin) for breakfast on a day when you have to be on your toes before lunch can help make you sharp as a tack.

Got an important lunch meeting? Order starches without fats or oils: pasta with fresh tomatoes and basil, no oil, no cheese; rice with veggies; rice with fruit. Your aim is to get the calming carbs without the high-fat food that slows thinking and makes you feel sleepy.

Eating Enough Food

Constant on-and-off dieting or even occasional crash dieting can rob your brain of energy without producing lasting weight control. Don't skip meals, don't eat anemic portions, and don't try to live on lettuce alone. Get the calories you need, with a mix of proteins, carbs, and fats, to keep your energy up and your brain sharp.

Eating Smaller Portions but More Often

Who says three scheduled large meals a day is right for you? Frequent smaller meals provide a continuous flow of energy to your brain. And by allowing yourself to eat before you're ravenously hungry, these grazing moments may enable you to keep from overeating, a risk you may face if you have hours between meals.

Choosing Foods That Turn into Energy Slower

Simple carbs, such as table sugar, pep you up fast and then let you down just as quickly. Your body metabolizes complex carbs, such as fruits and vegetables and whole grains, more slowly, so their effect on your brain's energy bank is smoother and lasts longer.

Reducing Your Belly Fat to Keep Your Brain in Shape

OK, this isn't specifically about food, but the result of too much of it. The human body stores extra fat in several well-defined places, and as the body ages, these fat deposits tend to expand. For men, it's shoulders and the abdomen, the large area between chest and pelvis commonly known as the belly. But belly fat may be hazardous to brain health, even when the body with the belly isn't overweight and its body mass index (BMI) is within normal range.

In 2008, data from a Kaiser Permanente study of nearly 7,000 volunteers, age 40 to 45, showed that people with big bellies are more likely than those with flat tummies to develop Alzheimer's disease later in life (Chapter 20 has more on this memory-robbing disease). Then, in 2010, researchers enlisted 733 men and women who agreed to a CT-scan of the abdomen and an MRI scan of the brain. What the picture showed was that the more deep fat around the belly, the lower the volume of the brain.

REMEMBER

Remember that healthy bodies come in all sizes and shapes. Holding to a brain-healthy shape definitely doesn't mean dieting to skeleton size. Doing that deprives your brain (and the rest of your body) of essential nutrients. In short, a sensible diet leads to a sensible body and a sensible brain.

Chapter **22**

Ten Ways to Boost Your Immune System

Vaccines are the best way to ward off potentially dangerous illnesses. But you can also take steps every day to make yourself less susceptible to illness, boosting your immune system, and making you better able to resist all kinds of bugs. Many of the changes you can make won't cost you anything and, as a bonus, will make you feel better every day of your life.

Getting Your Vaccinations

REMEMBER

If you browse the array of supplements that promise to boost your immune system at the pharmacy, you may find it hard to believe that getting vaccinated is the best immune system booster of all. But it's true: The best protection against diseases that used to be commonplace is getting vaccinated. While you can't be vaccinated against every disease, you can be vaccinated against many (Chapter 10 has info on vaccines based on your age). For diseases that don't have a vaccine yet, consider the rest of the suggestions in this chapter.

Decreasing Stress

Yes, stress can affect your immune system and make you more susceptible to getting sick. So how can you suffer from less stress when life is so stressful? The way you react to stressors — and everyone has them — can affect the way your immune system reacts.

WARNING

Some people go through life chronically angry — at everything. A car that pulls out in front of them, a long line at the grocery store, a perceived snub from a co-worker — everything generates a stress response. While it might seem like getting angry, yelling, and "getting it out of your system" would be a good thing, it really isn't. Staying in a continual "flight or fight" state triggers the release of chemicals such as cortisol that, over time, put a lot of stress on your immune system (Chapter 2 goes into some detail on this). In the short run, cortisol is beneficial, but if your levels are chronically high, you can produce fewer *lymphocytes* (white blood cells that help you fight off illnesses).

Learning to manage stress can take time and effort. Techniques that teach you to calm your breathing and certain types of exercise such as yoga, meditation, or prayer can help you get through stressful situations while keeping stress from becoming chronic. Take a look at Chapter 7 for more tips.

Eating Well

Micronutrients such as vitamins and minerals as well as macronutrients — protein, carbs, and fats — all help you maintain a healthy immune system. But the food you eat, and not any supplements you can find at the local health food store, is the best way to get the nutrients you need. Supplements can't overcome a poor diet, and too many supplements overpromise on their benefits.

Everyone has days where their diet falls off the nutritionally sound chart. Your goal should be to eat well most of the time. What does it mean to eat well?

>> First off, get enough protein. Protein is the building block for cells, and falling short can have serious side effects. Beef, fish, poultry, eggs, tofu, cheese, and nuts all supply protein.

>> You need carbohydrates too — but the right kind, in the right amounts. Complex carbohydrates, such as vegetables, beans, and whole grains, are good — a bag of chips, not so much. Refined sugars in large amounts can cause harm to many parts of your body, including your immune system.

>> Although fat has become a bad word in dietary terms, good fats are another essential part of healthy eating. Nuts, olive oil, fatty fish, and even dark chocolate can help boost your immune system.

REMEMBER

Eating well, with an adequate amount of fruits and vegetables along with protein and good fats, will usually supply the nutrients you need. Take a look at Chapter 4 for more nutrition pointers.

Maintaining a Healthy Weight

WARNING

Maintaining a healthy weight goes hand in hand with eating well (see the preceding section). Both overweight and underweight individuals can have immune system disruptions:

>> Excess weight can cause inflammation, which affects your immune responses in a number of ways, including by decreasing your white blood cell function and making you more susceptible to infection, as we have seen with COVID-19 and influenza.

>> Being underweight, particularly if you have a protein deficiency, can also affect your immune response, as seen with tuberculosis.

Keeping your weight within a normal range can help keep not only your immune system but all your major organs functioning well.

Getting Enough Sleep

Sleep is another area where falling short can have negative effects on your immune system. Too many things keep us from sleeping well and sleeping long enough and deeply enough to get into sleep states necessary for good health.

Disturbed or shortened sleep periods can cause inflammation and increased hormone stress levels. This can also disrupt some of our coordinated immune system responses. Some studies showed that restricted sleep can also decrease antibody production after vaccination.

WARNING

Taking sleeping pills every night can make sleep issues worse in the long run, so try to limit their use. Take a look at Chapter 8 for tips on getting good rest.

Exercising for Immunity

Walking half an hour a day, fast enough to get your heart rate up; bicycling; or working out at the gym three or four times a week can reduce your stress levels, which in turn can help your immune system. Regular exercise can also increase the way antibodies and white blood cells circulate through your body. Exercise can also help you control your weight, which in turn has benefits for your immune system.

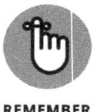
REMEMBER

Getting 150 minutes per week of moderate exercise, or 75 minutes of strenuous exercise, can pay big dividends toward boosting your immune system and making you feel better at the same time.

Saying No to Smoking

Smoking has an array of negative effects on your entire body, including your immune system. The numerous chemicals in tobacco, not just nicotine, can increase inflammation, particularly in your lungs, making you more susceptible to infection and tissue destruction. Smoking also has negative effects on your immune system's ability to respond to infection by decreasing white blood cell activity.

In some people, smoking can increase the risk of autoimmune diseases such as rheumatoid arthritis or multiple sclerosis. Smoking can cause a harmful overactive immune response that leads to these conditions and can lead to persistent chronic inflammation. Inflammation can lead to increased tissue destruction and more negative effects on cells that help keep your immune system in balance.

REMEMBER

One of the best things you can do for your immune system? Quit smoking — or don't ever start. Chapter 9 can help you get started.

Drinking Only in Moderation

Experts recommend no more than one drink per day for women and two for men.

WARNING

But the downside of alcohol consumption is that drinking to excess does a lot of harm to your immune system. Any more than that can disrupt your immune system, starting in your gastrointestinal (GI) tract (your digestive tract) after your first swallow. Alcohol decreases the number of healthy microbes in your GI tract, damages immune cells that line the intestine, and interferes with your body's healing processes. If you wonder if you're drinking too much, Chapter 9 can help you decide and know what to do next.

Staying Connected

Although it isn't yet clearly understood, and it may sound a little out there, there seems to be a definite connection between your mental state and your immune system. You've probably heard that "Happiness is a state of mind" or "You're only as happy as you make up your mind to be." While life circumstances can certainly steal joy from all of us, staying involved with life no matter what the circumstances may affect your immune system as well as your outlook.

Of course this isn't easy, or always possible. But some studies have shown a definite link between people's attitudes and involvement with other people and their immune system's functioning. So don't pooh-pooh the benefits of staying active, connected, and involved on your physical as well as your mental health.

TIP

Don't have family around? Look for other people to befriend or to get involved with. Develop hobbies that you can share with others. Volunteer somewhere. Talk to your neighbors when you're out walking. There's no reason to live a lonely, isolated life unless you're a person who really cherishes solitude. You don't have to be social every minute of the day, but maintain relationships that make you happy. Work on relationships that don't. And hopefully, your immune system will reward your efforts.

Considering Supplements

Okay, maybe all the tips earlier in this chapter sound like too much work. Why can't you just go to a store, pick up a few bottles of multivitamins, probiotics, and other heralded immune boosters, and call it good? While some supplements may have an effect on your immune system, most really don't. Others haven't been tested in any meaningful way — as in a well-designed clinical trial in humans, not small animals — in the amounts normally found in supplements. And the amounts used in the studies often exceed what's found in the average supplement.

However, if you want to add supplements to other methods of getting your immune system humming, there are a few you can try. Make sure to run anything you're taking past your healthcare provider:

>> **Vitamin D** deficiency is much more common than once thought. We spend less time outside, and sun exposure manufactures vitamin D in the skin. Those who have lower vitamin D levels are more at risk for respiratory infections, but unfortunately supplementing vitamin D doesn't always reduce infections. Because vitamin D is a fat-soluble vitamin, excess amounts are stored in the body and can be harmful, so check any supplements with your doctor. Be careful, as too much vitamin D can be dangerous.

>> **Vitamin C** is often thought to help the immune system fight off infections. Fruits such as oranges, tangerines, and strawberries and veggies such as spinach and kale supply you with vitamin C. Unfortunately, it won't necessarily keep a cold at bay. If you eat a balanced diet, you should have enough vitamin C. Talk to your doctor if you think a supplement might help you.

>> **Zinc,** when taken in proper quantities, helps boost immune cell development. Zinc deficiencies occur most commonly in the elderly, affecting as many as 30 percent, due to poor dietary intake or medications that decrease zinc absorption, such as diuretics. Talk to your doctor if you think you need more zinc in your diet.

>> **Vitamin B6** also plays a role in keeping your immune system working well. Beef, chicken, fish, and fortified cereal help meet your daily needs. Talk to your doctor if you think you might be deficient.

Chapter **23**

Ten Ways to Build Muscles in Minutes

Life's busier than ever — whether you're logging long hours, hunting for a new job, building a business, juggling kids' schedules, squeezing college and work into the same week, or finally tackling all the retirement activities you put off. No matter what's filling your days, finding time to work out can be tough.

But after reading this book, you know that adding activity to your lifestyle is a good way to feel better, sleep better, lose weight, improve the condition of your heart, and reduce your chances of developing the diseases that shorten men's lives. So what's a guy to do?

Don't worry — we've got you! In this chapter, we give you some pointers that help you squeeze in a quick strength-training workout when you don't have much time to spare. We also provide a 20-minute workout video so you can work out your whole body in just a few minutes, and we offer a super-fast workout when even 20 minutes seems impossible to commit to.

REMEMBER

Raising your heart rate and breaking a sweat for the good of your body doesn't have to be something you sacrifice because time feels tight.

Recognizing That Two Is Nearly as Good as Three

REMEMBER

For best results, weight train your entire body at least two to three times a week. Three times a week gives you faster results but takes more of your personal time. But when you're feeling time-crunched, take heart — studies show that if you train two days a week, you get 75 percent of the results you get from training three days a week.

So during the weeks that feel extra busy, you're still benefitting your body with just two strength workouts that week.

Fitting in a Short Workout When Time Is Tight

A strength-training workout doesn't have to be a dedicated routine you do specific days of the week. Here are some ways you can fit in a workout when your schedule is full but you're committed to getting or keeping a healthy body.

>> **Add on to your cardio workout.** Say you weight-train two days a week and hit the gym for three days a week. When you can't make it for your dedicated weight-training sessions, add a 20-minute quickie workout on the weight machines, after you finish your cardio-training.

>> **Divide your workout throughout the day.** Sometimes it's simply impossible to find more than a few spare minutes. Instead of giving up on strength training entirely, fit in a short workout in the morning and in the afternoon. You may even want to add another session at night. Three 10-minute workouts easily add up to 30 minutes of training.

>> **Do a daily quickie.** Maybe all you ever have time for during the week is a quickie workout. Until your life settles down and you find more time, schedule a daily quickie workout. Each day, target either your upper or lower body and your core. Take Friday off. On Saturday, fit in one total-body workout and rest on Sunday.

Keeping Muscles Moving When Your Week Is Packed

Even though two to three strength training sessions per week is the best way to get the body benefits you want, some weeks even two workouts seem impossible. Don't skip a training session entirely! Squeeze in one total-body conditioning workout that week. And to get more bang for your buck, try to make it a more intense workout than you'd normally do during your 2-3 weekly sessions.

Instead of doing nothing, keep your muscles stimulated and keep your motivation going with one full-body (and possibly more rigorous) workout.

Incorporating Workout Must-Do's

REMEMBER

Even when you're doing a quick training session, you need to keep in mind the basic weight-training principles explained in Chapter 6. Observe the following points each time that you train:

>> **Always warm up.** Even for a quick workout, you need to prepare your body for more rigorous work. Walk briskly for five minutes before you weight train. This warm-up can include walking quickly around the house, in the yard, or in the parking lot at the office.

>> **Work all major muscle groups.** Be sure to do exercises for your upper body, your lower body, and your core at least twice a week.

>> **Apply program variables.** Even for short workouts, training frequency, exercise selection, order, amount of weight, number of reps, number of sets, and rest periods are all still important components. The variety helps make sure all your muscle groups get attention and keeps you from getting bored. (Get all the info you need about reps and sets in Chapter 6.)

Making Sure Not to Sabotage Yourself with Dehydration

If you feel thirsty during your workout, you waited too long to take a sip of water and you're on your way to dehydration. Drink at least two 8-ounce glasses of water before starting your weight lifting routine and two to four glasses while working out. In order to work your muscles, you need water. Muscle is considered an active tissue, and water is found in the highest concentrations in active tissue. Your muscles are 72 percent water. If your body is only slightly dehydrated, your performance will decline, and you don't get the full benefits of your quick workout.

Signs and symptoms of dehydration include the following:

>> Dark yellow urine

>> Dry cough

>> Dry mouth

>> Fatigue

>> Headache

>> Lightheadedness

>> Loss of appetite

Getting Strategic with Your Sets and Stretches

Get the most out of a short workout by hitting all your muscle groups and squeezing in a solid stretch before you wrap. These tips can help you master the art of workout efficiency:

>> **Repurpose your waiting time to get more done, faster.** You can still rest your muscles between sets — remember, rest is as important as the reps. But make different use of the waiting time by alternating between upper- and lower-body exercises so that one part of your body rests while the other works. Save your core exercises for last.

>> **Mix in stretching exercises.** To be even more efficient, use your rest periods for stretches that target the muscle that you just worked. You can stretch your body all throughout the workout, and you won't need extra time for a stretching segment at the end.

Cooling Down Is Essential with Quickie Workouts

TIP

If you've done a fairly fast-paced weight workout, complete the workout with five minutes of slow cardio exercise. The cardio cool-down gives your pulse, blood pressure, and breathing a chance to slow down before you hit the showers. Ending your workout with an easy set also helps you cool down

Making the Most of a Minute

When you're trying to determine what you can fit into a specific workout window — say, 15 minutes — build your workout with one-minute sets.

In general, one set of a particular exercise takes approximately one minute. If each rep requires two seconds up, a brief pause, and two seconds down, plan on five to six seconds per rep. So, a set of 12 reps takes roughly one minute.

Getting In a Full-Body Burn Without Leaving the House

TIP

Check out this video for a total-body workout in just 20 minutes flat: www.dummies.com/go/weighttrainingfd4e. You can do this dumbbell workout in your bedroom, in your garage, or heck, even poolside — you only need enough space to lie down and to extend a leg behind you 3-4 feet.

Table 23-1 shows you the exercises covered in the video.

TIP

If you don't have any handheld weights, grab a couple of filled water bottles, canned goods, laundry detergent bottles, or books (particularly good when doing lunges and squats). And if you don't have a yoga mat, use a beach towel.

TABLE 23-1   20-Minute Video Circuit

Segment of Routine	Exercises
Warm-up	Squat side-to-side, skater jump, alternating back lunge, rope-a-dope
Shoulders	Shoulder press, plié with shoulder press, front raise, lateral raise
Arms	Biceps curl, triceps kickback, plié biceps curl
Legs	Side leg raise, inner-thigh raise, kneeling butt blaster, kneeling crossover
Abdominals and core	Hip lift with weights, bicycle crunch, bicycle with straight legs, oblique crunch
Shoulders	Shoulder press, plié press, front raise, lateral raise
Arms	Biceps curl, triceps kickback, plié biceps curl
Legs	Side leg raise, inner-thigh raise, kneeling butt blaster, kneeling crossover
Abdominals and core	Hip lift with weights, bicycle crunch, bicycle with straight legs, oblique crunch
Cool-down stretch	Pretzel quad stretch, sitting side reach, sitting triceps stretch, standing breath

Making Minutes Count with Body Weight Only

When you're really pressed for time, sometimes the best thing to do is plan a short workout for home that just uses your body weight. You'll still get plenty of resistance from just the weight of your body, especially if you're a beginner, but even seasoned gym rats will get a challenging workout depending on the number of reps you do. Check out Table 23-2 for an example.

TABLE 23-2   Ultra-Quick Body Weight Routine

Part of the Body	Exercise
Butt and legs	Squat, lunge
Back	Pelvic tilt
Chest	Push-up
Arms	Tricep dip
Abdominals	Basic abdominal crunch

If you have next to no time, do one set of reps for each exercise. If you have a little more time, do two sets of each, or do three sets of reps if you've got 15-20 minutes. Remember that some weight training exercise is better than none and helps you keep momentum when you're tempted to skip a session.

The following shows you how to perform a pelvic tilt and a bench dip. Check out Chapter 6 for instructions on performing the rest of these exercises.

Pelvic tilt

The pelvic tilt is a subtle move that focuses on your lower back but also emphasizes your abdominals. This is a good exercise to do if you have a history of lower-back problems. The pelvic tilt restores mobility to tight or stiff muscles and heightens body awareness of the muscles of the lower back. It's also a great warm-up exercise for more strenuous core training.

Getting set

Lie on your back with your knees bent and feet flat on the floor about hip-width apart. Rest your arms wherever they're most comfortable (see Figure 23-1a). Start with your pelvis in a level position with the natural curve in your lower spine.

The exercise

As you exhale, draw your abdominals in toward your spine and gently press your back down, tilting your pelvis backward. Don't tilt your head up and back or hunch your shoulders (see Figure 23-1b). As you inhale, return your pelvis to a level position. This is a small move that you feel as you tilt your pelvis.

Do's and don'ts

>> DO keep your head, neck, and shoulders relaxed.

>> DON'T lift your lower back off the floor as you tilt your pelvis up.

>> DON'T arch your back off the floor when you lower your hips back down.

Bench dip

The bench dip is one of the few triceps exercises that strengthen other muscles, too — in this case, the shoulders and chest. Figure 23-2 uses a bench, but you can substitute a sturdy chair, a stable edge like a couch, or even a staircase step.

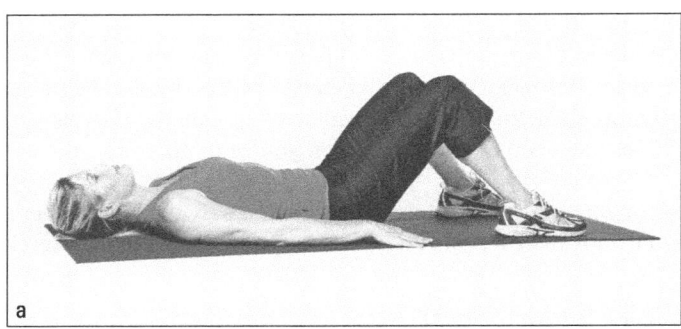

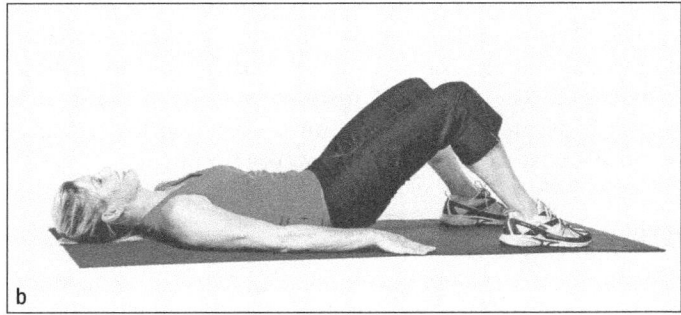

FIGURE 23-1:
Pelvic tilt.

Photo by Nick Horne

Be careful if you have wrist, elbow, or shoulder problems.

WARNING

Getting set

Sit on the edge of a bench with your legs together and straight in front of you, pointing your toes upward. Keeping your elbows relaxed, straighten your arms, place your hands so you can grip the underside of the bench on either side of your hips, and slide your butt just off the front of the bench so your upper body is pointing straight down (see Figure 23-2a). Keep your abdominals pulled in and your head centered between your shoulders.

The exercise

Bend your elbows and lower your body in a straight line. Hold for a few beats and then push yourself back up (see Figure 23-2b).

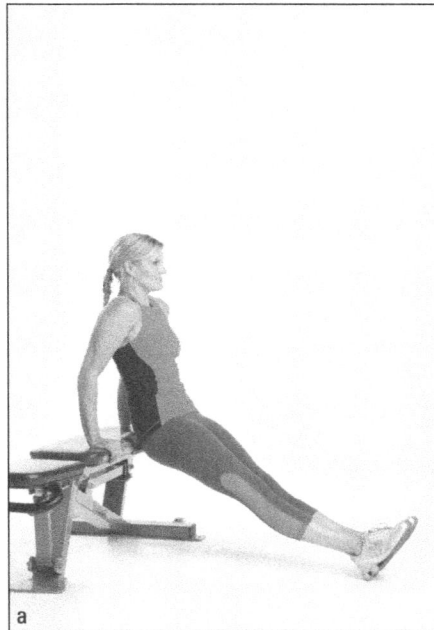 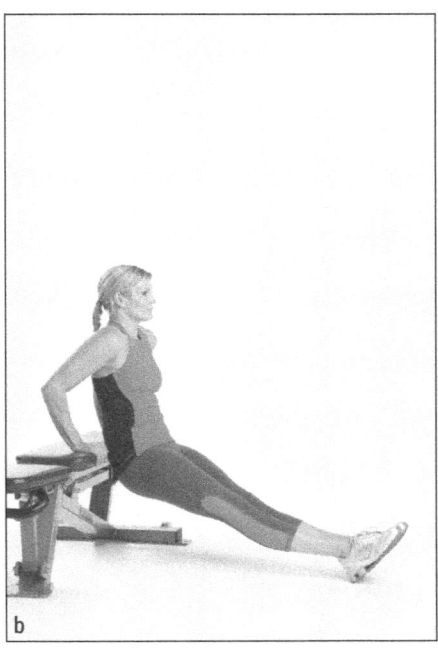

FIGURE 23-2:
Bench dip.

Photo by Nick Horne

Do's and don'ts

» DO try to keep your wrists straight rather than bent backwards.

» DO keep hips and back (as you lower) as close to the bench throughout the motion.

» DON'T simply thrust your hips up and down, a common mistake among beginners. Make sure that your elbows are moving.

Index

American Cancer Society, 287, 288

American College of Sports Medicine, 68

American Heart Association, 8

American Institute for Cancer Research, 51

antianxiety medication, 238

antibodies, 153

anticancer drugs, 272

antidepressants, 226, 238

antigens, 153

antiretroviral drugs (ART), 206

anxiety, 11, 87, 93

  behaving symptoms, 102–104

  feeling symptoms, 104

  overview, 102

  physical effects, 103

  seeking help for, 103–104

  thinking symptoms, 102, 104

ART. *See* antiretroviral drugs (ART)

artificial light exposure, 24–25

artificial sweeteners, 52

aspirin-induced asthma (AIA), 332

asthma, 319

  action plan, 334

  adult-onset asthma, 333

  airway congestion, 331

  airway constriction, 330

  airway edema, 331

  airway hyperresponsiveness, 330

  airway remodeling, 331

  allergic asthma, 333

  allergic (or atopic) asthma, 332

  aspirin-induced asthma (AIA), 332

  avoiding triggers, 335

  childhood-onset asthma, 333

  exercise-induced asthma, 332

  family history, 333

  food allergies, 333

  nonallergic asthma/nonatopic asthma, 332

  occupational asthma, 332

  prevalence, 329

  self-care, 335–336

  severity, 329

  symptoms of, 333–334

  triggering factors, 329

atherosclerosis/hardening of the arteries, 246, 311, 312

Atomic Habits (Clear), 31

AUD. *See* alcohol use disorder (AUD)

autoimmune diseases

  imbalance of hormones, 22

  type 1 diabetes. *see* type 1 diabetes

autonomic nervous system (ANS), 90–91

awareness, 31, 32

B

balanced hormones, 17

band lat pull-down

  do's and don'ts, 77

  getting set, 76

  steps to perform, 76–77

barbell biceps curl

  do's and don'ts, 81, 82

  getting set, 81

  steps to perform, 81

basal body temperature method, 194–195

basal cell carcinoma, 291

basic abdominal crunch

  do's and don'ts, 85

  getting set, 84

  steps to perform, 84

behavior therapy, 107

belly fat reduction, 363

bench dip, 377–379

benign prostatic hyperplasia (BPH), 286

benign (noncancerous) tumors, 270

biceps workout

  barbell biceps curl, 81–82

  one-arm dumbbell row, 77–78

biological therapy, 272

pre-exposure prophylaxis (PrEP), 206
serious risks, 205
symptoms, 206
timing your AIDS and STI talk, 213–216
transmission of, 205
treatment, 206
human papillomavirus (HPV), 201–202
hydraulic prosthesis, 234
hypersomnias, 122
hypothalamus-pituitary-adrenal (HPA)
    axis, 89, 90

I

imbalance of hormones
  autoimmune diseases, 22
  cardiovascular disease, 22
  chronic fatigue, 22
  digestive disorders, 22
  overweight, 18
  root causes of, 21
  visceral fat, 18
immune system boosting
  avoid smoking, 368
  decreasing stress, 366
  eating well, 366–367
  exercising, 368
  getting enough sleep, 367
  maintaining a healthy weight, 367
  maintain relationships, 369
  moderate drinking, 368–369
  supplements, 369–370
  vaccinations, 365
impaired mental health, sleep deprivation, 124
impotence. See erectile dysfunction (ED)
influenza vaccine, 156
insomnia, 122
insulin, 339
insulin resistance, 342, 344
intermediate level, weight training, 71
intermediate sleep, 110
internal condom, 192

interpersonal therapy, 107
intracerebral hemorrhage, 310, 313
intrauterine device (IUD), 188
ischemic stroke. See white stroke

J

Journal of the American College of Cardiology, 63

K

kilocalorie. See calories
"Knowing Weight-Routine Essentials," 68

L

lambskin condoms, 189
lateral raise
  do's and don'ts, 81
  getting set, 80
  steps to perform, 80–81
latex condoms, 189
levels of exercise
  extremely hard exercise, 60
  extremely light exercise, 60
  light exercise, 60
  somewhat hard exercise, 60
  very hard exercise, 60
  very light exercise, 60
Levitra (vardenafil), 233
Lewy body disease, 349
loneliness
  vs. aloneness, 100
  health problems, 99
  importance of human connection, 98
  long-term partnership, 98
  and pornography consumption, 99
  suggestions for making some connections, 101
long sleep, 114
long-term goals, 34
long-term memory, 351
low-density lipoprotein (LDL), 257
  levels, 257

lower-body workout
  lunge, 73–74
  squat, 72–73
lubricants, 190
lung cancer, 9, 271
  causes, 288
  diagnosis, 289
  non-small cell lung cancers (NSCLCs), 288
  overview, 287
  prevention, 290
  risk factors, 289
  signs and symptoms, 288
  small cell lung cancers (SCLCs), 288
  treatment, 289–290
lunge
  do's and don'ts, 74
  getting set, 73
  steps to perform, 73–74

M

macronutrients
  carbohydrates, 42
  definition, 42
  fat, 42
  protein, 42
Magnum condom, 190
maintenance of wakefulness test (MWT), 126
male infertility, 173
male menopause, 227
male organ. *See* penis
male reproductive system, 11
malignant tumors, 270
masturbation, 223
meatus, 163
meditation, 95
Mediterranean-DASH Intervention for
    Neurodegenerative Delay (MIND)
    diet, 360–361
Mediterranean diet, 13, 49–50
meiosis, 171–172
melanoma, 292
melatonin, 116

men's lifespan *vs.* women's lifespan, 18
menstruation, 179
mental health issues
  anxiety, 11
  chronic stress, 10
  depression, 11
  symptoms, 303
merkel cell carcinoma, 292–293
metabolic dysfunction, 21
metabolic issues, stress, 93
micronutrients
  minerals, 43, 366
  vitamins, 43, 366
microsleeps, 115
mild cognitive impairment (MCI), 349–350
mind-body practices, stress reduction, 96
mindset of making changes, 30–31
minerals, 43, 366
mini-laparotomy, tubal ligation, 184
moderate drinking, 13, 129, 141, 368–369
moderate exercise, 12, 60
moderate-intensity exercise, 264
moderate-intensity physical activity, 59
molluscum contagiosum, 210
morning-after pills. *See* emergency contraception
    pills (ECPs)
morning cure, 228
multiple sleep latency test (MSLT), 126
muscular endurance, 68
My Fitness Pal app, 43, 44

N

naloxone, 299
Narcotics Anonymous, 303
National Cancer Institute recommendations,
    quitting of smoking, 138
National Institute on Alcohol Abuse and
    Alcoholism, 274–275
National Safety Council, 298
National Sleep Foundation recommendations, 116
natural family planning, 193–194
nature's flavor enhancers

R

radiation therapy, 272, 275, 290

recommended dietary allowances (RDAs) of nutrition, 44

  based on your age, 45–46

  for minerals for healthy men, 45, 46

  nutrition labels, 44–45

  for vitamins for healthy men, 45

red stroke, 314

  combined with white, 315

  intracerebral hemorrhage, 310, 313

  other names, 311

  subarachnoid hemorrhage, 314–315

red wine, benefits and risks of, 139

refined sugar, 53

regular inactivity, 23

repetitions and sets, weight training, 68–69

reproduction

  Cowper's fluid, 178

  egg journey, 178–179

  embryo, 179

  fertilization process, 178

  fetus, 180

  giving birth process, 180

  pregnancy confirmation, 180

  sexual intercourse, 178

  sperm-egg meet-up, 177

  sperm's journey, 178

resting energy expenditure (REE), 48

restless legs syndrome (RLS), 123

resveratrol, 139

reverse crunch

  do's and don'ts, 85

  getting set, 85

  steps to perform, 85, 86

risks of smoking

  with cancer and other diseases, 131

  and heart disease, 130

  secondhand smoke, 131

S

"safe" drinking limits of alcohol, 140

safer sex, 211–212

saturated and trans fats, 53

scrotum, 169

secondhand smoke, 131

selective serotonin reuptake inhibitors (SSRIs), 226

semen, 172

seminal vesicles, 277

sensation-seeking, 301, 302

sexual health

  contraceptives. *See* contraceptives

  male reproductive system, 11

  sexually transmitted infections (STIs)/sexually transmitted diseases (STDs). *see* sexually transmitted infections (STIs)/sexually transmitted diseases (STDs)

sexual intercourse, 176, 179. *See also* reproduction

sexually transmitted infections (STIs)/sexually transmitted diseases (STDs), 12

  avoiding self-prescribe medication, 201

  candidiasis, 211

  Centers for Disease Control and Prevention, 200

  chlamydia, 202–203

  cost of treatment, 207

  genital warts, 201–202

  Golden Rule, 213

  gonorrhea, 203

  hepatitis B, 207

  herpes, 207–210

  human immunodeficiency virus (HIV), 205–207

  human papillomavirus (HPV), 201–202

  molluscum contagiosum, 210

  overview, 199–200

  pubic lice/crabs, 210

  risks minimization, 216–217

  seeking medical help, 201

  syphilis, 204

  timing your AIDS and STI talk, 213–216

  trichomoniasis, 210

About the Authors

We would like to thank the following contributors to this work:

Christine Adamec; Kimlin Tam Ashing, PhD; Simon Atkins, MD; William E. Berger, MD, MBA; LaReine Chabut; Megan Coffee, MD, PhD; Patricia Corrigan; Sarah Densmore; Charles H. Elliott, PhD; Humberto M. Fagundes, MD; Kevin Felner, MD; Kristin Ferguson-Wagstaffe; Marshalee George, PhD, MSPH, MSN, AOCNP®, CRNP; Mary Kenan, PhD; Lane Kennedy; Mark Edwin Kunik, MD, MPH; Clete A. Kushida, MD, PhD; Paul H. Lange, MD; Pierre A. Lehu; Alan P. Lyss, MD; Isabella Mainwaring, CDP, QLS, OCN; John R. Marler, MD; Sarah McKay, PhD; Tamar Medford; Liz Neporent; Sharon Perkins, RN; Dr. Simon Poole; Carol Ann Rinzler; Amy Riolo; James M. Rippe, MD; Alan L. Rubin, MD; Suzanne Schlosberg; Meg Schneider; Patricia Burkhart Smith; Laura L. Smith, PhD; Richard W. Snyder, DO; Michael Wasserman, MD; Dr. Ruth K. Westheimer; and Tonya A. Winders, MBA.

Publisher's Acknowledgments

Executive Editor: Tracy Boggier

Compiling Editor: Kristin Ferguson-Wagstaffe

Development Editor: Dan Mersey

Technical Editor: Dr Jennifer Fildes

Production Editor: Magesh Elangovan

Managing Editor: Murari Mukundan

Illustrator: Kathryn Born

Cover Image: © donskarpo/Getty Images